Therapeutic Change

An Object Relations Perspective

APPLIED CLINICAL PSYCHOLOGY

Series Editors:
Alan S. Bellack
Medical College of Pennsylvania at EPPI, Philadelphia, Pennsylvania
Michel Hersen
Nova University School of Psychology, Fort Lauderdale, Florida

---

A Continuation Order Plan is available for this series. A continuation order will bring
deliver of each new volume immediately upon publication. Volumes are billed only upon
actual shipment. For further information, please contact the publisher.

Therapeutic Change
An Object Relations Perspective

Sidney J. Blatt
Yale University
New Haven, Connecticut
and

Richard Q. Ford
Austen Riggs Center, Inc.
Stockbridge, Massachusetts

In Collaboration with

William H. Berman, Jr.
Barry Cook
Phebe Cramer
and
C. Edward Robins

PLENUM PRESS • NEW YORK AND LONDON

Library of Congress Cataloging-in-Publication Data

Blatt, Sidney J. (Sidney Jules)
    Therapeutic change : an object relations perspective / Sidney J.
Blatt and Richard Q. Ford ; in collaboration with William H. Berman,
Jr., ... [et al.].
        p.   cm. -- (Applied clinical psychology)
    Includes bibliographical references and index.
    ISBN 0-306-44601-4
    1. Personality change--Case studies. 2. Object relations
(Psychoanalysis)--Case studies. 3. Psychodynamic psychotherapy-
-Case studies. 4. Psychiatric hospital patients--Case studies.
I. Ford, Richard Q. II. Berman, William H., 1954-   . III. Title.
IV. Series.
    [DNLM: 1. Mental Disorders--therapy--case studies.
2. Psychological Tests--case studies. 3. Therapeutic Community-
-case studies. 4. Treatment Outcome--case studies. 5. Object
Attachment--case studies.   WM 40 B644t 1994]
RC489.025B58   1994
616.89'1--dc20
DNLM/DLC
for Library of Congress   93-51011
                                                                 CIP

ISBN 0-306-44601-4

© 1994 Plenum Press, New York
A Division of Plenum Publishing Corporation
233 Spring Street, New York, N.Y. 10013

Printed in the United States of America

To the patients and staff of the Austen Riggs Center
who, with courage and fortitude, have wrestled with
the demons

No one who, like me, conjures up the most evil of those half-tamed demons that inhabit the human breast, and seeks to wrestle with them, can expect to come through the struggle unscathed.

SIGMUND FREUD (1905 [1901])

Foreword

Dynamic psychotherapy research has become revitalized, especially in the last three decades. This major study by Sidney Blatt, Richard Ford, and their associates evaluates long-term intensive treatment (hospitalization and 4-times-a-week psychotherapy) of very disturbed patients at the Austen Riggs Center. The center provides a felicitous setting for recovery—beautiful buildings on lovely wooded grounds just off the quiet main street of the New England town of Stockbridge, Massachusetts. The center, which has been headed in succession by such capable leaders as Robert Knight, Otto Will, Daniel Schwartz, and now Edward Shapiro, has been well known for decades for its type of intensive hospitalization and psychotherapy. Included in its staff have been such illustrious contributors as Erik Erikson, David Rapaport, George Klein, and Margaret Brenman. The Rapaport–Klein study group has been meeting there yearly since Rapaport's death in 1960. Although the center is a long-term care treatment facility, it remains successful and solvent even in these days of increasingly short-term treatment.

Sidney Blatt, Professor of Psychology and Psychiatry at Yale University, and Richard Ford of the Austen Riggs Center, and their associates assembled a sample of 90 patients who had been in long-term treatment and who had been given (initially and at 15 months) a set of psychological tests, including the Rorschach, the Thematic Apperception Test, a form of the Wechsler Intelligence Test, and the Human Figure Drawings. This test battery was the one assembled by David Rapaport and used at the Menninger Foundation, as well as at the Austen Riggs Center and other centers. The data analyses also involved independent and carefully controlled ratings of the narrative clinical case records prepared at the same two points in the treatment process.

The amount of change (both psychological and behavioral), based on independent ratings made on the clinical case records and psychological tests at the beginning of treatment and again 15 months later, is impressive. The most impressive changes were: decreased frequency and/or lessened severity of clinical symptoms, better interpersonal relations, increased intelligence, decreased thought disorder, and decreased fantasies about unrealistic interpersonal relations.

These results are congruent with the findings of a follow-up study conducted a number of years after discharge (Plankun, Burkhardt, & Muller, 1985) with a similar and partially overlapping sample (20% psychotic, 53% severe personality disorder, 27% major affective disorder). The Average Global Adjustment Scale (a version of the Health–Sickness Rating Scale, Luborsky, Diquer, Luborsky, McLellan, Woody, & Alexander, 1993) at admission was only 34, but at follow-up it was 64.4, indicating that while the patients at follow-up showed some functional difficulty in several areas, there was generally adequate functioning with some meaningful interpersonal relationships (Endicott, Spitzer, Fleiss, & Cohen, 1976). Such a change at a 13-year follow-up is impressive. Even without a comparison group, the changes very likely represent the benefits of the treatment provided.

This study of change in clinical records and psychological tests is special in several ways. It is one of the few systematic studies of change in long-term, inpatient treatment with seriously disturbed patients—patients who have had considerable prior outpatient treatment (over 2 years on average) and several brief prior hospitalizations (1.32 hospitalizations for 4.5 months, on average), neither of which proved very successful. The study used systematic procedures for transforming detailed, narrative, clinical case reports into quantitative data in two major realms: the assessment of clinical symptoms and the quality of interpersonal behavior. Relatively new procedures were used to evaluate diagnostic psychological tests (TAT, Human Figure Drawings, intelligence tests, and the Rorschach) as measures of therapeutic change. These assessments of clinical case records and of psychological test protocols were conducted in a carefully constructed, methodologically rigorous research design to assure the independence of the various ratings. A basic clinical distinction was made between two fundamental configurations of psychopathology, anaclitic and introjective patients; the results indicate that these two types of patients come to treatment with different needs, problems, and strengths, and that they change in different ways. Many of the findings of therapeutic change are linked to this innovative clinical distinction.

The study also evaluated the efficacy of aspects of Rorschach responses at admission as prognostic indicators of therapeutic response. The patients who manifested greater therapeutic change over 15 months of treatment were those patients who initially were more able and/or willing to communicate disrupted thinking and images of destructive and malevolent interactions, but who at the same time had indications of a greater capacity for interpersonal relatedness (their Rorschach responses contained human forms that were more differentiated, articulated, and integrated).

It is a major advance to evaluate therapeutic change in terms of the innovative distinction between anaclitic patients, who have disturbances primarily in forming satisfying interpersonal relationships, and introjective patients, who show disturbances mainly in self-definition, autonomy, self-worth, and identity. Both types of patients showed benefits from the treatment, but change in anaclitic patients occurred largely in the quality of their interpersonal relationships. Introjective patients changed mainly in their manifest symptoms of psychosis, neurosis, and affective disturbances, as well as in their cognitive processes. The main changes that occurred in each group, therefore, appeared to be consistent with their personality organization. The importance of this difference in personality organization has also been shown by Blatt (1992) in his reanalysis of the data of the Menninger Psychotherapy Research Project, which indicated that anaclitic patients did significantly better in supportive psychotherapy and introjective patients in psychoanalysis. A further lead worth following in future studies is the suggestion that anaclitic patients might show greater long term gain if they were helped in establishing supportive social networks.

The results of this study are a landmark; the size of the benefits implies that the intensive, long-term treatment program is very effective. These systematic empirical findings should have substantial impact on the current debate about the value of long-term, intensive, psychoanalytically informed treatment for seriously disturbed patients. The results are consistent with much clinical evidence, although there is not much clinical-quantitative *comparative* evidence based on studies of short-term versus long-term treatments in randomized samples. But such comparative evidence will come, and the results very likely will support the value of what is called here long-term treatment, although it should rather be called "time appropriate" treatment, since some patients need long-term treatment. Indirect quantitative support for such a conclusion comes from a recent report by Shea et al. (1992), revealing that a very high percentage of patients who completed short-term treatment in the NIMH depression collaborative study (Elkin et al., 1989) afterwards sought further treatment, presumably to make up for the insufficiency of the brief (16 session) treatment they received.

This Riggs study, the Menninger study (e.g., Wallerstein, 1986), and the Penn study (Luborsky, Crits-Christoph, Mintz, & Auerbach, 1988) are similar in two major ways: their assessment measures and naturalistic design, in which patients who apply to the facility are given the treatment that is clinically indicated. The alternative design is to randomly assign patients to alternative treatments. But, as Howard, Krause, and Orlinsky (1986) point out, the randomized comparison design loses some patients because they will not accept the randomization and it places some patients in treatments that may be less than suitable for them. The Riggs, Menninger, and Penn studies all demonstrate that much can be learned from the naturalistic design. The Riggs study especially shows the value of this approach in analyses based on the anaclitic versus introjective distinction, together with analyses of other factors that may influence outcome (e.g., Luborsky, Crits-Christoph, Mintz, & Auerbach, 1988; Miller, Luborsky, Barber, & Docherty, 1993). We at Penn now intend to apply some of the analyses conducted in the Riggs study.

LESTER LUBORSKY

University of Pennsylvania

REFERENCES

Blatt, S. J. (1992). The differential effect of psychotherapy and psychoanalysis on anaclitic and introjective patients: The Menninger Psychotherapy Research Project revisited. *Journal of the American Psychoanalytic Association, 40*, 691–724.

Elkin, I., Shea, M. T., Watkins, J. T., Imber, S. D., Sotsky, S. M., Collins, J. F., Glass, D. R., Pilkonis, P. A., Leber, W. R., Dockerty, J. P., Fiester, S. J., & Parloff, M. B. (1989). NIMH Treatment of Depression Collaborative Research Program: General effectiveness of treatments. *Archives of General Psychiatry, 46*, 971–983.

Endicott, J., Spitzer, R. L., Fleiss, J. L., & Cohen, J. (1976). The Global Assessment Scale: A procedure for measuring overall severity of psychiatric disturbances. *Archives of General Psychiatry, 33*, 766–771.

Howard, K., Krause, M., & Orlinsky, D. (1986). The attrition and the attrition dilemma: Toward a new strategy for psychotherapy. *Journal of Consulting and Clinical Psychology, 54*, 106–110.

Luborsky, L., Crits-Christoph, P., Mintz, J., & Auerbach, A. (1988). *Who will benefit from psychotherapy? Predicting therapeutic outcomes.* New York: Basic Books.

Luborsky, L., Diquer, L., Luborsky, E., McLellan, A. T., Woody, G., & Alexander, L. (1993). Psychological health-sickness as a predictor of outcomes in dynamic and other psychotherapies. *Journal of Consulting and Clinical Psychology, 61*, 542–548.

Miller, N., Luborsky, L., Barber, J., & Docherty, J. (1993). *Psychodynamic treatment research: A handbook for clinical practice.* New York: Basic Books.

Plankun, E., Burkhardt, D., & Muller, J. (1985). 14-year follow-up of borderline and schizotypical personality disorders. *Comprehensive Psychiatry, 26*, 448–455.

Shea, M. T., Elkin, I., Imber, S. D., Sotsky, S. M., Watkins, J. T., Collins, J. F., Pilkonis, P.

A., Beckham, E., Glass, D. R., Dolan, R. T., & Parloff, M. B. (1992). Course of depressive symptoms in the Treatment of Depression Collaborative Research Program. *Archives of General Psychiatry, 49,* 782–787.

Wallerstein, R. (1986). *Forty-two lives in treatment—A study of psychoanalysis and psychotherapy.* New York: Guilford Press.

Preface

This book is about a 15-month period in the lives of 90 very troubled young adults. We undertook this project to evaluate how such persons, so seriously disturbed as to require hospitalization, might change when undertaking long-term, intensive, psychodynamically oriented treatment on an inpatient basis.

We evaluated change from multiple perspectives, using systematic analyses of detailed clinical case reports prepared both at the beginning of the treatment process and then much later, and using a range of psychological assessment procedures administered at these same two times: the Wechsler Intelligence Test, the Thematic Apperception Test, Human Figure Drawings, and the Rorschach test—applying to this last several different conceptual models. We sought to understand more fully the nuanced and subtle ways patients might reveal their readiness to relinquish the safeties of troubled and troubling behaviors. We indeed succeeded in identifying significant patterns of change that occur across types of observations and in different kinds of patients.

The seriously disturbed patients in our study usually had over 2 years of prior outpatient psychotherapy as well as at least one brief psychiatric hospitalization of several months duration before they decided to undertake long-term, intensive inpatient treatment. This latter treatment, on average, lasted approximately 2 years. Our assessment of change took into account, on average, the first 15 months.

A 2-year period of hospitalization is a relatively short time, merely a beginning, in the struggles of these seriously troubled individuals to revise decades of distortions, both real and imagined, which have massively blocked the progress of their psychological development. But such a period is a very long time, and very expensive, to those in positions of political and economic authority charged with the care of the mentally ill—and now tasked, in today's world of spiraling health care costs, to reduce that expenditure drastically.

This book was not conceived with these stresses in mind; yet we believe it makes an important contribution to the contemporary debate on health care costs. It represents a scientifically sophisticated documentation of the effectiveness of long-term, inpatient, psychodynamic treatment of severe mental illness. It bolsters the proposition that this expensive care is effective care. It provides data to support the concept that doing something once slowly and carefully may turn out in the long run to be less expensive than doing it quickly many times—or not doing it at all.

Such documentation is hard to come by. The particular feeling states of very troubled persons, which result in imaginings and behaviors difficult to comprehend for both participant and observer, must, in the conventions of modern social science, be reduced to numbers: means, correlation matrices, and other statistical methods of considerable complexity. We offer here a description of change in troubled persons, but a description built on numbers. Readers at home with these conventions, which so elegantly shift the nuances of reality into the bin of numbers, will not need the following paragraphs. They may at once begin reading, as we so often do, from the concluding chapter back to the research design and back again to the conclusions. But others may find it helpful, before starting out, to have a summary of our findings unencumbered by the details of the careful research techniques, the sometimes novel conceptualizations, and the lengthy statistical analyses essential to this kind of science.

Even with this accommodation, the reader will here find no evocation of the journey of a single individual through the vicissitudes of terror, panic, extraordinary loneliness, confusion, lack of purpose, and systematic undermining of hope that so often characterize the experience of severely troubled persons. We deal instead with summaries of summaries, with vast reductions in that particular universe of imaginings and behaviors lodged within 90 persons across 15 months of an intensive therapeutic experience.

Missing also are all the others who have contributed to that experience. Only by inference are those persons present who have entered into the personal struggle of each individual patient. The setting for this study is the Austen Riggs Center, a private, voluntary psychiatric hospital at the crossroads of a Norman Rockwell village located in the Berkshire hills of western Massachusetts. A patient coming into this setting is engaged by artists, other patients, drama coaches, psychiatric workers, nurses, social workers, nursery school teachers, psychotherapists, physicians, and many others led over the decades by psychoanalyst–scholars such as Robert Knight, David Rapaport, Erik Erikson, Otto Will, and Daniel Schwartz. The results reported here suppose, but barely hint at, the energetic presence of all these people.

We document first that the work done in this setting is effective. But a caveat is in order. It is not possible to answer the popular question, "Does psychotherapy work?"—or, in this context, "Does psycho-dynamically oriented inpatient treatment work?" No one knows how to isolate fully the effects of treatment, or, better, that skein of largely interpersonal interactions called "treatment," from all of the other effects impinging on any individual across time. But we do show that people in this inpatient setting change, largely for the better.

Troubled persons, as we all do to some degree, create imaginative worlds divorced from reality in an effort to reduce pain and discover safety. Their disturbed and disturbing behaviors most often represent disguised efforts to achieve this result. We used psychological tests to access and then understand and evaluate these imaginings, that is, how patients conceive of themselves and others, and how these imaginings compare with observed behaviors: isolation, impulsivity, longing, exciting initiative, helplessness, and the like. To evaluate change in behavior we made independent assessments of detailed clinical case reports prepared on each patient as part of routine procedures. Two groups of researchers were assembled and then carefully kept apart. One group, not knowing the work of the other, evaluated the imaginings; the other group assessed the behaviors. Each studied the patients twice, once at the beginning of treatment and once 15 months or so later. Their findings were then compared.

Within each level of observation—behavioral accounts and assessment of psychological processes—we used several types of evaluations. In behavioral accounts, we assessed change in the extent and severity of clinical symptoms as well as in the quality of interpersonal relatedness within the clinical context—the relationships established with other patients, with the wide range of clinical staff, and within the intense relationship with the therapist. We also made multiple independent observations of psychological change using several well-established procedures—the Rorschach, the Thematic Apperception Test (TAT), Human Figure Drawings (HFDs), and an intelligence test (the Wechsler–Bellevue). But with each of these well-established procedures, we used relatively new methods for evaluating responses. Our approach was based on an interest in assessing representational processes, that is, those cognitive–affective schemas or templates that indicate both the developmental level and the ways of conceptualizing self and others. The assessment of these representational structures, particularly on the Rorschach, enabled us to make important observations about the nature of psychopathology and the processes of therapeutic change.

Most impressive was the agreement among the various observations made through independent assessments of these behavioral and psychological dimensions. Assessments of change in clinical symptoms and interpersonal behavior were consistent with the results from the evaluation of change obtained from a wide range of psychological test assessments. These latter assessments evaluated changes in cognitive processes on the intelligence test and on the Rorschach; changes in the potential for both distorted and adaptive interpersonal relations on the Rorschach; changes in the predominant psychological defenses expressed in stories about personal feelings and thoughts told to the interpersonal themes of TAT cards; and changes in the organization of representations of self and others expressed in drawings of the human figure. All these procedures indicated substantial change, in theoretically expected ways, in the total group of patients over the course of the treatment process. These various independent indications of significant behavioral and psychological change toward the end of inpatient treatment are highly congruent with estimates of improvement reported by an independent group of investigators who conducted a follow-up study with many of these patients, years after these patients had left the therapeutic program.

At the outset of this research, we made a critically important innovation in those research techniques regularly used to address the question of change during treatment. We assumed that different persons, at least early on in their inpatient experience, change in different ways. This assumption has proved exceedingly productive. Indeed, one of us (Blatt, 1992) has in a different context shown that a reanalysis of the findings of another major investigation of psychotherapy outcome, the Menninger Psychotherapy Research Project, is considerably enhanced by this assumption. Put simply, we assume that severely troubled persons are more or less preoccupied with one, and only one, of the two major tasks of emotional development: either the work of coming close to another person or the work of defining oneself as separate from another person.

We found that these two types of interpersonal orientation can be readily discerned and that their adherents indeed change in different ways. Those inpatients preoccupied with coming close to and remaining attached with another person reveal positive change, as judged by their later behaviors and imaginings, primarily in a progressive giving up of their detailed but unrealistic fantasies about other persons. By contrast, those inpatients concerned primarily with their own separate identity and their own self-esteem manifest positive change, again evaluated through their later behaviors and imaginings, mainly by relinquishing fantasy efforts to mix together and then meld concepts that in reality need first to be kept separate and then put into relationship.

These two types of patients tended to maintain their separate strategies for safety; during the 15-month period of the study, their routes to change remained largely independent of the other group. Had we not consistently distinguished those persons who early in treatment focused on attachment from those who focused on separateness, many of our most important findings would have been blurred together and lost.

Finally, using a relatively new statistical technique in psychological science to assess the direction of change, we describe some of the imaginative qualities identified in patients early in treatment that turn out to predict subsequent improved behavior. These predictors fall into two areas: what is imagined and how it is imagined. At first, these results seem surprising indeed. In the area of *what* one imagines, the results were as follows: Seriously disturbed inpatients who early in the treatment imagined interactions as disrupted, malevolent, destructive, and unilateral appear later in treatment to be more constructively engaged with others. In a somewhat similar—and also surprising—vein, the greater the disordered thinking at the beginning, the less frequent and severe the clinical symptoms are later on. In the area of *how* one imagines, the results were as follows: The degree to which patients were able at the beginning of treatment to imagine human figures who were more fully human, more elaborated and well-articulated with physical and functional attributes, portrayed in congruent and appropriate action and interaction—to that extent they later demonstrated more appropriate interpersonal behavior. In sum, we show that those patients who later demonstrate greater positive change in behavior were, at the beginning of treatment, better able to communicate both their experience of destructive relationships and their disordered thinking, while at the same time indicating a relatively greater capacity to interact appropriately with others.

These findings, seemingly straightforward in summary, represent the work of more than a dozen investigators over an equal number of years. Having learned patience, we are now excited at the size and rare quality of the fish we have caught. Those who have themselves tried to ply these uncertain waters will readily appreciate the pleasure we feel at here presenting the results of our endeavor.

Our evaluations of change in these seriously disturbed patients participating in an intense, therapeutic, inpatient treatment program were based on clinical case records and psychological test protocols established as part of extensively defined but routine clinical procedures. Thus we are indebted to the wide range of clinical staff at the Austen Riggs Center for systematic and detailed clinical observations and for psychological test protocols precisely administered and carefully recorded. Across the years of this project, colleagues have made invaluable contributions. We are especially indebted to our collaborators, Drs. William H. Berman, Jr., Barry Cook, Phebe Cramer, and C. Edward Robins. We are also grateful to Drs. Sally Bloom–Feshbach, Dianna Hartley, Roslyn Meyer, Robert H. Spiro, and Alan Sugarman for their essential work, especially in the early phases of this project, and to Dr. Steven Tuber for his assistance in the basic scoring of the Rorschach protocols. Ms. Barbara Conway effectively managed the data processing and analyses, and David S. Blatt, Judith B. Casey, Julie Sugarman, Madeline Wagner, and Christine Whalen carefully scored and collated data gathered from the clinical case records and the various psychological test protocols. And "The Joans" (Cricca and Scarveles) provided dedicated secretarial services in preparing the final manuscript.

We are also indebted to Dr. Otto A. Will, Jr., former medical director of the Austen Riggs Center, who invited us to use the clinical files at the Austen Riggs Center for research, and to Dr. Daniel P. Schwartz, who, as subsequent medical director, provided continued support for this endeavor. We are grateful to many members of the clinical staff at the Austen Riggs Center for their cooperation and many helpful suggestions and criticisms, especially to Dr. William J. Richardson, former director of research, and Dr. Martin Cooperman, former associate medical director, both of whom provided critical support and encouragement at difficult times in the course of this work. This project was funded by a grant from the John D. and Catherine T. MacArthur Foundation and a bequest from the estate of Joseph P. Chassell, M.D., Ph.D.; we are grateful to them for the support that made this investigation possible.

SIDNEY J. BLATT
RICHARD Q. FORD

Contents

Figures and Tables

CHAPTER 1

Theoretical and Methodological Issues in the Study of Therapeutic Change

INTRODUCTION

The clinical research presented in this book was initiated with several goals. First, we sought to assess systematically the effects of the therapeutic process with seriously disturbed patients hospitalized in an intensive, long-term, open inpatient treatment facility that offered psychodynamically informed treatment, including psychotherapy four times weekly.

In evaluating therapeutic change, we were particularly interested in assessing change in psychological and behavioral dimensions that occurred in individuals toward the end of their participation in the treatment program but prior to their discharge. We believe that the vast proportion of studies that evaluate therapeutic change and progress by assessing adaptation in a broad social context several months or even years subsequent to treatment usually conflate several different domains of change. Social adaptation subsequent to hospitalization and treatment is a very complex phenomenon that depends only partly on the patient's progress in the treatment process. Such adaptation is influenced substantially by the social support systems available to the patient subsequent to the termination of treatment—that is, support provided by the patient's family and friends and/or by the clinical facility (Blatt, 1975). Thus, it seems important to distinguish different types or levels of therapeutic change. In this study we are primarily interested in assessing the psychological and behavioral effects of the treatment process before these dimensions begin to interact with a host of potentially confounding external factors. We believe an essential first step in studying the effects of long-term treatment is to establish whether a treatment program results in significant change within the treatment context. If therapeutic gain can be convincingly demonstrated at the end of treatment, then subsequent research should be directed to the complex questions of how, to what degree, and in what ways constructive psychological and behavioral changes in different types of patients within the therapeutic process contribute to broader forms of adaptation in the complex social matrix beyond the treatment setting. An essential first step in studying therapeutic change, however, is to demonstrate that treatment results in substantial change within the treatment context and to specify precisely the nature of that change for different types of patients.

As a second goal, we sought to evaluate the contributions of diagnostic psychological tests, especially the Rorschach but also the Thematic Apperception Test, Human Figure Drawings, and the Wechsler Intelligence Test, to the assessment of change in cognitive, affective, and interpersonal dimensions during the treatment process. We were particularly interested in new methods of evaluating the nature and quality of object relations and mental representations on the Rorschach (Blatt, 1990a) and their potential contributions to assessment of therapeutic change. We use these procedures in this research, not primarily for idiographic clinical evaluation of individual patients but for establishing precisely defined, empirical variables that capture essential psychological dimensions that can contribute to assessing systematically the effects of the treatment process across a large group of patients. The empirical variables used for evaluating psychological test protocols in this investigation had been developed in prior cross-sectional and/or longitudinal research, with both clinical and nonclinical samples, that demonstrated both their reliability and validity as measures of psychological organization and psychopathology. In this investigation, we sought to evaluate the utility of these variables in assessing the effects of a long-term, intensive treatment process with seriously disturbed inpatients.

As a third goal, we sought to test the validity of theoretical formulations (Blatt, 1974, 1990b, 1991; Blatt & Blass, 1990; Blatt & Shichman, 1983) that propose a distinction between two fundamental configurations of personality development and psychopathology: (1) an anaclitic configuration that includes disorders occupied primarily with interpersonal relationships while defensively avoiding issues of a sense of self and in which primarily avoidant defenses of denial and repression are used (e.g., infantile or dependent and hysterical disorders) and (2) an introjective configuration that includes disorders occupied primarily with establishing and maintaining a sense of self-definition as separate, autonomous, independent, and functional while defensively avoiding issues of interpersonal relatedness and in which primarily counteractive defenses such as projection, intellectualization, rationalization, and overcompensation are used (e.g., paranoia, obsessive–compulsive disorders, guilt-laden depression, and phallic narcissism). We were interested in evaluating whether this distinction could be made reliably from clinical case records and if it facilitated our understanding of therapeutic change in the seriously disturbed inpatients who provided the data for this study.

Fourth, paying particular attention to Rorschach indicators of the quality of the object relations and object representation, we also sought to identify the variables at the beginning of the treatment that proved able to predict the effectiveness of the treatment process as assessed from evaluations of clinical functioning provided independently by members of the clinical treatment staff.

THEORETICAL CONSIDERATIONS: TWO CONFIGURATIONS OF PSYCHOPATHOLOGY

Early in the history of psychoanalysis, the individual was viewed essentially as a closed system; theory focused primarily on innate biological forces. Interest was directed initially toward understanding the impact of biological drives, especially infantile sexuality, on the maturation of the psychic apparatus. Also of interest was how the intensity of these drives contributed to the development of psychopathology. Subsequently, the focus was extended to an interest in the modulating or control functions of the ego—the defenses—and their interaction with the drives. This interest in the defensive functions of the ego, initially conceptualized as biological thresholds that regulate the expression of the drives, was later broadened to include the ego's external, reality-oriented, adaptive functions, which were also seen as modulating factors between drive impulses and reality adaptation. Many of the psychoanalytic ego psychologists from 1940 to 1960, who were interested in the metatheory of psychoanalysis (the economic, topographic, and structural models of the mind) and studied autonomous ego functions such as impulse–defense configurations, affect regulation, and the organization of thought processes and other adaptive ego functions, still had a basic biological orientation. Even as late as 1960, many psychoanalysts continued to view the individual as a *closed system* (Loewald, 1960) and continued to focus primarily on biological forces of discharge and defense (thresholds) and innate, inborn ego structures. They were interested in how these basic biological predispositions unfolded in normal personality development and how disruptions of the equilibrium between drive, defense, and other ego functions could result in psychological disturbance.

Based partly on Freud's interest in cultural phenomena, psychoanalytic theory began to extend its primary interest in innate biological predispositions to include interests in the cultural context and how these factors also influence psychological development. Interest in the superego as the internalization of cultural prohibitions and standards led to a fuller appreciation of the family as the mediating force in the transmission of cultural values. Greater emphasis was placed on the role of parents in shaping psychological development. Beginning around 1960, major movements in both England and the United States began to consider psychological development as occurring in an *open system* in which there was a complex transaction between the unfolding biological predispositions of the child and the patterns of care provided by caring agents. The infant's biological predispositions of impulse and defense were now seen as profoundly influenced by the interaction with the care-giving patterns provided by significant figures in the environment. Object relations theorists in England, such as Donald Winnicott, John Bowlby, Michael Balint, Ronald Fairbairn, John Sutherland, and Harry Guntrip, and ego psychologists in the United States, such as Margaret Mahler, Edith Jacobson, and Selma Fraiberg, as well as Anna Freud in London, began to consider the important role of parents in shaping psychological development. The emphasis in personality development on the modulation of the impetus toward instinctual discharge and gratification was now supplemented by an appreciation of the infant's powerful need for object relatedness. As Mahler (1960, p. 551) noted, "Only object relationship with the human love object, which involves partial identification with the object, as well as cathexis of the object with neutralized libidinal energy, promotes emotional development and structure formation."

Increasingly, psychoanalysts came to view psychological development as the result of the complex interaction between the child's evolving libidinal and aggressive drives, the development of modulating and adaptive ego functions, and the interpersonal matrix of the family and culture. Interpersonal interactions with significant care-giving figures are now considered by many psychoanalysts to be a major factor in the formation of cognitive–affective structures, defined primarily in terms of evolving concepts or mental representations of the self and of others in the object world (Jacobson, 1964). Psychological development occurs in relationships with significant care-giving figures through the processes of internalization (Behrends & Blatt, 1985) that result in the formation of intrapsychic structures that can best be understood in terms of the quality of the representations of self and others (Blatt, 1974; Blatt, Wild, & Ritzler, 1975; Meissner, 1981; Schafer, 1978).

Over the last three decades, a number of psychoanalysts have sought to integrate traditional concepts of psychoanalysis with a broadened, psychodynamically based developmental theory, concepts of object relations, and beginning attempts to develop a systematic psychology of the self (Blatt & Lerner, 1983, 1991). "Experience-distant" metapsychological concepts of energies, forces, and structures— concepts used to describe the functioning of the mind based on a closed system model derived partly from the natural and biological sciences— were being replaced by a more "experience-near" (Klein, 1976) clinical theory concerned with concepts of the self and others in a "representational world" (Jacobson, 1964; Sandler & Rosenblatt, 1962). The consideration of personality development as an open system required the development of a new scientific method concerned with systematically assessing the construction of the meaning of psychological events and the articulation of motives rather than trying to explain psychological functioning as the result of changes in energies, forces, and counterforces (Holt, 1967; Home, 1966; Klein, 1976; Schafer, 1978). This new emphasis in psychoanalytic theory gives fuller recognition to the development of the individual's construction of his reality—his conceptions of himself in interaction with his object world. These symbolic constructions of the representational world evolve out of interpersonal experiences, and they, in turn, organize and direct subsequent behavior. These representational constructions become increasingly structured and integrated with development.

The recent emphasis in psychoanalytic theory on the development of the representational world captures two dimensions that are unique and fundamental to the human condition: (1) that we evolve and function in a complex interpersonal matrix and (2) that we are primarily a symbolizing species. The representational world is our symbolic construction of significant interpersonal experiences. It is important to note that this interest in the representational world in psychoanalytic theory is consistent and convergent with recent trends in cognitive theory, developmental psychology, and attachment theory and research, which also address the importance of the development of representation as a major psychological process.

Psychoanalytic theory is in a particularly good position to provide insight into the vicissitudes and subtleties of the interpersonal matrix that lead to the development of cognitive–affective structures of the representational world throughout the life cycle. It has a unique vantage point for appreciating how experiences at various critical nodal points in the life cycle, from the initial infant–mother matrix to senescence, affect the development of the representational world. We can define some of the universal qualities that occur at each major developmental nodal point and how the psychological qualities of particular figures in the individual's life, and the relationships established with them at these various nodal points, contribute to the individual's construction of his or her unique representational world.

The content and structure of the representational world that develop at these various nodal points in the life cycle can be defined in a number of different ways. Concepts of self and of others and their actual and potential interactions constitute one of the primary dimensions of the representational world. Representations of self and others refer to the conscious and unconscious mental schema, including their cognitive, affective, and experiential components, that evolve out of significant interpersonal encounters. Beginning as vague, diffuse, variable, sensorimotor experiences of pleasure and unpleasure, schema gradually develop into differentiated, consistent, relatively realistic representations of the self and significant others. Earlier forms of representations are based on action sequences associated with need gratification, intermediate forms are based on specific perceptual and functional features, and higher forms are more symbolic and conceptual (Blatt, 1974). Deriving from significant interpersonal relationships, concepts of the self and of others are essential components of the representational world that are organized at different developmental levels at various points in the life cycle. Thus, personality development involves two fundamental tasks: (1) the establishment of stable, enduring, mutually satisfying interpersonal relationships; and (2) the achievement of a differentiated, consolidated, stable, realistic, essentially positive identity.

These two developmental tasks delineate two primary developmental lines (A. Freud, 1963, 1965a,b) that normally evolve as a complex dialectical process. Development in either line is contingent on this dialectical interaction: The development of the concept of the self is dependent on establishing satisfying interpersonal experiences, and, likewise, the continuation of satisfying interpersonal experiences is contingent on the development of more mature concepts of the self in interaction with others. Meaningful and satisfactory interpersonal relationships contribute to an evolving concept of the self, and, in turn, new levels of the sense of the self, or of identity, lead to more mature levels of interpersonal relatedness (Blatt, 1990b, 1991, in press; Blatt & Blass, 1990; Blatt & Blass, in press; Blatt & Shichman, 1983).

These two primary developmental lines evolve throughout the life cycle. The establishment of stable and meaningful interpersonal relatedness defines an "anaclitic" developmental line. The development of a consolidated and differentiated identity and self-concept defines an "introjective" developmental line. These two developmental lines evolve from more primitive to more integrated modes of organization. In normal development, these two developmental lines evolve in a reciprocal, synergistic way. Most formulations usually consider personality development as a linear sequence. Some theories emphasize primarily the development of the capacity to form meaningful interpersonal relationships, whereas other theories emphasize primarily the development of the self as the central issue in personality development (Blatt & Blass, 1990). But these two developmental lines normally evolve throughout the life cycle in a reciprocal interaction or dialectic transaction. In normal personality development, these two developmental processes evolve in an interactive, reciprocally balanced, mutually facilitating, synergistic fashion from birth through senescence (Blatt, 1974, 1991; Blatt & Blass, 1990; Blatt & Shichman, 1983).

These formulations are consistent with a wide range of personality theories ranging from fundamental psychoanalytic formations to basic empirical investigations of personality development that consider relatedness and self-definition to be two basic dimensions of personality development. Freud (1930), for example, observed in *Civilization and Its Discontents* that "the development of the individual seems . . . to be a product of the interaction between two urges, the urge toward happiness, which we usually call 'egoistic,' and the urge toward union with others in the community, which we call 'altruistic' (p. 140). . . . The man who is predominantly erotic will give the first preference to his emotional relationship to other people; the narcissistic man, who inclines to be self-sufficient, will seek his main satisfactions in his internal mental processes" (pp. 83–84). Freud (1914, 1926) also distinguished between object and ego libido and between libidinal instincts in the service of attachment and aggressive instincts necessary for autonomy, mastery, and self-definition. Loewald (1962, p. 490) noted that the exploration of "these various modes of separation and union . . . [identify a] polarity inherent in individual existence of individuation and 'primary narcissistic union'—a polarity that Freud attempted to conceptualize by various approaches but that he recognized and insisted upon from beginning to end by his dualistic conception of instincts, of human nature, and of life itself." Bowlby (1969, 1973), from an ethological viewpoint, considered striving for attachment and separation as the emotional substrate for personality development. Michael Balint (1959), from an object relations perspective, also discussed these two fundamental dimensions in personality development—a clinging or connectedness (an oconophilic tendency) as opposed to self-sufficiency (a philobatic tendency). Shor and Sanville (1978), based on Balint's formulations, discussed psychological development as involving a fundamental oscillation between "necessary connectedness" and "inevitable separations" or between "intimacy and autonomy." Personality development involves a "a dialectical spiral or helix which interweaves the[se] two dimensions of development."

The dialectic, synergistic development of concepts of self and of relationships with others can be illustrated by an elaboration of Erikson's epigenetic model of psychosocial development. Erikson's (1950) model, although presented basically as a linear developmental process, implicitly provides support for the view that normal personality development involves the simultaneous and mutually facilitating development of self-definition and interpersonal relatedness. If one includes in Erikson's model an additional stage of cooperation versus alienation (occurring around the time of the development of cooperative peer play and the initial resolution of the oedipal crisis at about 4 to 6 years of age), and places this stage at the appropriate point in the developmental sequence, between Erikson's phallic–urethral stage of "initiative versus guilt" and his "industry versus inferiority" of latency (Blatt & Shichman, 1983), then Erikson's epigenetic model of psychosocial development illustrates the complex transaction between interpersonal relatedness and self-definition that occurs in normal development throughout the life cycle.

Erikson initially emphasizes interpersonal relatedness in his discussion of trust versus mistrust, followed by two stages of self-definition, autonomy versus shame and initiative versus guilt. This is followed by the new stage of interpersonal relatedness, cooperation versus alienation, and then by two stages of self-definition, industry versus inferiority and identity versus role diffusion. The following stage, intimacy versus isolation, is again clearly a stage of interpersonal relatedness, followed by two more stages of self-definition, generativity versus stagnation and integrity versus despair (Blatt & Shichman, 1983). As indicated in Figure 1.1, Erikson's epigenetic model of psychosocial crises provides thematic content that elaborates the development of self and object representation at different stages of the life cycle (Blatt, 1974; Blatt & Blass, in press).

This reformulation of Erikson's model (Blatt, 1990b; Blatt & Blass, 1990, in press; Blatt & Shichman, 1983) corrects the deficiency noted by a number of theorists (e.g., Franz & White, 1985) that Erikson's model is primarily an identity theory that tends to neglect the development of interpersonal attachment. The fuller articulation of an attachment devel-

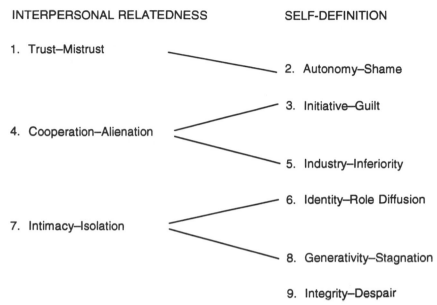

INTERPERSONAL RELATEDNESS   SELF-DEFINITION

1. Trust–Mistrust

2. Autonomy–Shame

3. Initiative–Guilt

4. Cooperation–Alienation

5. Industry–Inferiority

6. Identity–Role Diffusion

7. Intimacy–Isolation

8. Generativity–Stagnation

9. Integrity–Despair

FIG. 1.1. The dialectic interaction of interpersonal relatedness and self-definition implicit in Erikson's Psychosocial Model. (Adapted from Blatt, 1990b.)

opmental line broadens Erikson's model and enables us to note more clearly the dialectic transaction between relatedness and self-definition implicit in Erickson's developmental model. Relatedness and individuality (attachment and separation) both evolve through a complex interactive developmental process. The evolving capacities for autonomy, initiative, and industry in the self-definition developmental line proceed in parallel with the development of a capacity for relatedness. This capacity for relatedness progresses from a capacity to engage with and trust another, to cooperate and collaborate in activities with peers (e.g., play), to achieve a close friendship with a same-sex chum, and to eventually experience and express feelings of mutuality, intimacy, and reciprocity in an intimate, mature relationship. In normal development, there is a coordination between the evolving capacities along these two developmental lines. For example, one needs a sense of basic trust to venture in opposition to the need-gratifying other in asserting one's autonomy and independence, and later one needs a sense of autonomy and initiative to establish cooperative and collaborative relationships with others (Blatt, in press; Blatt & Blass, in press).

Numerous other personality theorists, using a variety of different terms, have also discussed interpersonal relatedness (or attachment) and self-definition (or individuation) as two central processes in personality development. Angyal (1951) discussed surrender and autonomy as two basic personality dispositions. Surrender for Angyal (1951) is the desire to seek a home, to become part of something greater than oneself, while autonomy represents a "striving . . . (to be) an autonomous being . . . that asserts itself actively instead of reacting passively. . . . [Autonomy is] a striving for freedom and for mastery" (pp. 131–132). Bakan (1966) similarly defined communion and agency as two fundamental dimensions in personality development. Communion for Bakan (1966, pp. 14–15) is a loss of self in a merging and blending with others and the world. It involves participating in a larger social entity and feeling in contact or union with others. In contrast, agency defines a pressure toward individuation and emphasizes feeling comfortable with isolation, alienation, and aloneness. The basic issues in agency are separation and mastery.

Other theorists, from a variety of theoretical perspectives, have discussed two similar dimensions in personality development such as the importance of motives for affiliation (or intimacy) (e.g., McAdams, 1980, 1985) as compared with achievement (e.g., McClelland, 1980, 1986; McClelland, Atkinson, Clark, & Lowell, 1953) or power (Winter, 1973). McAdams (1985) discussed extensively the interplay between power and intimacy in personality organization. In studies of life narratives, McAdams (1985) found that two central themes defined two dominant clusters in his data: (1) themes of intimacy (such as feeling close, warm, and in communication with others) and (2) themes of power (such as feeling strong and of having a significant impact on one's environment). Wiggins (1991), an empirically based personality investigator, argued that agency and communion should serve as primary conceptual coordinates for the measurement of interpersonal behavior and as the fundamental coordinates of a trait language for describing personality functioning. Wiggins noted that circumplex and five-factor models of personality that have been useful in the conceptualization and measurement of interpersonal acts, traits, affects, problems, and personality disorders are "derived from the meta-concepts of agency and communion." Although agency and communion may not by themselves capture the broad spectrum of individual differences that characterize human transactions, Wiggins (1991) concluded that they "are propaedeutic to the study of [the] . . . determinants of interpersonal behavior."

These various theoretical positions concur that normal personality organization involves an integration of these two basic dimensions: a capacity for interpersonal relatedness and the development of self-definition (Stewart & Malley, 1987). Angyal (1951, pp. 135–136), like Bakan (1966), stressed that the major task in life is to achieve a compromise and balance between these two forces such that they are both represented fully in one's experiences. Increased autonomy, mastery, and a capacity to govern one's life and environment are best accomplished by understanding and respecting laws and rules of the social matrix. Similarly, an intimate relationship requires a capacity for relinquishing one's autonomy to some degree, but it also requires a capacity for mastery of one's environment, resourcefulness, and self-reliance, without which a relationship is in danger of deteriorating into helpless dependency and possessiveness. McClelland (1986) discussed the most mature form of power motive as based on an essential integration of autonomy and affiliation. Kobasa, Maddi, and Kahn (1982) also discussed the importance of a blend of communion and agency, of intimacy and power needs, as central to the development of psychological well-being and hardiness.

While normality can be defined ideally as an integration of interpersonal relatedness and self-definition, many individuals place a relatively greater emphasis on one of these developmental processes over the other. This relative emphasis on interpersonal relatedness or self-definition delineates two basic personality configurations, each with experience, preferred modes of cognition, defense, and adaptation (Blatt, 1974, 1990b, 1991; Blatt & Shichman, 1983). As Bakan (1966) noted, individual differences in personality style and motivational disposition can be understood in part according to which of these two tendencies an individual gives priority (Maddi, 1980).

Individuals who place a relatively greater emphasis on interpersonal relatedness are generally more figurative in their thinking and focus primarily on affects and visual images. Their thinking is usually characterized more by simultaneous rather than by sequential processing. The emphasis is on reconciliation, synthesis, and integration of elements into a cohesive unity rather than on a critical analysis of separate elements and details (Szumotalska, 1992). In terms of cognitive style, these individuals tend to be repressors and levelers (Gardner, Holzman, Klein, Lipton, & Spence, 1959; Gardner, Jackson, & Messick, 1960), and their predominant tendency is to seek fusion, harmony, integration, and synthesis. These individuals are primarily field dependent and very aware of and influenced by environmental factors (Witkin, 1965). Their primary goal is to seek harmony, peace, and satisfaction in interpersonal relationships (Luthar & Blatt, 1993). Thinking is much more intuitive and determined by feelings and personal reactions than by facts, figures, and other details. Their primary mode is more libidinal than aggressive, and they value affectionate feelings and the establishment of close, intimate relationships (Blatt, Quinlan, Chevron, McDonald, & Zuroff, 1982; Blatt & Zuroff, 1992).

In individuals focused primarily on self-definition, thinking is much more literal, sequential, linguistic, and critical. Issues of action, overt behavior, manifest form, logic, consistency, and causality are attended to rather than feelings and interpersonal relationships. Thinking is highly valued, and emphasis is on analysis rather than synthesis, on the critical dissection of details and part properties rather than on achieving an integration and synthesis (Szumotalska, 1992). Attention is focused on details and contradictions, logic and consistency, cause and effect, and responsibility and blame. These individuals tend to be sensitizers or sharpeners and to be field independent (Witkin, 1965; Witkin, Dyk, Faterson, Goodenough, & Karp, 1962). Their experiences and judgment are determined primarily by internal appraisal rather than by environmental events. Spontaneity and expressions of feelings are carefully controlled; the individual's primary goal is self-assertion, control, autonomy, power, and prestige rather than relatedness. The primary instinctual mode of these individuals involves assertion and aggression in the service of differentiation and self-definition rather than affection and intimacy (Blatt & Shichman, 1983; Blatt & Zuroff, 1992).[1]

In their discussion of the anaclitic/introjective personality styles, Blatt and Shichman (1983) noted that different types of psychological defenses or coping styles are integral to these two basic personality types. Defenses can be discussed as specific mechanisms (e.g., denial, repression, isolation, intellectualization, reaction formation, overcompensation), or individual defenses can be considered as specific examples of several broad categories of defense. A more generic classification of defenses is the differentiation of avoidant versus counteractive defenses (Blatt & Shichman, 1983) or repression versus sensitization (Byrne, Barry, & Nelson, 1963). Both avoidant and counteractive defenses attempt to keep aspects of painful and conflict-laden issues out of awareness, but they do so in very different ways. Denial and repression are avoidant defenses; they seek to avoid recognizing and acknowledging the existence of conflictual issues. In contrast, counteractive defenses (e.g., projection, intellectualization, reaction formation, and overcompensation) do not avoid conflicts but rather transform them into an alternative acceptable form. Reaction formation and overcompensation are examples of counteractive defenses in which an impulse is transformed into its opposite (Blatt, 1990b; Blatt & Shichman, 1983). Repression and sensitization (Byrne et al., 1963), or disengaged and engaged coping styles, are examples of avoidant and counteractive defenses, respectively.

The research of Byrne et al. (1963) on two primary types of defenses, repression and sensitization, offers support for the distinction of two primary personality configurations. Repressors tend to be more concerned with interpersonal relations and tend to maintain a more positive and optimistic outlook about themselves and others. They tend to have a more global cognitive approach (Hamilton, 1983) and avoid contradiction and controversy. They have difficulty expressing anger and personal conflicts. Although they try to avoid conflict and interpersonal difficulties, they have more conflictual relationships (Graziano, Brothen, & Berscheid, 1980) and are less aware of feelings about themselves and others that might disrupt their relationships. They try to avoid conflictual themes and report few negative childhood experiences (Davis & Schwartz, 1987), but their speech has a greater frequency of disruptions than other groups. Although they report little awareness of contradiction and conflict (Beutler, Johnson, Morris, & Neville, 1977; Byrne et al., 1963; Rofe, Lewin, & Padeh, 1977; Tempone & Lambe, 1967), they are physiologically responsive to emotionally stressful situations (Epstein & Fenz, 1967; White & Wilkins, 1973). Repressors have a marked discordance between their subjective experiences and their physiological responses. Although repressors report low levels of anxiety (Slough, Kleinknecht, & Thorndike, 1984; Sullivan & Roberts, 1969), they have high levels of physiological arousal (Weinberger, Schwartz, & Davidson, 1979).

Sensitizers, in contrast, are preoccupied with issues of self-worth, self-control, and identity and are overly critical of themselves and others. They have more negative views of themselves and are more aware of contradiction and conflict. They are ruminative, autonomous, independent, less influenced by the judgment of others (Zanna & Aziza, 1976), introspective, and self-critical.

Thus, two broad categories of defense processes, avoidant (repression) and counteractive (sensitization), parallel particular modes of thinking, feeling, and behaving that are an integral part of two primary personality or character styles. Avoidant defenses, such as denial, repression, and displacement, are typical of the character style that emphasizes interpersonal relatedness, while counteractive defenses, such as intellectualization, reaction formation, and overcompensation, are typical of the character style that emphasizes self-definition and identity. In the extreme, these two types of defenses and types of personality styles are also an integral part of two different configurations of psychopathology (Blatt, 1974, 1990b, in press; Blatt & Shichman, 1983).

Biological predispositions and disruptive interpersonal events can interact in complex ways to disturb this integrated developmental process and lead to exaggerated preoccupation with one developmental line to the neglect of the other. Psychopathology is the consequence of impairments in development that interfere with the reciprocal development of satisfying interpersonal relations and a meaningful concept of the self. Psychopathology is characterized by a lack of flexibility and a loss of the opportunity to change as a consequence of new experiences. Rigid, fixed concepts of the self restrict the opportunity to establish new types of interpersonal experiences, and repetitive types of interpersonal interactions and experiences restrict and seriously limit further modification, revision, and growth of the self.

In our view, individuals cope with severe developmental disruptions by exaggerated and distorted attempts to achieve equilibrium either by establishing a preoccupation with maintaining interpersonal relatedness (an anaclitic preoccupation) or by maintaining a consolidated concept of the self (an introjective preoccupation). Most psychopathological disorders are expressions of extreme exaggerations of one of these two primary developmental lines and the defensive avoidance of the other line. The determination of which developmental line (the concept of the self or the mode of interpersonal relatedness) (introjective or anaclitic) becomes the primary focus of compensatory maneuvers, and symptomatic expression in psychopathology is influenced by a host of possible parameters. These parameters include biological predispositions such as gender, specific environmental factors and events such as the phase of development in which the disruptions occur, the specific conflictual issues involved, the cultural and family matrix, the character style of the primary caregivers, and the values of the individual and the family. Disruptions of developmental processes can be relatively mild or severe. The earlier and the more extensive the disruptions, the greater the exaggerated emphasis of one developmental line at the defensive avoidance of the other and the greater the possibility of psychopathology.

Most forms of psychopathology can be considered as distorted exaggerations of either the anaclitic or the introjective developmental line. As illustrated in Figure 1.2, exaggerated and distorted preoccupation with establishing satisfying interpersonal relations that interferes with the development of a consolidated concept of self defines the psychopathologies of the anaclitic configuration. This would include the infantile personality, anaclitic depression, and hysterical disorders. Exaggerated and distorted preoccupation with establishing and maintaining the definition of the self that interferes with establishing meaningful interpersonal relations defines the psychopathologies of the introjective configuration. This would include paranoid, obsessive–compulsive, introjective depressive, and phallic–narcissistic disorders (Blatt & Shichman, 1983).

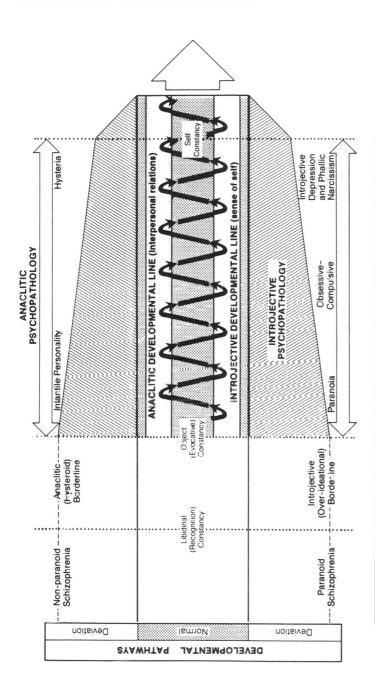

FIG. 1.2. A model of normal and psychopathological development. (Adapted from Blatt & Shichman, 1983.)

Psychopathologies within the *anaclitic configuration* are interrelated and share a preoccupation with libidinal and interpersonal issues such as conflicted attempts to establish satisfying interpersonal relations with feelings of trust, intimacy, cooperation, and mutuality. Predominant in the psychopathologies of the anaclitic configuration (the infantile personality, anaclitic depression, and hysteria) are preoccupations about the dependability of interpersonal relationships and the desire to be close and intimate and to give and receive care and love. Intense concern about these issues can be expressed in a form most relevant to an early developmental level—at the level of the basic dependent, unilateral, caring mother–child dyad—or at the more mature, complex, reciprocal, oedipal level where there are conflicts about giving as well as receiving love. Depriving, rejecting, inconsistent, unpredictable, or overindulgent relationships have led to conflicts around libidinal issues of care, affection, love, and sexuality. These intense and exaggerated concerns about interpersonal relatedness interfere with the development of a sense of self. Defenses in anaclitic psychopathology are primarily avoidant maneuvers—denial, repression, and displacement.

Psychopathological disorders within the *introjective configuration* are interrelated and share a basic focus on issues of aggression and struggles for self-definition. As illustrated in Figure 1.2, excessive preoccupation with issues of self-definition, autonomy, self-control, self-worth, and identity is expressed in primitive form in paranoia, in somewhat more advanced form in obsessive–compulsive personality disorders, and at higher developmental levels in introjective (guilt-laden) depression and phallic narcissism. All of these forms of introjective psychopathology are exaggerated and distorted attempts to establish and maintain a sense of self-definition and identity at the expense of interpersonal relatedness. The individual seeks to achieve separation, definition, control, independence, and autonomy from controlling, intrusive, punitive, excessively critical, and judgmental figures. These struggles for individuation are also expressed in conflicts around the management and containment of affect, especially aggression directed toward others and the self. These excessive preoccupations with autonomy and self-definition interfere with the capacity to establish intimate and meaningful interpersonal relationships. Defenses in introjective psychopathology are basically counteractive. Projection (splitting, externalization, disavowal, and reversal), doing and undoing, reaction formation, isolation, intellectualization, rationalization, introjection, identification with the aggressor, and overcompensation are all attempts to control, modify, and transform impulses.

Psychopathologies within the anaclitic configuration have a better

capacity for affective bonding and a greater potential for the development of meaningful interpersonal relations. In the psychopathologies of
the introjective configuration, ideational processes are more valued and
there is greater potential for the development of logical, rational
thought. Although most forms of psychopathology are organized primarily around one configuration or the other, there also may be some
patients who have features from both the anaclitic and introjective dimensions and whose psychopathology derives from both configurations.

In each of these two configurations of psychopathology, there are
several evolving levels of organization ranging from more primitive to
more integrated attempts to establish meaningful interpersonal relations
and a consolidated self-concept. Psychopathologies at higher levels of the
anaclitic and introjective configurations, such as hysteria or introjective
depression and phallic narcissism, are likely to be considered oedipal
disorders, whereas psychopathologies at the lower levels of the configurations, such as the infantile personality or paranoid and obsessive–
compulsive disorders, would often be thought of as pre-oedipal disorders. Many patients, however, will range across the entire spectrum of a
configuration, and their disorders will have a complex mixture of both
oedipal and pre-oedipal features.

There are a number of important consequences of identifying two
primary configurations of personality organization and psychopathology. First, this approach provides a basis for integrating a wide variety of
symptomatic expressions of psychological disturbance into a unified developmental model in which there are two major configurations of psychopathology, each of which can range over several levels of organization, from more primitive and undifferentiated to more mature and
integrated. Second, the various forms of psychopathology within each
personality configuration are considered in dynamic relationship to one
another. Within a single configuration there are dynamic and structural
relationships among more and less primitive expressions of psychopathology. The various forms of psychopathology are no longer considered as isolated disease entities but rather as interrelated modes of adaptation organized along two basic dimensions: interpersonal relatedness
or self-definition. Third, the dynamic relationships among the various
forms of psychopathology within each configuration define potential
lines of regression and progression along which individuals may
change. Each of the forms of psychopathology within the personality
configuration represents impairments at a particular phase in the developmental sequence. The various phases within each developmental line
define nodal points at which particular individuals may experience diffi-

culty. Thus, individuals can be identified as having difficulties predominantly within one or the other personality configuration, with a primary organization at a particular developmental level, and with the potential to regress or progress to other levels of the configuration, depending on particular situations and circumstances and the nature of their psychopathology (Blatt & Shichman, 1983).

The distinction of two primary configurations of psychopathology has important implications for understanding aspects of the therapeutic process. There may be fundamental differences in the nature of the transference encountered with patients with psychopathology in each of these two configurations. In the anaclitic configuration, transference themes may center more on libidinal and affective dimensions and the patient's struggle with issues of dependency, intimacy, loss, abandonment, envy, and jealousy. In the introjective configuration, themes of aggression, self-definition, and self-worth may dominate the therapeutic relationship as patients struggle with issues of power, control, autonomy, criticism, and competition. Likewise, different types of countertransference issues may be stimulated within the therapist by patients whose pathology is predominantly anaclitic or introjective. One might also expect that the nature of the therapeutic process would be different in some respects for these two types of patients, and that, initially at least, these two different types of patients might be more responsive to different aspects of the treatment process and change in different ways and along different dimensions.

Rather than searching for universal measures of change, it might be more productive to consider the possibility that different types of patients may change in different ways. Grouping all patients together may cancel out effects that are predominant in one group and irrelevant in other types of patients. The distinction between these two broad types of psychopathology—the anaclitic and introjective configurations—may provide a way of investigating differential expressions of change in the intensive treatment of seriously disturbed young adults.

METHODOLOGICAL ISSUES IN THE ASSESSMENT OF THERAPEUTIC CHANGE

Research in psychotherapy has usually addressed issues such as the evaluation of long-term outcome, the relative effectiveness of different forms of treatment, and the identification of variables characteristic of the patient, the therapist, and/or the therapeutic process that affect the treatment process. Most of these studies consider all patients as the same, expecting them to change in similar ways. In addition, most studies use economic or pragmatic criteria of social adjustment, rather than psychological variables, to evaluate change. In contrast, the present study sought to identify important psychological dimensions and to explore whether different psychological variables change in different types of patients after a substantial period of treatment.

One of the primary difficulties in psychotherapy research has been the development of reliable, independent measures of psychological change. The lack of such measures places serious constraints on the capacity to discern potential expressions of therapeutic change. Thus, a primary task in studies of therapeutic change is to identify reliable measures that can assess a number of relevant psychological dimensions along which different patients might change. In this study, we use two levels of observation of therapeutic change: (1) data from a clinical perspective describing clinical symptoms and disruptions of manifest social behavior and (2) data from independent assessments of cognitive, affective, and interpersonal dimensions through the use of psychological tests, especially the Rorschach but also the Thematic Apperception Test (TAT), Human Figure Drawings (HFDs), and an intelligence test.

Several central methodological issues need to be considered in the use of procedures for the systematic assessment of therapeutic change. First, the measures must have demonstrated reliability and validity. Measures of change must be stable, consistent, and related to aspects of psychological well-being and adaptive functioning as well as to aspects of psychopathology. Second, one must specify precisely the methods of assessment and the domains being assessed. Third, the methods and domains of assessment need to be relevant to the goals of treatment to ensure that the measures have some relationship to the nature of the interventions. Fourth, one must consider the relationship of the nature of change being assessed to the types of patients being evaluated.

Reliability and Validity

The importance of developing valid and reliable measures of change has been highlighted by a comprehensive and systematic review of psychotherapy research conducted by Smith, Glass, and Miller (1980). By reducing a wide range of research measures to standardized scores, Smith et al. conducted a "meta-analysis" of 475 studies of counseling and psychotherapy. They found large effect sizes, demonstrating the overall effectiveness of psychotherapy. They also found, however, a relationship between effect size and a particular quality of outcome measures—what they termed the measure's "reactivity." "Highly *reac-*

tive instruments are those that reveal or closely parallel the obvious goals or valued outcomes of the therapist or experimenter; which are under control of the therapist, who has an acknowledged interest in achieving predetermined goals; or which are subject to the client's need and ability to alter his scores to show more or less change than what actually took place. Relatively nonreactive measures are not so easily influenced in any direction by any of the parties involved" (Smith et al., 1980, pp. 66–67). In a commentary on this work, Cohen (1984, pp. 334–335) noted that Smith et al. found that "group versus individual (psychotherapy), length of treatment, therapist experience, and virtually anything else except for the reactivity of the outcome measure have no demonstrable effect on outcome."

The American Psychiatric Association's comment on the book by Smith et al. (1980) was particularly blunt: "The largest (although still relatively small) correlation with Effect Size was something called reactivity of outcome indicator ($r = .18$). This implies that the more easily an outcome indicator can be faked (that is, the more obvious the social desirabilities of the items), the larger the effects reported in the investigation" (APA Commission on Psychotherapies, 1982, p. 138). Thus, across 475 studies of psychotherapy outcome, the single, most important variable associated with the demonstrated effectiveness of psychotherapy is the susceptibility of the outcome measure to influence by the hopeful expectations and demand characteristics of the therapist and/or the patient. The findings by Smith et al. (1980) clearly indicate that if psychotherapy research is to progress, we need to develop more sophisticated and comprehensive methods for assessing psychological changes that are independent of influence of the participants in the treatment process.

Methods for assessing change, and their corresponding specific state-of-the-art technologies, have been delineated in a comprehensive survey based on conferences sponsored by the National Institute of Mental Health (NIMH) (Waskow & Parloff, 1975). The editors divided the entire range of potential assessment methods into four categories: (1) patient measures (tests and inventories, direct self-reports, behavioral measures, physiological measures, interviews and speech measures, cognitive and perceptual measures, projective techniques); (2) therapist measures (therapists' assessments and measures of outcome); (3) relevant others' measures (i.e., the use of estimates by relatives and other significant informants besides therapists and independent clinical evaluators); and (4) independent clinical evaluations. Luborsky (1975b, p. 233) noted that "independent clinical evaluations have an obvious advantage over the patient and therapist as judges of therapeutic outcome; as nonparticipants, they have little stake in the outcome of treatment and, hence, less reason to be biased."

Most commentators routinely urge the use of multiple outcome criteria. Working with severely disturbed patients, for example, McGlashan (1984b, p. 588) warned specifically against relying solely on patient self-report measures. Following an extended commentary on methodological issues, McGlashan compared findings on 155 borderline and schizophrenic patients based on both self-assessment and interview–assessment ratings using the same rating scales. He found that "patients scored themselves as significantly healthier on several less concrete or specifiable outcome dimensions such as social functioning, psychopathology, and global functioning." McGlashan (1984a, p. 575) concluded that "although self-assessments might be a valid reflection of the patient's perspective, that perspective should not constitute the only source of information concerning outcome."

Luborsky (1975b, p. 234), in a review of the methods for conducting independent clinical evaluations, included measures based on interviews and diagnostic psychological tests conducted by an independent investigator—someone not directly involved in the treatment process. Thus, Luborsky moved psychological test assessment, including "projective techniques," out of the category of "patient measures" and placed it more appropriately as a method of evaluation by an expert, independent, external observer. Despite the evident value of psychological tests as providing potentially independent evaluations of the treatment process, most psychotherapy outcome studies have been reluctant to use these assessment procedures. Even Luborsky (1975b), who stressed the importance of independent assessment, did not include traditional projective techniques, specifically the Rorschach and TAT, among his recommended methods of expert, external observation, primarily because of the time and expense involved in using these methods. Based on criteria for the value of an assessment method, including the economy of time and effort, meaningfulness, reliability, and validity, Luborsky (1975b) proposed a battery relying largely on moderately structured interviews.

In his other recommendation, Luborsky offered his Health–Sickness Rating Scale (HSRS; Luborsky, 1975a), a unidimensional, clinically anchored rating scale designed to apply to the entire range of mental health, not necessarily requiring a specifically structured interview, that can be applied to highly diverse data. Commenting on the HSRS, Kernberg (1984, p. 249) wrote, "One rather unexpected finding of the Menninger Foundation's Psychotherapy Project was that a relatively simple, qualitative measure of outcome—namely, the health–sickness rating scale—correlated so highly with paired comparisons of variables drawn from the major qualitative write-ups of change (involving multiple, individualized criteria) that the costly and tedious paired comparison method was largely superfluous. We had thought, on theoretical grounds, that psychotherapy outcome implied change along various dimensions which could not be integrated into one global measure of improvement; our findings convinced us that an integrated and quantified measure of improvement (the HSRS) was a reasonable reflection of change." Despite Kernberg's high praise for this single-scale ranking of all levels of psychopathology and normalcy, Luborsky (1975b, p. 238) noted possible shortcomings: "(The HSRS) probably should have more differentiation (by further specification of distinctions) at the schizophrenic level, as well as in the high-normal and super-normal range."

Even though ratings by independent experts were reduced to the use of a single scale that is noted to have limitations, especially at either end of the scale, Luborsky, like many others, seemed reluctant to include psychological tests among the methods recommended for independent assessment. One of the major problems with psychological assessment as a method for independent assessment is the time, effort, and skill involved in using these procedures. But psychological tests have the important advantage of potentially providing truly independent assessments of change because the data can be fully disguised and judges can be asked to rate pre- and postassessment protocols without being influenced by the knowledge that these protocols were part of a study of therapy outcome or that a particular protocol was obtained early or late in the treatment process. Ratings of treatment protocols, in contrast, can often be potentially influenced by the rater's awareness that the assessment is part of a posttreatment evaluation. Thus, psychological assessment procedures, especially methods for evaluating projective techniques that provide reliable and valid measures of important psychological dimensions, could potentially serve as valuable independent assessments of treatment outcome.

Domain of Change

Depending on the types of patients being studied and the nature of the treatment process, different aspects of the patient's functioning need to be assessed. Severely disturbed patients have particular symptoms in comparison with more integrated patients, and they have impairments in certain areas and involving particular functions. In the study of change in psychotherapy, careful attention needs to be given to the domains being assessed. A fair amount of research has been conducted on the assessment of change in severely disturbed inpatients, that is, those in the borderline and schizophrenic range of psychopathology. Drawing from the work of Hughlings Jackson, and following distinctions first presented by Strauss, Carpenter, and Bartko (1974), Keith and Matthews (1984, pp. 70–71) clustered clinical symptoms in serious psychopathology (borderline states and schizophrenia) into three groups: problems associated with positive symptoms, negative symptoms, and disorders of personal relationships. "Positive symptoms refer to symptoms present in schizophrenia such as hallucinations and delusions; negative symptoms refer to symptoms characterized by their absence such as a lack of goal directed behavior, blunting of affect, verbal paucity, and so forth; disordered personal relationships refer to patterns of asociality, withdrawal, and lack of close personal ties" (Strauss et al., 1974).

As noted by Keith and Matthews (1984, p. 72), the data of Strauss et al. (1974) supported the conclusions that positive symptoms develop over a short period of time, are a reaction to biological or socioenvironmental causes, and have minimal prognostic importance. Negative symptoms develop over an extended period of time and are considered either the source of chronicity or the result of it. Disordered personal relationships, in contrast, develop over the long term, are considered the consequence of an interactive process of uncertain etiology, and are viewed as prognostically important for productive functioning as well as in the development of negative and positive symptoms. Keith and Matthews (1984) cited an imposing array of well-designed, rigorous clinical trials of neuroleptic medications that demonstrated that such medications effectively control positive symptoms in severe pathology. Such drugs, however, do not affect negative symptoms and disordered personal relationships, and relatively little progress has been made in developing methods of estimating change in these latter two categories in the treatment of seriously disturbed patients. Clearly, the domains of change need to be specified in the study of seriously disturbed patients, and methods of assessment must be selected that are particularly sensitive to aspects of these domains in which change is expected to occur.

Measures Relevant to Domain of Change

A variety of measures are often used in psychotherapy research, but frequently they seem to be chosen on the basis of the ease of assessment rather than whether they are particularly relevant to the domains considered most salient for the types of difficulties being experienced by the patients included in the study. Since Luborsky's (1975b) recommendations, almost all research studies have used independent clinical evaluations but have usually eschewed projective tests as a method of assessment. More psychodynamically oriented studies have used either global measures modeled on the HSRS or other forms of ratings based on structured interviews. Such interviews are often used to rate the need for posttreatment psychotherapy, hospitalization, or medications; to rate aspects of social functioning including employment, social activity, and level of interpersonal intimacy; or to rate more clinically oriented dimensions such as the level of psychopathology, symptoms, and global functioning. More behaviorally oriented studies have relied on ratings of specifically observed or reported behaviors. In a survey of 216 outcome studies published in the *Journal of Consulting and Clinical Psychology* between 1976 and 1981, Lambert, Christensen, and DeJulio (1983, p. 11) found that of the 106 studies using trained observers, more than half showed a preference for rating specific behaviors.

A more recent study of individual psychotherapy with seriously disturbed inpatients, considered by many (e.g., Karon, 1984; Klerman, 1984; May, 1984; Parloff, 1984) to be representative of the state of the art in the field, is the Boston Psychotherapy of Schizophrenia Project initiated by Stanton et al. (1984) and completed by Gunderson et al. (1984). This 10-year-long, ambitious, and complex project compared the effectiveness of two forms of psychotherapy, supported by medication, with schizophrenics of midlevel severity of psychopathology. Out of a vast array of data gathered in this study, a noteworthy comment can be made about the efficacy of outcome measures.

The researchers tapped a wide range of outcome variables. In the process of organizing their data, they derived 15 "outcome clusters" from about 95 discrete variables (Stanton et al., 1984, p. 545). These 95 variables came from three sources: interview instruments, projective tests, and patient self-reports. Ten of the 15 "outcome clusters" were derived almost entirely from the interview instruments, two exclusively from the Rorschach, one largely from the TAT, and two from reports by the patients and by a significant other. Gunderson et al. (1984, p. 580) noted that the researchers had originally planned to have 60 patients in each of the two treatment conditions used in the study, but because of a high attrition rate they were able to maintain only about 20 patients in each group for the 2-year period of the study. Of the 15 "outcome clusters," they found nine were significantly correlated ($p<.05$) with outcome measures. Four of the nine significant correlations were obtained with variables derived exclusively from the Rorschach (Holt's measures of primary process thinking and adaptive regression). It is noteworthy that the investigators as well as several reviewers (e.g., Klerman, 1984, p. 611; May, 1984, p. 606) did not give as much credence to the "outcome clusters" derived from psychological tests as they did to several discrete behavioral variables involving "days employed full-time," "units of productive activity," and "occupational level reached." Although these discrete behavioral variables are of value for assessing capacity for social adaptation, it is important to ask why these reviewers placed so little emphasis on the significant changes noted on the independently assessed dimensions measured by psychological tests.

The data of the Boston Psychotherapy of Schizophrenia Project suggest that the Rorschach, along with interviewing techniques and the assessment of manifest social behavior, can provide sensitive measures of change in severely disturbed patients. This suggestion must be considered against several decades of skepticism about the reliability and validity of data gathered through "projective procedures" and their potential contribution to research. Much of the myth about the supposed limited contribution of projective techniques in research is based either on studies that have used the test procedures in mechanical ways without sufficient regard for the clinical and theoretical rationale for analyzing the data or on studies that have examined the relationship of this type of data to inappropriate criteria (Blatt, 1975). Appelbaum (1977, Chapter 7), using data from 39 cases of the Menninger Psychotherapy Project, demonstrated that ratings derived from psychological tests (especially the Rorschach) agreed significantly more often with the external criteria ("global diagnostic impression, treatment recommendations, and specific treatment predictions") than did psychiatric ratings. Support for the contribution of projective test data in clinical research is far from disheartening if one considers studies in which clinically relevant differentiations are related to reasonably well-specified and controlled criteria (Blatt, 1975). The Rorschach has been particularly effective in recent investigations of several important dimensions of severe psychopathology including the study of thought disorder (e.g., Blatt & Ritzler, 1974; Harrow & Quinlan, 1985; Holt, 1962, 1977; Johnston, 1975; Johnston & Holzman, 1979; Quinlan, Harrow, Tucker, & Carlson, 1972) and aspects of object relations and object representation (Blatt, Brenneis, Schimek, & Glick, 1976b; Kavanaugh, 1982, 1985; Mayman, 1967; Mayman & Krohn, 1975; Schwager & Spear, 1981). It is important to stress that these new approaches to the Rorschach view it not as a "perceptual test" (e.g., Beck, 1945; Exner, 1974) based on theories dominant in psychology in the first half of the 20th century, but as a procedure for assessing representational structures and processes. Cross-sectional research using these new approaches to the Rorschach (e.g., Blatt & Berman, 1984; Blatt & Ritzler, 1974; Lerner & St. Peter, 1984; Lerner, Sugarman, & Barbour, 1985; Wilson, 1982, 1985) indicate that two primary representational dimensions, thought disorder and the quality of object representation, are important for understanding aspects of severe psychopathology. These findings also suggest that representational dimensions could be assessed on other test procedures such as the TAT and Human Figure Drawings and that these dimensions may be of particular relevance for assessing therapeutic change in seriously disturbed patients.

Another major methodological issue in the study of therapeutic change has been the assumption that all patients are expected to change along the same dimensions. Almost all studies of therapeutic change use universal measures of change that are applicable to all patients. Studies usually fail to discriminate among different types of patients and to allow for the possibility that different types of patients may change in very different ways.

As discussed earlier, theoretical formulations (Blatt, 1974, 1990b; Blatt & Shichman, 1983) suggest that there are two major configurations of psychopathology that are distinctly different from each other, each containing several types of disordered behavior that range from relatively severe to relatively mild forms of psychopathology. Based on a number of developmental and psychodynamic considerations, Blatt and Shichman (1983) differentiated between what they call "anaclitic" and "introjective" disorders. As discussed earlier (pp. 14–18), these two broad configurations of psychopathology seem to define two different types of patients with different types of personality organization, who have different needs and preoccupations and who use different types of defenses. One might expect these two different types of patients to come to treatment with very different needs and possibly to change in different ways.

In summary, our study of therapeutic change is unique in at least two basic regards. Based on substantial prior cross-sectional research, we developed reliable procedures for the analysis of Rorschach responses, TAT stories, and aspects of HFD, which assess representational dimensions that have provided important cross-sectional differentiation among seriously disturbed patients. In the present study, we use two independent sources for the clinical evaluation of change during the intensive treatment of seriously disturbed inpatients: the new methods outlined above for the evaluation of psychological tests and previously established procedures for assessing clinical case records that focus on manifest symptoms and the quality of interpersonal relating. We also differentiate two broadly defined but very different types of personality organization. We then use our various methods for analyzing clinical case records and psychological test protocols to assess whether different patterns of change occur in these two different types of patients.

NOTES

1. Spiegel and Spiegel (1978) propose a similar distinction in their formulations of Dionysian and Apollonian personality styles. There may also be some correspondence between the differentiation of the anaclitic and introjective personality configurations and psychophysiological observations such as different functions attributed to the two cortical hemispheres (Galin, 1974; McKinnon, 1979) and to cortical versus limbic functions (Lapidus & Schmolling, 1975).

CHAPTER 2

Methods for Assessing Therapeutic Change in Clinical Case Reports

CLINICAL CONTEXT OF THE STUDY

A major aspect of the present research is the clinical context in which the treatment was conducted. The Austen Riggs Center, a relatively small, private, intensive, inpatient, open treatment facility, is dedicated to the long-term clinical care of seriously disturbed late adolescents and adults. There is an excellent patient–staff ratio and all patients are seen in intensive psychotherapy at least four times weekly. Considerable attention is also given to the therapeutic community. An extensive array of educational and recreational activities and other support services is provided. In many ways, the Austen Riggs Center approaches the ideal long-term treatment facility; for some time now, throughout the mental health field, it has been considered as offering clinical care of the highest quality. In addition, most patients in the present study came from families of at least middle socioeconomic status and usually had access to reasonable levels of material support both during and following hospitalization. Hospital costs, however, of a significant number of the patients were covered, at least to some degree, by third-party payment.

Conducting research at the Austen Riggs Center possibly limits the extent to which findings can be generalized about the efficacy of treatment in other clinical settings. But the large number of well-trained and highly qualified staff and the relative absence of external limitations on the conduct of the treatment (e.g., restrictions in institutional resources or frequent premature curtailment because of patient finances) maximize the opportunity for studying the effects of treatment in a setting in which treatment could be maximally effective. In a real sense, this research investigates the possibility of therapeutic change in an almost ideal context.

For over 40 years, the Austen Riggs Center has maintained detailed clinical files including extensive clinical evaluations made at intake, yearly, and at discharge, as well as psychological test and retest protocols, obtained annually. An extensive and intensive admission evaluation is conducted on each patient based on clinical interviews with the family and with the patient during the first 6 weeks of hospitalization. The various data from these interviews are gathered and integrated in a lengthy and detailed case report, which is discussed at an admission conference with the entire clinical staff. This initial case report includes family history (the history of the parents, sibling[s], spouse, and children, if any), the developmental history of the patient, a description of the present illness and its onset, the course of any previous therapy, current and past medical evaluations, a description by nurses and activities staff of the patient's initial behavior in the hospital, and a detailed account of the first 6 weeks of the psychotherapeutic interaction. This material is written from primarily a behavioral and phenomenological orientation, describing in detail the patient's various experiences, both current and past, without the imposition of explicit theoretical formulations. Table 2.1 summarizes the various sources of material used in preparing the case records.

TABLE 2.1
Sources of Data Used in Clinical Case Reports

Time 1 (Between 4 and 8 weeks of admission)	Time 2 (After at least 1 year of treatment)
Case identification	Additional family history
Statement of the problem	Additional developmental history
Evaluation of informants' reliability	Additional physical data
Family history	Therapist's monthly progress notes on course of therapy
Developmental history and present illness	Nurses' report
Physical data	Activities report
Clinical examination	Current case formulation
Nurses' reports	Current diagnosis
Activities reports	Current prognosis and recommendations
Course in the hospital	
Case formulation	
Diagnosis	
Recommendations and prognosis	

During the course of treatment and hospitalization, notes are made monthly by the therapist, summarizing patient–therapist interaction. A yearly evaluation follows, and a detailed case report, similar to the initial case report, is prepared in which much more attention is given to direct, firsthand accounts of experiences with the patient in the various treatment modalities rather than to prehospital history. As with the initial case report, this detailed annual report is presented at a conference of the entire clinical staff. At both the admission and the annual evaluation conference, the deliberations are recorded and transcribed, including a final consensus of diagnostic formulations.

There is little difference among case reports prepared over the past 4 decades. Although there have been changes in the debates around theoretical issues and the various concepts used in diagnostic formulations, there is impressive continuity and similarity in the rich array and detailed phenomenal and behavioral accounts contained in these case reports over 4 decades. These two documents, the clinical case reports and conference discussions at admission and about a year later, provided the observational data on which ratings were made, including the assessment of clinical symptoms, interpersonal behavior, and social adjustment.

In addition, coordinated with both the first case report and the annual case re-presentation, an extensive battery of diagnostic psychological tests is administered to the patients, including the Rorschach, Thematic Apperception Test (TAT), Wechsler Intelligence Test, and, in some cases, Human Figure Drawings (HFDs).

NATURE OF THE SAMPLE

Approximately 1200 patients were admitted to the Austen Riggs Center between 1953 and 1975. Two hundred and fifty of these patients had both remained at the Riggs Center for longer than one year and been given an initial and a second set of psychological tests later in the treatment process. Patients who did not stay longer than a year had been either discharged or transferred to another clinical facility because they were unable to tolerate the demands of the open hospital setting. In addition, some patients who remained longer than a year were not given a second set of psychological tests because of a request made by the therapist.

Thus, 250 patients had remained in treatment for at least a year and had been given psychological tests both early and later in the treatment process. To select a relatively homogeneous sample of patients who were dealing with similar life issues, we chose from among the 250 patients all those who were between the ages of 18 and 29 at the time of admission. These 100 patients had been given a full set of psychological tests including the Rorschach, the TAT, and an intelligence test, both at admission and a year or more later during their hospitalization. There were no patients in this sample who had a total, full-scale IQ of less than 80 or definite indications of central nervous system damage. All patients included in the sample had 200 or more sessions of individual, psycho-analytically oriented psychotherapy between testings. Ninety of these 100 patients had psychological test protocols that were written in a suffi-ciently legible form, so they could be used in research. These 90 patients constitute the sample of this study.

These patients had an average of 28.45 months of prior outpatient treatment, and 57% of these patients had previously been admitted, at least once, to a psychiatric hospital (an average of 1.32 prior admissions) for a total average prior hospitalization of 4.75 months. In terms of traditional diagnostic nomenclature (DSM-IIIR), approximately 20% ($n =$ 29) of the sample were considered psychotic, 70% ($n = 50$) as severe personality disorders (including borderline and narcissistic disorders), and 10% ($n = 11$) as primarily depressed. The average Global Assess-ment Score (GAS; Endicott, Spitzer, Fleiss, & Cohen, 1976) of a compara-ble sample was 34 (Plakun, 1989), indicating major impairments in work, family relations, judgment, thinking, and/or mood, or some impair-ments in reality testing or communication (e.g., obscure, illogical, or irrelevant speech) or a serious suicide attempt. Most of the patients came from families of at least the middle socioeconomic class and were reasonably well educated and of at least average intelligence. They were a relatively homogeneous sample demographically. Prior research (As-trachan, Brauer, Harrow, & Schwartz, 1974; Heffner, Strauss, & Grisell, 1975) indicates that such a group of patients is most likely, given their level of severe disturbance, to respond constructively to intensive thera-peutic interventions.

The 45 women and 45 men in the sample ranged in age from 18 to 29 with an average age at intake of 20.94 years. They were hospitalized on average for 26 months, and there was an average of 15 months between the initial evaluation and the second assessment. The second assess-ment was conducted on average 10.9 months prior to discharge and usu-ally was not viewed by staff or patients as part of the discharge process.

RESEARCH DESIGN

Patients were evaluated at two points in time, approximately 6 weeks after admission and after at least 1 year of intensive treatment. At

TABLE 2.2
Schematic of Research Design

Time 1	Time 2
Case record (CR 1)	Case record (CR 2)
Test record (TR 1)	Test record (TR 2)

both points in time, we rated aspects of manifest clinical symptoms, interpersonal behavior, and social adjustment based on material available in the clinical case reports. We also assessed variables derived from the psychological test protocols gathered at these two points in time. The ratings on the clinical case records and the psychological test protocols were made by separate research teams, and even within the psychological test protocols, separate research teams rated the TAT stories, the HFD, and several different conceptual systems applied to the Rorschach protocols (e.g., thought disorder and the concept of the human object). The analyses of these independent sources of data (clinical case records and psychological test protocols) enabled us to develop measures for the evaluation of the extent and nature of therapeutic change. Table 2.2 is a schematic presentation of this basic research design.

Rating of the Clinical Case Records

The development of reliable procedures for assessing manifest clinical symptoms and social behavior from the clinical case records was an essential step in our attempt to study change during long-term intensive treatment of seriously disturbed adolescents and young adults.

To control for halo effect and rater bias in the scoring of the clinical case records, two judges (an MSW social worker and an advanced graduate student in clinical psychology) independently rated the case records. After initial training and establishment of adequate interrater reliability, these two judges worked independently. The initial case reports were randomly split in half, and each half was rated at Time 1 by a separate judge. After each judge rated half of the cases at Time 1, he or she rated the other half of the case records at Time 2, without knowledge of the other judge's ratings at Time 1.

The analysis of in-depth narrative clinical descriptions from multiple observers (e.g., psychiatrists, psychologists, social workers, nurses, activities personnel) called for scales specifically designed to fit such data. We could not optimally use, for example, scales designed to rate focused information gained from several hours of interview, such as

Gunderson's Psychotherapy Outcome Interview (Gunderson & Gomes–Schwartz, 1980); nor did we consistently have the refined data from the therapist to use Schulz's Self and Object Differentiation Scale (Schulz, in Gunderson & Mosher, 1975). We were able, however, to find scales for rating clinical variables appropriate to the quality and time frame of the extensive data we had available in the clinical files.

Clinical Symptoms

Most researchers agree on the need to evaluate overt symptomatology and impairment in functioning when studying change. The experience of the Menninger Psychotherapy Research Project, for example, indicates the importance of rating clinical symptoms. Factor analyses of 10 of their 12 ratings of clinical dimensions derived from psychodynamic concepts yielded one factor that correlated between .85 and .90 with several ratings of severity of symptomatology (McNair, in Spitzer & Klein, 1976, p. 58). Because observation of clinical symptoms is standard in most studies, a number of different scales were readily available.

Because our ratings were based on narrative clinical case reports following 6 weeks of evaluation and again after a year or so of hospitalization and treatment, we were not able to use procedures developed for rating a single clinical interview such as the Current and Past Psychopathology Scales (CPPS) (Endicott & Spitzer, 1972) or the Schedule for Affective Disorders and Schizophrenia (SADS) (Endicott & Spitzer, 1979). We chose instead a rating scale developed specifically as a standardized method for abstracting information about symptoms and social functioning directly from case records. Strauss and Harder (1981) designed a Case Record Rating Scale (CRRS) to maximize reliability of ratings across a wide range of symptoms reported in the typical case history record. Strauss and Harder chose items to provide data on 32 symptom dimensions originally derived from factor analysis, modified by clinical judgment, and subsequently used and revised in several studies. Items are rated for absence or presence of a symptom (score of 0 or 1, respectively) and whether it is continuous and/or severe (score of 2). Our judges were able to achieve acceptable levels of reliability (Item Alpha >.65) for rating these clinical symptoms in a case record.

Based on a replicated factor analysis of clinical characteristics in a representative sample of first psychiatric admissions, Strauss, Kokes, Ritzler, Harder, and Van Ord (1978) identified several highly stable clusters of symptoms that did not correspond to usual diagnostic typologies. Based on an orthogonal four-factor solution with varimax rotation, Strauss et al. (1978) found the following four factors: a "psychosis" factor that accounted for 20.6% of the variance, a "neurosis" factor that accounted for 11% of the variance, and "bizarre-retarded" and "bizarre-disorganized" factors that accounted for 8% and 6.5% of the variance, respectively. Strauss et al. reported that these four factors significantly differentiated among several diagnostic groups (schizophrenics, affective disorders, psychotics, and neurotics).

The symptoms on the psychotic factor include delusions of control, reference, grandeur, religion, and sex; visual, auditory, tactile, and olfactory hallucinations; suspiciousness; derealization; and depersonalization. Symptoms on the neurotic factor included depression, restlessness, somatic complaints, anxiety, obsessions, and withdrawal, as well as some insight into one's problems. The bizarre-retarded factor consisted of symptoms of retarded movement and speech, flat affect, and bizarre behavior. The bizarre-disorganized factor included symptoms of incomprehensibility, unkempt appearance, bizarre behavior, nonsocial speech, and incongruent and labile affect. Because very few of our patients had "bizarre behavior," we changed the name of these last two factors to "flattened affect" and "labile affect" to indicate that the primary difference between these last two factors in our sample was primarily in affect tone. Strauss et al. (1978) commented that the first two factors (psychosis and neurosis) were particularly robust and stable. These four scales (Psychosis, Neurosis, Flattened Affect, and Labile Affect) were rated for all patients at Time 1 and Time 2. We conducted factor analyses on our ratings of these four Strauss–Harder scales in an attempt to reduce the four scales to one or two primary factors. Despite the use of several iterations and different types of rotations, no clear factor structure emerged. Thus, each of the four symptoms scales, as originally defined by Strauss and Harder, was treated in the data analyses as an independent criterion of clinical symptomatology. These scales are presented in detail in Appendix 1.

Social Behavior

We also sought to evaluate dimensions of social behavior based on descriptions in the clinical case records that were prepared by members of the nursing and activities staff and other members of the clinical team. We sought to evaluate patterns of behavior drawn from observations of the patients' day-to-day interactions with other patients and staff. We were especially interested in rating interpersonal communication and patterns of social behavior and involvement.

Several measures we considered were less than optimal because they confounded symptom ratings with ratings of social adjustment (e.g., Ellsworth, 1970; Honigfeld, Gillis, & Klett, 1966; Lorr, 1961; Lorr & Klett, 1966). Most of the scales we found were not designed to rate clinical case records; rather they often required highly detailed daily or weekly observations and were not attuned to broader patterns across time that were often reported in our clinical case records. We found two scales that used dichotomous ratings to rate more general dimensions of social and interpersonal behavior: the Ward Behavior Inventory (Burdock & Hardesty, 1968) and the Ward Behavior Rating Scale (Fairweather et al., 1960). Both seemed appropriate for rating social behavior from clinical case reports. We chose the latter because it seemed to provide somewhat more comprehensive items.

Fairweather and his colleagues (1960) developed a procedure for rating changes in ward behavior in an inpatient therapeutic setting over a long period as part of a study of the relative effectiveness of therapeutic programs for psychotic patients. In part, Fairweather et al. were interested in the changes in social behavior of chronic psychotic patients in an inpatient therapeutic setting. The Fairweather Ward Behavior Rating Scale is a dichotomous, forced-choice rating scale with each set of items designed to assess a specific adaptive behavior and its corresponding maladaptive counterpart (e.g., "The patient participates in the activities around him" and "The patient ignores the activities around him"). The scale consists of 76 items related to ward behavior. Items are grouped on an *a priori* basis into three areas: interpersonal communication, self-care, and participation in work and recreational activities. We were particularly interested in the first area, interpersonal communication, and used the subset of the Fairweather Scale, consisting of 28 items, designed to assess this dimension. Two judges were able to achieve an acceptable level of reliability (Item Alpha >.65) in rating this scale. A high score is indicative of poor interpersonal involvement. A copy of the Fairweather Scale for interpersonal communication is included in Appendix 2.

Interpersonal Relations

Some investigators have argued that symptom amelioration (or a reduction in manifest symptoms) is a measure of psychopathology or of personality change that is superior to ratings based on psychodynamic constructs. Symptoms are often believed to be reliable and valid measures because they are simpler to judge (e.g., McNair, in Spitzer & Klein, 1976; Mintz, 1981). Mintz (1981) posed this classic debate in the form of a question: "Should our criteria (for evaluating treatment) stick to observable behavior, or is there need for sophisticated clinical judgment to come to a meaningful psychodynamic understanding of overt behavior change?" (p. 503). Based on a review of relevant research literature, he concluded that "if a patient's initial symptoms do not improve, there will in general be a good consensus that treatment has not been successful. . . . When the initial symptoms improve, dynamic assessments of treatment outcome and symptomatic assessments do not diverge" (p. 506). Kernberg, in contrast, based on his experiences with the Menninger Psychotherapy Research Project, commented, "For future research on long-term psychoanalytic psychotherapy, a design focusing on the combined impact of patient and treatment variables should include Ego Strength, particularly in three areas: the severity of symptoms, including the initial level of anxiety, the quality of object-relations . . . and nonspecific aspects of ego strength such as anxiety tolerance, impulse control, and sublimatory effectiveness" (in Spitzer and Klein, 1976, pp. 35–36).

To assess dimensions such as ego strength, the quality of object relationships, and the capacity for sublimation, we considered Bellak's procedures for rating ego functions (Bellak, Hurvich, & Gediman, 1973). We found, however, that our judges could not rate these scales reliably because the Bellak Scales assess a very broad range of functioning (from high levels of integrated adaptation to severe psychopathology) over a seven-point scale and therefore these scales had little range and differentiation at the lower end of the continuum on which to rate very disturbed patients. Bellak et al. (1973), in their original development of this scale, did not attempt to make differentiations among severely disturbed patients; rather, they developed their procedures primarily to distinguish across a very broad spectrum—from schizophrenia to normality. We found the same difficulty with the well-established Health–Sickness Rating Scale (Luborsky, 1962). This scale provides a unitary and global rating of a patient's general mental health on a scale ranging from 0 to 100. It was designed as an interval scale with a range that extends into high levels of normal adaptive functioning. Again, our judges were unable to achieve acceptable reliability because there was an insufficient number of differentiations at the more disturbed level of the continuum.

Our judges, however, were able to use effectively several of the example-anchored, 100-point rating scales developed by the Menninger Psychotherapy Research Project. These scales were designed specifically to make differentiations among more disturbed patients based on written clinical descriptions. Michael Harty and his colleagues at the Menninger Foundation, based on the experience of the Psychotherapy Research Project, developed twelve 100-point rating scales (Harty, 1976; Harty et al., 1981) for rating more global clinical dimensions.

In discussing psychotherapy research, Kernberg (1976, 1984) especially called for measures of the quality of object relations, including antisocial features (partially assessed as Superego Integration), measures of impulse control, and sublimatory effectiveness. Prior research by Kernberg (1976, 1984) and by Harty et al. (1981) suggested that 5 of the 12 scales were most appropriate for our study: Motivation for Treatment, Social and Sublimatory Effectiveness, Impulsivity, Superego Integration, and Quality of Object Relations. Harty et al. (1981) found that these five scales had high factor loadings on a single factor that accounted for 36% of the variance in the ratings of 32 scales attempting to evaluate data on hospital intake. Harty et al. (1981) noted that psychiatric symptoms "are evidence of the person's efforts to come to terms with personal dilemmas. . . . 'The problem,' as distinct from the symptoms, is always in some sense a relationship problem, involving needs and fears having to do with acceptance or rejection, intimacy or isolation, power or weakness, autonomy or dependency in relation to others" (Harty et al., 1981). We expected that the behavioral dimensions of interpersonal relatedness, as assessed by these five scales, would be essential elements of change during the course of long-term treatment. Judges were able to rate these five scales (Motivation for Treatment, Social and Sublimatory Effectiveness, Impulsivity, Superego Integration, and Quality of Object Relations) at acceptable levels of reliability (Item Alpha >.65, except for Impulsivity, which was .62). These scales are presented in detail in Appendix 3.

Factor analysis of the ratings on these five Menninger scales on the case records of our 90 subjects at admission identified two primary orthogonal factors. The first factor accounted for 46.95% of the total variance, and four of the five scales had significant loadings on this factor: Motivation for Treatment, Social and Sublimatory Effectiveness, Superego Integration, and Quality of Object Relations. The factor loadings of these four scales on this first factor were .83, .59, .73, and .88, respectively. Scores on these four scales were transformed to standard (z) scores and then combined for each subject to get a score for this first factor, which we labeled Capacity for Interpersonal Relatedness. Impulsivity had only a minimal loading (−.003) on this factor. The second factor, composed of the Impulsivity Scale with a factor loading of .95, accounted for 24.49% of the total variance. The other four scales had factor loadings less than .50 on this second factor. These two factors, especially Factor I, along with the Fairweather Scale of Interpersonal Communication, were our primary measures of the quality of interpersonal relatedness.

Summary of Case Record Ratings

Ratings of clinical and social behavior at admission and after at least 1 year of intensive treatment consisted of the following seven scales:

1. The Strauss–Harder rating of four different types of clinical symptoms
2. The Fairweather Scale for assessing interpersonal communication
3. The two Menninger factors for assessing manifest social behavior based on a factor analysis of the ratings at Time 1
   a. Capacity for Interpersonal Relatedness (Factor I)
   b. Impulsivity (Factor II)

These seven criteria of clinical functioning, derived from the clinical case records, were relatively independent at Time 1. The intercorrelations at Time 1 of the four Strauss–Harder symptom scales ranged from .25 to .42. The Menninger Factor I score was minimally correlated with the Menninger Factor II score but was highly correlated with the Fairweather Scale ($r = -.64$). Menninger Factor I and the Fairweather Scale were only moderately correlated with the four Strauss–Harder scales ($r = .17$ to .45). And Menninger Factor II was independent of the four Strauss–Harder scales ($r = .03$ to .18).

CHAPTER 3

Methods for Assessing Therapeutic Change in Psychological Test Protocols

Coordinated with the preparation of the clinical case reports after the first 6 weeks of hospitalization and again much later in the treatment process (after at least 1 year of treatment), all patients were administered an extensive battery of diagnostic psychological tests, including the Rorschach, the Thematic Apperception Test (TAT), a Wechsler Intelligence Test, and, in some cases, the Human Figure Drawing (HFD) test. This testing was conducted by advanced, postdoctoral fellows in clinical psychology who were committed to diagnostic psychological testing and supervised by senior clinical psychologists. The test procedures were administered using a standard, well-specified format and a consistent theoretical orientation (Rapaport, Gill, & Schafer, 1945). The test protocols were all recorded verbatim and parallel the quality of the clinical records in detail and thoroughness. These psychological test protocols provide the data for independent evaluations of a number of important psychological dimensions. In addition to regular scoring procedures, newly developed conceptual schemes were used to score various aspects of these protocols.

There has been considerable concern about the reliability and validity of data gathered through "projective tests" and about their potential contribution to research. One of the major limitations to the systematic use of the Rorschach in clinical research has been the large number of discrete, yet interrelated, scoring categories and ratios that have been developed over the years. Certainly, differences in the location, determinants, content, and qualitative features of Rorschach responses express important psychological dimensions. Furthermore, subtle distinctions within many of these scoring categories often add vital refinements that are very useful for fine-grain analyses of the Rorschach in the clinical context. But such a plethora of variables creates considerable difficulty in research. Unless a research study is directed toward the investigation of the relationship of specific Rorschach variables to highly select phenomena, the excessive number of scores that can be generated from the Rorschach usually overwhelms the investigation with a multitude of variables that are difficult, if not impossible, to manage conceptually and statistically. In addition, the traditional scoring of the Rorschach produces a myriad of isolated variables and ratios, many of which have undemonstrated reliability and validity. The empirical and conceptual relationships among many of these scores are unclear, and the interpretation of many of the scoring categories is often based on untested assumptions. Frequently, the interpretive rationale for many of these isolated variables is based more on clinical lore than on systematic evidence or theory. In addition, the many separate and fragmented scores and categories stand in isolation without a cohesive personality theory or a conceptual model for their integration. These issues place serious limitations on the use of the Rorschach in research.

One way to reduce the overwhelming number of variables derived from the Rorschach would be to examine the relationships among all the various Rorschach variables through a process such as factor analysis. But there have been very few factor-analytic studies of the Rorschach because the large number of variables derived from a Rorschach protocol would demand very large samples in order to conduct a factor analysis. Given the time required to administer and score a Rorschach protocol, most investigators have found such a large sample size prohibitive. Since Murstein's 1960 summary of some 20 factor-analytic studies of the Rorschach, there have been eight additional multidimensional analyses of the Rorschach, including Cooley and Mierzwa (1961), Schori and Thomas (1972), Ewert and Wiggins (1973), Haggard (1978), and Schaffer, Duszynski, and Thomas (1981). As Schaffer et al. (1981) pointed out, other than for Haggard and their own work, almost all the factor-analytic studies fail to control for response productivity (R). This is of particular consequence because many Rorschach variables are summation scores, clearly influenced by total R. Also, many of the factor-analytic studies used Rorschach protocols collected from different sources, administered under different conditions, and scored according to different scoring systems. Thus, most of these attempts to reduce the Rorschach to a select number of dimensions have been only partially effective.

Schaffer et al. (1981), after partialing out the effect of R, identified seven primary factors in both individually and group-administered Rorschachs. The first four factors were consistent with findings previously reported by Haggard (1978). These seven factors were whole responses, human movement responses, controlled affect (color and shading) responses, animal responses, large and rare detail, color dominance, and R. While one might disagree with the interpretation Schaffer et al. gave to their findings, the congruence of these seven factors with Haggard's earlier findings indicates that there is some consistency among a number of discrete scoring categories on the Rorschach that lead to the identification of a meaningful factor structure.

Another way to reduce the vast number of scores generated from conventional Rorschach scoring procedures, in addition to multidimensional analysis, is to evaluate Rorschach responses using broad, integrative, conceptual models. Weiner (1977) discussed the value of a more conceptual approach to the Rorschach in contrast to the use of empirical signs, clusters and configurations, or an analysis based on global clinical judgments. Several recent approaches to the Rorschach have taken this more conceptual orientation and have integrated numerous isolated Rorschach scores into more concise and overarching variables. It is important to stress that many of these new approaches to the Rorschach are often not based on a theory of the Rorschach per se but rather use implicit or explicit personality theories as broad conceptual models for integrating traditionally separate and independent Rorschach scores into more molar variables. A number of these conceptual approaches to the Rorschach, based on theoretical models about aspects of psychological processes rather than aspects of test theory, generate more comprehensive variables that can be scored with acceptable levels of reliability and that are related to important personality dimensions. These recently developed conceptual schemes extend beyond many of the current procedures for evaluating Rorschach responses. Most contemporary procedures for evaluating Rorschach responses (e.g., Beck, 1945; Exner, 1974, 1978) are based on a view of the Rorschach as a "perceptual test." These views of the Rorschach as a perceptual test are now outdated because they are derived primarily from theories of sensation and perception that were dominant in psychology in the first half of the 20th century. With the development of the "cognitive revolution" (Gardner, 1985) in psychology, beginning around 1960, research with the Rorschach must move to considering the Rorschach not as a "test of perception" but as an experimental procedure for evaluating mental representations. Evaluations of Rorschach protocols in research need to articulate new conceptual models that consider Rorschach responses as part of representational rather than perceptual processes (Blatt, 1990a). In these new approaches, personality theories can provide the conceptual basis for scoring the representational dimensions of Rorschach responses as well as for integrating the multitude of scores into meaningful composite variables that capture major dimensions of personality organization. Recent findings indicate that these more molar variables can be scored with acceptable levels of reliability and that they are often related to important personality dimensions.

Athey, Fleischer, and Coyne (1980), using a more conceptual approach to the Rorschach, conducted a "dimensional analysis." They attempted to restrict the range of variables conceptually, by defining three primary domains on the Rorschach: thought organization, affect organization, and object relations. Based on a conceptual model, they assigned 15 to 17 traditional Rorschach variables to each of these three domains. The scores of the Rorschach responses of 50 addicted patients with different degrees of psychopathology were subjected to a principle components factor analysis with varimax rotations for each of the three domains. Within each domain, Athey et al. (1980) were able to extract several factors.

Within the thought organization domain, the first two factors were thought disorder and productive integrative fantasy. The affect domain contained factors such as affect tolerance and control, and anxiety tolerance. Finally, factors reflecting general interests, muted and strong motives, and dehumanized representations emerged from the object relations domain. Additional multivariate analyses were performed on these three domains, but they did little to clarify further the dimensional structure or its interpretation. The three domains as a whole were unrelated to independent aspects of diagnostic profiles and minimally related to independent estimates of the treatment process. The extent of thought disorder, however, was negatively related to long-term psychological change, and, paradoxically, long-term psychological change was positively related to an absence of human object representations. Despite the lack of major statistical findings, Athey et al. (1980) tentatively concluded that it would be productive to conduct future Rorschach-based research with broad conceptual domains and configurations of Rorschach scores rather than with isolated, fragmented variables.

Blatt and Berman (1984) considered yet another way to reduce the vast number of scores generated from conventional Rorschach scoring procedures. They evaluated Rorschach responses within three broader conceptual frameworks based more on cognitive or representational models that integrate numerous isolated Rorschach scores into a few more concise and consolidated variables. Blatt and Berman (1984) used three broader conceptual approaches to the Rorschach that assessed (1) thought organization and process, (2) the quality of object representation (the concept of the human object), and (3) thought disorder. They used multivariate techniques to study the organization of scores derived from these three conceptual systems, as well as several conventional composite Rorschach scores that have been found to reflect significant aspects of psychological functioning (e.g., F+%, experience balance, the weight sum of color and shading responses, and the number of human movement responses (Allison, Blatt, & Zimet, 1968/1988; Rapaport, Gill, & Schaffer, 1945).

Based on a factor analysis of 18 variables derived from both traditional dimensions and several new conceptual approaches to the Rorschach, Blatt and Berman (1984) identified seven orthogonal factors that accounted for 73.6% of the total variance of the measures used. These seven factors represented a wide range of important cognitive and affective functions that can be measured with the Rorschach. High factor loadings of single variables on each of the seven factors suggested that individual variables, rather than composite factor scores, could be used to assess each of the seven factors. Correlations among these seven variables were consistently low, and these seven variables significantly discriminated among a sample of opiate-addicted patients, a matched nonaddicted community sample, and a group of psychiatric inpatients. None of these seven Rorschach variables correlated significantly with IQ, and several of these variables correlated significantly with overall level of ego functioning as assessed on the Bellak Ego Functioning Interview (Bellak, Hurvich, & Gediman, 1973) and Loevinger's (1976) measure of level of ego development. The seven individual variables that assess salient psychological dimensions include two traditional Rorschach variables (F+% and experience balance) and five variables derived from three relatively recent conceptual approaches to the Rorschach developed by Robert Holt (1962, 1966, 1977) and by Blatt and his colleagues (Blatt & Ritzler, 1974; Blatt, Brenneis, Schimek, & Glick, 1976a).

Robert Holt (1962, 1966, 1977), based on Freud's (1900) concepts of primary and secondary process thought, developed a complex manual for assessing thought organization by evaluating the extent and nature of primitive thinking on the Rorschach and the effectiveness with which this type of thinking is integrated into appropriate, reality-oriented responses. Holt (1977) and others demonstrated that these variables are related to independent assessment of creative thinking and complex cognitive activity. Blatt and Ritzler (1974) developed a procedure for assessing qualitative features of Rorschach responses (Rapaport, Gill, & Schafer, 1945) for the extent of thought disorder based on the severity of disruptions of the boundaries between independent percepts, concepts, and events. The severity of boundary disturbances, as assessed in thought-disordered responses, differentiated among different types of psychiatric patients (Blatt & Ritzler, 1974; Lerner, Sugarman, & Barbour, 1985; Wilson, 1985) and was related to independent assessments of a wide range of clinical dimensions (Blatt & Ritzler, 1974). Blatt and his colleagues (Blatt, Brenneis, Schimek, & Glick, 1976a, 1976b; Blatt & Lerner, 1983; Blatt, Schimek, & Brenneis, 1980), based on developmental psychological principles (Piaget, 1954; Werner, 1948; Werner & Kaplan, 1963), also developed procedures for assessing the quality of object representation. This analysis of Rorschach responses assesses the developmental level of total and partial human and quasi-human figures. These various dimensions develop longitudinally from early adolescence to adulthood, effectively differentiate between normals and patients, and are related to independent estimates of the severity of psychopathology (Blatt et al., 1976a).

THOUGHT ORGANIZATION

Robert Holt (1962, 1966, 1977) developed a complex conceptual procedure for using the Rorschach to assess (1) the extent and type of drive-laden, illogical, and unrealistic thought (defense demand), and (2) the effectiveness with which drive-laden, nonlogical primary process thinking is integrated into appropriate, reality-oriented responses (defense effectiveness).

Holt differentiated two types of primary-process thinking: (1) content primary process, which assesses the degree that Rorschach responses contain drive-related content (e.g., oral, anal, sexual, exhibitionistic, voyeuristic, homosexual, and aggressive themes), and (2) formal primary process, which assesses the degree to which responses contain nonlogical thinking. Nonlogical thinking includes the types of primary-process thought described by Freud (1911/1958) (condensation, displacement, substitution, and symbolization), such as thinking in which there is a relative lack of conjunctive, casual, temporal, and other relationships; or thought that is unrealistic and nonlogical, involving logical contradiction, unlikely activities, and verbal condensations. Content and formal primary-process scores are combined into a single score called defense demand (DD), which indicates, in part, the intensity and primitiveness of the content and the extent to which responses deviate from logical, orderly, realistic thinking. DD is scored for each response on a 6-point scale, and the total amount of DD in the record is divided by the total number of responses (Sum DD/Rt).

The Holt (1962, 1966, 1977) system also assesses the degree to which responses that contain DD (drive-laden, nonlogical thinking) are realistic and understandable. Holt termed this integration of drive content and illogical elements into realistic and understandable form defense effectiveness (DE). This variable is assessed, in part, by the degree to which the image corresponds to the properties of the card (form level), the degree to which the response is placed in appropriate contexts (e.g., literary, aesthetic, temporal, cultural), the degree to which the individual derives pleasure from the response, and the extent to which subsequent responses remain realistic and appropriate. Various other criteria, such as indications of defensiveness or disruption, failure to give expected features (movement, color, or shading), and changes in form level are also included in the rating of DE. The summary score of DE is the sum of all DE ratings on a 6-point scale, divided by the number of responses that contained primary-process thinking (Sum DE/Rp).

The Holt system also includes a measure called "adaptive regression," a composite measure of DD and DE that assesses the degree to which drive content and nonlogical thinking are expressed in appropriate and adaptive form in the total Rorschach record. The amount of DD in each response (ranging from 1 to 6) is multiplied by the DE of that response (-3 to $+2$), and these products are summed for the entire Rorschach and divided by the total number of Rorschach responses (Sum DD × DE/Rt). Because DE is scored on a 6-point scale from -3 to $+2$, including a zero score, some scores can be ambiguous. High scores on adaptive regression indicate that the Rorschach protocol contains a fair amount of primary-process material that is integrated effectively into meaningful and realistic responses. Low scores on this measure indicate extensive primary-process material that is poorly integrated. Intermediate scores are more ambiguous, however, and can reflect smaller amounts of primary-process thinking with good integration or a large amount of primary-process thinking with inconsistent integration that is poor on some responses and effective on others. To attempt to correct for this ambiguity, we converted the DE scale to range from 1 to 6, without a zero point. Holt's adaptive regression measure, however, both in its original form and in this modified form, did not emerge as a separate independent dimension in the factor analysis. This is consistent with the conclusions reached earlier by Blatt, Allison, and Feirstein (1969) that Holt's DE measure may be a better measure of integrative capacity than the more complex measure of adaptive regression.

Reliability estimates ($n = 76$) of the scoring of these variables, consistent with prior reports (Blatt & Feirstein, 1977) were at acceptable levels (Item Alpha $>.70$).

THOUGHT DISORDER

Thought disorder (degree of disruption of the differentiation and integration of boundaries) is often considered as one of the primary dimensions in most conceptualizations of psychosis. Empirical research studies with the Rorschach (Blatt & Ritzler, 1974; Harrow & Quinlan, 1985; Johnston, 1975; Johnston & Holzman, 1979) confirm earlier reports (Powers & Hamlin, 1955; Rapaport, Gill, & Schafer, 1945/1946; Watkins & Stauffacher, 1952) that not only do thought disorder measures on the Rorschach differentiate psychotic from other clinical samples, but different types of thought disorder also differentiate within the psychotic range (e.g., nonparanoid and paranoid schizophrenia, borderline disorders, and manic and depressive psychosis) (Lerner, Sugarman, & Barbour, 1985; Wilson, 1985).

Blatt and Ritzler (1974) proposed a conceptual model that integrates the three major forms of thought disorder on the Rorschach (contamination, confabulation, and fabulized combination) along a developmental continuum defined by the degree of disturbance of the differentiation and integration of boundaries. On the basis of concepts from developmental psychology (e.g., Piaget, 1954; Werner, 1948) and psychoanalytic theory (e.g., Jacobson, 1964; Mahler, 1968), these three types of thought disorder can be considered as indicating different degrees of disturbance in the articulation of boundaries. The most severe boundary disturbance is reflected by the contamination response, in which independent concepts or images lose their identity and definition. Boundaries are so unstable that independent representations cannot be consistently maintained, and they merge, or tend to merge, into a single distorted unit. An example of a contamination response is "rabbit hand," given as a response to the lower detail of Card X of the Rorschach, in which the images of a "rabbit" and a "hand" lose their separateness and merge into a single, distorted, idiosyncratic response. The next major thought disorder on the continuum indicating difficulties in maintaining boundaries is the confabulation response. In this type of response (e.g., a diabolic bat), an initially accurate perception becomes lost in extensive, unrealistic, grandiose, personal elaborations and associations. In confabulatory thinking, ideas and images do not merge and fuse as in a contamination; rather, the extensive, unrealistic elaboration indicates a loss of the distinction between the external perception and personal associations and reactions to it. The third major, but less severe, level of boundary disturbance is indicated by the fabulized combination response. In these responses, the separate definition of independent objects or concepts is maintained, as is the distinction between the perception and reactions to it. But unrealistic thinking is expressed by establishing illogical, arbitrary relationships between independent and separate percepts or concepts. Two separate percepts are interrelated simply because they are spatially or temporally contiguous (Holt, 1962; Rapaport, Gill, & Schafer, 1945/1946). Spatial or temporal contiguity is taken as indicating a real relationship, even though an arbitrary and unrealistic one. In a response such as "Prairie dogs standing on a butterfly" to Card VIII, spatial juxtaposition is taken as indicating a real relationship, even though an arbitrary and unrealistic one.

We distinguished between two types of fabulized combinations, one in which there is an arbitrary relationship established between two well-defined and independent objects (e.g., dogs standing on a butterfly) (fabulized combination-regular) and the other in which the arbitrary relationship occurs within the definition of a single object (e.g., a bear with a rabbit's head) (fabulized combination-serious). This latter type of fabulized combination is considered more serious and more like a contamination because there is a tendency for two disparate parts to blend into a single idiosyncratic figure.

An overall estimate of thought disorder was developed for the Rorschach by differentially weighting these different types of thought disorder based on the severity of boundary disturbance (Blatt & Ritzler, 1974). Differential weighting of these three types of thought-disordered responses gives a composite measure of the extent and severity of thought disorder on the Rorschach. This composite measure of severity of thought disorder was derived from full expressions of the three types of thought disorder with boundary disturbance (contamination, confabulation, and fabulized combination) as well as milder manifestations of each type of thought disorder discussed by Allison, Blatt, and Zimet (1968/1988) and Rapaport, Gill, and Schafer (1945) as thought disorder tendencies.[1] Based on the conceptual system developed by Blatt and Ritzler (1974), the various types of thought disorder were combined into a single thought disorder measure (Blatt & Berman, 1984). The differential weighting given to each type of thought disorder for this composite thought disorder measure is presented in Table 3.1. The composite thought disorder score is the weighted sum of each of the different types of thought disorder, covaried for total number of Rorschach responses as a way of controlling statistically for the effects of overall response productivity. Higher scores indicate more extensive thought disorder. Interjudge reliability for two raters for the total measure of thought disorder was satisfactory (Item Alpha $>.70$), consistent with reliability figures reported by Blatt and Ritzler (1974) and Wilson (1985).

Blatt and Ritzler (1974) found that the severity of thought disorder

TABLE 3.1

Weighting of Various Types of Thought Disorder for
Composite Thought-Disorder Score on the Rorschach[a]:
Degrees of Boundary Disturbance in Thought Disorder

	Weighting for severity
1. Contamination	6
2. Contamination tendency	5
3. Fabulized combination-serious	5
4. Confabulation	4
5. Confabulation tendency	3
6. Fabulized to confabulation	3
7. Fabulized combination-regular	2
8. Fabulized combination tendency	1

[a]The composite thought-disorder score is the weighted sum of thought-disorder scores, covaried for total number of Rorschach responses.

based on different types of boundary disruption in seriously disturbed inpatients was significantly related to the severity of psychopathology, independently assessed impairments of complex cognitive functions such as object sorting and intelligence test performance, the capacity for reality testing, indications of difficulty with affect modulation, disturbed representations of human figures, the degree of involvement in interpersonal relationships, and the degree of constructive response to therapeutic intervention. In addition, Blatt and Ritzler (1974) found, in two independent samples, that the two extreme ends of the boundary disturbance continuum (contamination and fabulized combination-regular) rarely occur together (in only 1.5% of patients). Patients generally tend to have one type of thought disorder. When there is more than one type of thought disorder in a Rorschach protocol, it is most often types of thought disorder that are next to one another in the boundary disturbance continuum. A more detailed description of each type of thought disorder is presented in Appendix 4.

CONCEPT OF THE OBJECT

The development of the concept of the object has been an important issue in developmental psychology (e.g., Piaget, 1954; Werner, 1948; Werner & Kaplan, 1963) and in psychoanalytic theory (e.g., Jacobson, 1964; Mahler, 1968). The concept of the object has been studied in normal development (Scarlett, Press, & Crockett, 1971; Signell, 1966), and it has been investigated in psychopathology in children and adults (Bannister & Salmon, 1966; Blatt, 1974; Blatt, Wild, & Ritzler, 1975; Blatt & Wild, 1976; Reker, 1974; Whiteman, 1954). Mahler (1968), Searles (1965), and others, for example, have discussed the schizophrenic patient's difficulty in maintaining the distinction between human and nonhuman and how this important dimension in psychosis is related to the child's failure to differentiate himself or herself and mother as "whole and separate objects" (Searles, 1965, p. 670).

The structure of the concept of the object has been discussed in terms of developmental principles (Werner, 1948; Werner & Kaplan, 1963) of differentiation, articulation, and integration (Crockett, 1965), and in terms of dimensions of cognitive organization (Bieri, Atkins, Briar, Leaman, Miller, & Tripodi, 1966; Todd & Rappoport, 1964; Warr & Knapper, 1968). Others have approached the concept of the object as an issue in "person perception," and Kelly's Personal Construct Theory and the Role Repertory Test (Kelly, 1955) and Osgood's Semantic Differential (Osgood, Suci, & Tannenbaum, 1957) have figured prominently in this research.

Another potentially important, but neglected, source of data in the study of the concept of the object is the human response given to the Rorschach stimuli. The importance of the human response on the Rorschach has been noted in a variety of contexts but generally with a minimum of theoretical elaboration. For example, McFate and Orr (1949), using the Berkeley Longitudinal data (Macfarlane, 1971), and Ames (1966) report a significant increase in the number of human responses through adolescence. It also has been reasonably well established that the appearance of the human response varies directly with cognitive development and social maturity (Draguns, Haley, & Phillips, 1967), is consistent over time for the same subject (Schimek, 1968), and occurs frequently in the records of well-adjusted normal adults (Barry, Blyth, & Albrecht, 1952; Rapaport, Gill, & Schafer, 1945). Also, prior research (Friedman, 1953; Hemmendinger, 1960) indicated that Rorschach human responses generally become increasingly complex and integrated with age and psychological health. In addition, there is a congruence between the content of the human responses and characteristic modes of interpersonal adaptation (Beck, Beck, Levitt, & Molish, 1961; Kelly & Fiske, 1951; Mayman, 1967).

Correspondence between the quality of human response and psychopathology has been examined by a number of investigators. Parker and Piotrowski (1968) showed that schizophrenics have a favorable reaction to dehumanized and unreal figures, and Blatt and Ritzler (1974) found that distorted human responses, particularly human–inanimate blends, increase in frequency across seriously disturbed inpatients as severity of pathology increases. Mayman (1967) demonstrated that the content of the human responses correlated with independent clinical assessments of severity of symptoms, motivation for change, and the quality of interpersonal relations. These results with normal as well as clinical samples suggest that the human response on the Rorschach is a valuable way of assessing an individual's concept of the object.

Based on a theoretical conceptualization derived from developmental psychology (Werner, 1948; Werner & Kaplan, 1963), Blatt, Brenneis, Schimek, & Glick (1976b) developed an extensive procedure for evaluating the developmental level of human responses on the Rorschach. Three developmentally derived, primary dimensions of human responses were considered: differentiation, articulation, and integration. Differentiation was defined as the nature of the response with human content; articulation was defined as the degree to which the response was elaborated in terms of its perceptual and functional characteristics; and integration was defined as the way the concept of the object was integrated into a context of action and interaction with other objects.

The concept of the human object is assessed on all responses that have any humanoid features. These humanoid responses are considered in terms of the *degree of differentiation* (whether the figure is a full human, a full quasi-human, or a part feature of a human or quasi-human figure); the *degree of articulation* (the extent to which the figure is elaborated in terms of manifest physical and/or functional attributes); the *motivation of action* (the degree to which the action attributed to the figure is internally determined—unmotivated, reactive, or intentional action); the *integration of the action* (the degree to which the action is congruent with the role of the figure, i.e., fused, incongruent, nonspecific, or congruent); *the content of the action* (the degree to which the action is malevolent or benevolent and constructive); and *the nature of any interaction with another figure* (the degree to which the interaction is active–passive, active–reactive, or active–active, in which mutual, reciprocal relationships are established). In each of these six categories (differentiation, articulation, motivation of action, integration of the object and its action, the content of the action, and the nature of the interaction), responses are scored along a developmental continuum. This developmental analysis is made for those human responses that are accurately perceived (F+) and for those that are inaccurately perceived (F−) (see Table 3.2).

Differential weighting for scores within each of the six categories assessing the concept of the object reflects the developmental progression, with higher scores indicating higher developmental levels. Score values are as follows:

TABLE 3.2
Concept of the Object on the Rorschach[a]

---

1. *Differentiation*
   1. Quasi-human detail
   2. Human detail
   3. Quasi-human figure
   4. Human figure
2. *Articulation*
   1. Perceptual features (size or physical structure, clothing or hair style, posture)
   2. Functional (age, sex, role, specific identity)
3. *Action*
   1. Unmotivated
   2. Reactive
   3. Intentional
4. *Integration of object and action*
   1. Fused
   2. Incongruent
   3. Nonspecific
   4. Congruent
5. *Content of action*
   1. Malevolent
   2. Benevolent
6. *Nature of interaction*
   1. Active–passive
   2. Active–reactive
   3. Active–active

Composite Scores

1. *Capacity for establishing appropriate and meaningful interpersonal relationships (object representation +) (OR+)*
   a. The degree to which *accurately perceived* (F+) human responses to the Rorschach are well-articulated, fully human figures, seen as engaged in intentional, highly congruent, and benevolent activity, as well as in mutually active interactions with others.
2. *Investment in inappropriate, unrealistic, possibly autistic types of relationships (object representation −) (OR −)*
   a. The degree to which *inaccurately perceived* (F−) human responses to the Rorschach are well-articulated, fully human figures, seen as engaged in intentional, highly congruent, and benevolent activity, as well as in mutually active interactions with others.

---

[a]From Blatt, S. J., Brenneis, C. B., Schimek, J., & Glick, M. (1976a).

Differentiation: a quasi-human detail (Hd) = 1, a human detail Hd = 2, a full quasi-human figure (H) = 3, a full human figure H = 4.
Articulation: perceptual attributes = 1, functional attributes = 2.
Motivation: unmotivated = 1, reactive = 2, intentional = 3.
Integration of object and action: fused = 1, incongruent = 2, nonspecific = 3, congruent = 4.

Content of action: malevolent = 1, benevolent = 2.
Nature of interaction: active–passive = 1, active–reactive = 2, active–
active = 3.

A detailed presentation of this scoring system is available in Appendix 5.
Reliability estimates for the scoring of these six categories for F+ and F−
responses in both clinical and normal samples are at acceptable levels
(Item Alpha >.70), consistent with prior reports that range from .86 to
.97.

To reduce the number of variables measuring the concept of the
object, a factor analysis was conducted on the 12 object representations
(OR) scores obtained for each subject. A weighted sum for each of the six
categories was obtained for F+ and F− responses separately. Each of
these 12 weighted sums was corrected by covariance for total response
productivity. The residualized scores for each of these 12 variables (six
categories each for F+ and F− responses) were subjected to a common
factors (SAS Institute, 1979) factor analysis with commonalities less than
or equal to 1.00. Using the lambda criterion of ≥1.00, two factors were
retained and rotated for an orthogonal varimax solution. These two
factors accounted for 53.52% of the total variance. The factor analysis
yielded two primary factors: the developmental level of accurately perceived responses (OR+) (percent total variance = 27.19) and the developmental level of inaccurately perceived responses (OR−) (percent total
variance = 26.33). All six OR+ scoring categories had factor loadings on
factor 1 that exceeded .70, and all six OR− scoring categories had factor
loadings on factor 1 that were less than .20. All six OR− scoring categories
had factor loadings on factor 2 that exceeded .53, whereas the loadings
of the OR+ categories did not exceed .20 on this factor. All six residualized scores for OR+ scoring categories are standardized and summed
to give a total residualized weighted sum score for accurately perceived
responses. The same is done for all six OR− scores. The residualized
weighted sum of accurately perceived human responses (OR+) is
viewed as indicating the capacity for investment in satisfying interpersonal relationships. The residualized weighted sum of inaccurately perceived human responses (OR−) is viewed as an indication of the tendency to become invested in autistic fantasies rather than realistic
relationships. These two dimensions of the quality of human responses
on the Rorschach (OR+ and OR−) emerged as two of the seven factors
in the factor analysis conducted by Blatt and Berman (1984).

In addition to the weighted sum of OR+ and OR−, an average
(mean) developmental level was obtained for each of the six categories
for F+ and F− responses. These six mean developmental level scores for
F+ responses were standardized and combined into a total mean devel-

opmental level score. The same was done with F– responses. The mean developmental level for accurately perceived (F+) responses is viewed as another measure of the capacity to become engaged in meaningful and realistic interpersonal relations. The mean developmental level of inaccurately perceived (F–) responses is viewed as another measure of the tendency to become involved in unrealistic, inappropriate, possibly autistic types of relationships. The manual for scoring the concept of the object is presented in Appendix 5.

Using this conceptual model for evaluating human responses to the Rorschach, Blatt et al. (1976b), using data from the Berkeley Longitudinal Project (Macfarlane, 1971), examined the development of human responses in a study of normal subjects over a 20-year period from early adolescence to young adulthood. Thirty-seven normal subjects had been given the Rorschach at ages 11 to 12, 13 to 14, 17 to 18, and 30, and these protocols were analyzed in a repeated measure design. The results indicated that these formal properties of the human responses show consistent changes with development. In normal development, from pre-adolescence (age 11 to 12) to adulthood (age 30), there was a marked increase in the number of well-differentiated, highly articulated, and integrated human figures that were accurately perceived. There was a significant increase with age in the degree to which the attribution of activity was congruent with important characteristics of the figures and the degree to which the object was seen as involved in constructive and positive interactions with others. Likewise, differentiation of the object, fuller articulation of attributes, fuller integration of action, and the representation of interactions that were reflective, motivated, purposive, and benevolent all significantly increased with age (Blatt et al., 1976b).

Prior research (Blatt et al., 1976b) also investigated the nature of the human response in the Rorschach protocols of a hospitalized sample ($n = 48$) of seriously disturbed adolescents and young adults. In a sample of 48 patients hospitalized in a long-term, intensive treatment facility, there were no significant relations between the severity of pathology as assessed by degree of thought disorder on the Rorschach and any aspects of accurately perceived human responses (OR+). However, more seriously disturbed inpatients, as compared with less seriously disturbed patients and normals, gave significantly more inaccurately perceived human responses (OR–). These responses were more fully articulated, had more unmotivated and nonspecific action, and involved interactions containing both benevolent and malevolent content that were primarily active–passive and active–reactive. Although there were no significant relationships between severity of pathology and aspects of accurately perceived figures (OR+), significant positive relations were found in seriously disturbed inpatients between severity of psychopathology and increased elaboration of aspects of inaccurately perceived human figures (OR−) (Blatt et al., 1976b).

TRADITIONAL RORSCHACH VARIABLES

Two additional factors emerged in the factor analysis conducted by Blatt and Berman (1984) that are assessed by conventional scoring categories (F+% and experience balance). F+% assesses the degree of accuracy of the form of responses given to the Rorschach—the degree to which the responses correspond to the form of the stimulus. The F+% is considered to reflect the capacity for reality testing. Experience balance is a ratio of the number of human movement responses to the weighted sum of the responses that are either fully or partially determined by the chromic colors of the Rorschach cards. A ratio in which the human movement is dominant is assumed to reflect an inner-directed, ideational orientation in contrast to a color-dominated ratio, which is assumed to reflect a more externally directed, experiential, and affective orientation (Allison, Blatt, & Zimet, 1968/1988).

These seven Rorschach dimensions defined in the factor analysis, two traditional variables, and five variables derived from new conceptual approaches appear to capture a wide range of important dimensions on the Rorschach: the degree of reality testing (F+%), the primary mode of experience (action or ideation) (experience balance), the degree of access to more primitive modes of thought (DD), the extent to which these primitive modes of thought are integrated effectively (DE), the degree of the investment in appropriate (OR+) and inappropriate interpersonal relationships (OR−), and the severity of pathological thinking (thought disorder). These seven dimensions or factors represent empirically independent orthogonal factors that can be accurately assessed by single variables. Providing a comprehensive assessment of a broad range of psychological processes, these seven variables also supplied the basis for differentiating among several clinical groups and for understanding some of the unique personality characteristics of different types of patients. A number of these dimensions, in addition, were significantly correlated with independent assessments of ego functions and ego development conducted with very different procedures (a clinical interview and a sentence completion test) (Blatt & Berman, 1984).

In summary, the findings of Blatt and Berman (1984) suggest that there may be considerable advantage in using new approaches to the Rorschach, at least in research, that generate higher-order variables based on conceptual models of personality development and organization that integrate the diversity of observations that can be made on the Rorschach. These results also suggest that it is important to explore these new approaches to the Rorschach based on theories of cognition and representation rather than remaining with an approach based primarily on a theory of perception (Blatt, 1990a). Using theoretical approaches to the Rorschach based on explicit theories of personality organization and functioning and viewing the Rorschach as an experimental procedure for assessing mental representations may provide creative and productive ways of integrating the diversity of observations that can be made as individuals respond to the ambiguity of the Rorschach stimuli.

It is important to stress, however, that these new approaches are not, and should not, be considered as independent of traditional scoring procedures. The Holt analysis is based partly on traditional Rorschach scores, but these various scores are integrated in new and creative ways based on the psychoanalytic theory of thinking. Likewise, the analysis of object representation on the Rorschach developed by Blatt et al. (1976b) uses traditional distinctions about human responses on the Rorschach, but these distinctions are extended based on developmental psychological principles derived from Heinz Werner and Jean Piaget. The analysis of thought disorder, based on conceptualization of degree of boundary disruption (Blatt & Ritzler, 1974; Blatt & Wild, 1976; Blatt, Wild, & Ritzler, 1975), derives from a psychoanalytic model of psychopathology (Rapaport et al., 1945), particularly of psychotic and borderline functioning. These new approaches to the Rorschach, using personality theories to develop theoretical models to assess representational processes, seem to provide ways of more effectively managing what is often experienced as a confusing and overwhelming array of isolated scores and ratios, thus making the Rorschach more useful for the systematic investigation of a wide range of clinical phenomena.

In the present investigation, we attempted to use the variables derived from each of the seven factors defined by Blatt and Berman (1984) (defense demand and defense effectiveness [Holt, 1967], weighted thought disorder [Blatt & Ritzler, 1974], the concept of the object [OR+, OR−] [Blatt et al., 1976a,b], accuracy of reality testing (F+%) [Korchin & Larson, 1977], and experience balance) to study therapeutic change. Experience balance, however, is a ratio of the number of human movement responses to the weighted sum of color responses (Allison, Blatt, & Zimet, 1968/1988; Rapaport, Gill, & Schafer, 1945) in which the numerator and/or denominator can be zero. Because such a ratio score is difficult to deal with statistically, we evaluated separately the components of the experience balance: the number of accurately and inaccurately perceived human movement responses (M+, M−) and the weighted sum of color responses (Sum C).

Because the Holt assessment of DD and DE is a labor-intensive and demanding scoring procedure, we assessed the value of these seven variables to evaluate therapeutic change on the first 24 patients in our total sample of 90 patients. The Holt DD and DE variables were omitted from subsequent analysis because they failed to provide any consistent indication of therapeutic change. In addition, Blatt and Berman (1984) note that Holt's score of DD was correlated significantly ($p<.001$) with thought disorder ($r = .54$) and Holt's score of DE was correlated significantly with F+% ($r = .44$). Both of these correlations are easily understandable, since thought disorder and F+% each play a central role in the assessment of DD and DE, respectively. The remaining five variables, however, appeared to be effective in evaluating therapeutic change in the first 24 patients and thereafter were scored for the entire sample of 90 patients.

MUTUALITY OF AUTONOMY (MOA)

In addition to scoring the Rorschach protocols for these variables (thought disorder, OR+, OR−, F+%, M+, M−, and Sum C, and experience balance), we also scored the Mutuality of Autonomy (MOA) scale (Urist, 1973). The MOA scale was developed as part of the research group at the University of Michigan, where Martin Mayman and his colleagues (Krohn and Mayman, 1974; Mayman, 1967; Ryan, 1973; Urist, 1973) developed procedures for evaluating the content of object representations. This research group demonstrated that the content of dreams, early memories, TAT stories, and Rorschach responses can be scored with a high degree of reliability and provide important information about the quality of the interpersonal relationships to which an individual is predisposed. Mayman and his colleagues focused primarily on the content dimensions of the human responses (e.g., inanimate, destructive, decaying, malformed, weak, or warm, friendly, and mutually cooperative), in contrast to Blatt et al. (1976b) who, in their research on the concept of the object, focused on the more structural aspects of the human representation (differentiation, articulation, and integration). Mayman and his colleagues evaluated human representations in terms of the degree of humanness or dehumanization, the degree of intactness versus fragmentation or fusion, the warmth and vitality, the ease of empathy with the inner world of feelings and emotions, and the degree of empathy and differentiation with which human figures are perceived

(Mayman & Krohn, 1975). They found that relatively inexperienced clinical judges could make reliable ratings of these dimensions and that these ratings related significantly to health–sickness ratings (Luborsky, 1975a) in a posttreatment psychiatric evaluation and to other clinical criteria (Krohn, 1972; Urist, 1973).

Urist (1977; Urist & Shill, 1982) developed the MOA scale derived in part from Mayman's formulations, to assess the thematic content of interactions on the Rorschach by rating all human, animal, and inanimate relationships (stated or implied) in a protocol along a continuum ranging from mutual empathic relatedness (1) to themes of malevolent engulfment and destruction (7). Using the theoretical perspective of ego states and focusing on the thematic content, the MOA scale systematically evaluates the degree to which interactions between humans, animals, and/or objects on the Rorschach range from depictions of calamitous violence and destructiveness to portrayals of mutual empathic relatedness. These distinctions can be scored with acceptable levels of interrater reliability ($p>.70$) and have been found to correlate significantly ($p<.05$) with measures of interpersonal and clinical functioning in a variety of populations. Scale points 1 and 2, the most adaptive scores in the scale, refer to themes of reciprocal acknowledgment and benign parallel interactions, respectively. As an example, a score of 1 is given to the response to Card II of "two people having a heated political argument." An example of a score of 2 is "two animals climbing a mountain" on Card VIII. Scale points 3 and 4 indicate an emerging loss of autonomy in interaction in which the "other" exists solely either to be leaned on (a score of 3) or to mirror oneself (a score of 4). An example of a score of 3 is a response to Card I of "two men leaning on a mannequin." A score of 4 is given to the response "a tiger looking at its reflection in the water" to Card VIII. Points 5, 6, and 7 reflect an increasing malevolence and loss of control over one's separateness. A score of 5 is given to responses characterized by themes of coercion, hurtful influence, or threat. An example is "a witch casting a spell on someone" to the top large detail of Card IX. A score of 6 indicates violent assault and destruction of one figure by another—for example, "a bat impaled by a tree" to Card IV. Finally, a score of 7 represents a larger than life destructiveness imposed usually by inanimate, calamitous forces as depicted, for example, in the response to Card X, "a tornado hurtling its debris everywhere."

To reflect a subject's range or repertoire of interactions, Urist (1977) also recommended using each subject's single highest (most pathological) and single lowest (most adaptive) MOA score as an indication of the range of an individual's representational repertoire. The MOA scale is presented in greater detail in Appendix 6.

Urist (1977) reported significant positive correlations of the MOA scale with independent ward staff ratings of interpersonal relationships and with aspects of autobiographical descriptions of interpersonal experiences of adult inpatients. He stressed that individuals have a range of object representations that define the limits of their capacity for interpersonal relations. Calculating a mean MOA score, as well as the single most disrupted score and the single most adaptive score, Urist also found that individuals' capacities to give at least one response at the more integrated end of the MOA scale correlated significantly with ratings of constructive interpersonal behavior on the ward, whereas the tendency to give at least one response at the more disrupted end of the scale correlated significantly with ratings of disrupted relationships in autobiographical narratives. In a second study, Urist and Shill (1982) used comprehensive case records to assess the quality of interpersonal relationships of 60 adolescent patients. Developmental and family history reports, as well as clinical progress and nursing staff notes, were assessed with a version of the MOA scale adapted for rating clinical records. Ratings of the clinical case records correlated significantly with the mean and the single most disrupted MOA score on the Rorschach. The single most adaptive MOA scores on the Rorschach, however, did not correlate with any ratings derived from clinical case records.

Harder, Greenwald, Wechsler, and Ritzler (1984) found that the MOA scale correlated significantly with ratings of severity of psychopathology derived from both complex symptom checklists and independent diagnostic assessments according to the *Diagnostic and Statistical Manual of Mental Disorders* (3rd ed. [DSM-III]; American Psychiatric Association, 1980). The mean MOA score derived from only four Rorschach cards (Cards I, II, VI, and VIII) differentiated among schizophrenic, affective, and nonpsychotic conditions. More severe psychiatric disorders were associated with a more disrupted mean MOA score. Spear and Sugarman (1984), using a modified version of the MOA scale, identified differences among infantile borderline patients, obsessive/paranoid borderline patients, and schizophrenics. Kavanagh (1982, 1985), in an analysis of the test protocols from the Menninger Psychotherapy Research Project, compared pre- and posttreatment Rorschach protocols of 33 patients receiving either psychoanalysis or psychotherapy. Kavanagh found no difference between admission and termination Rorschach protocols either for the mean MOA score or for the single most disrupted or most adaptive MOA score. Based on an independent clinical judgment of subjects' MOA level, however, Kavanagh reported a significant relationship with degree of improvement at the end of treatment for patients treated both in psychoanalysis and in psychotherapy. Because the

MOA scale rates the nature of interactions on the Rorschach between animal and inanimate percepts as well as between human figures, it has also been useful in the study of object representations in young children (Coates & Tuber, 1988; Ryan, Avery, & Grolnick, 1985; Tuber, 1983; Tuber & Coates, 1989). Thus, the Urist MOA scale seems to be a reliable and useful measure with adults, adolescents, and children in both clinical and nonclinical samples. MOA ratings correlated significantly with independent assessments of interpersonal behavior from clinical case records (Spear & Sugarman, 1984; Urist & Shill, 1982), ward staff ratings of social interactions (Urist, 1977), psychiatric symptomatology in adults and in children (Harder et al., 1984; Tuber & Coates, 1989), and ratings of interpersonal behavior in a nonclinical context (Ryan et al., 1985). Blatt, Tuber, and Auerbach (1990), however, noted that the MOA scale appears to be a broad-gauge measure that correlates significantly with clinical symptoms and thought disorder as well as with independent estimates of the quality of object relations. The mean MOA score appears to assess primarily the severity of clinical symptoms (impaired reality testing and thought disorder) and secondarily impaired interpersonal relationships.

SCORING PROCEDURES FOR THE RORSCHACH

Rorschach test protocols were scored by two judges specifically trained to score the various dimensions of the Rorschach protocols. The judge who did the basic scoring of the Rorschach, as well as for the thought-disorder and MOA measures, was an experienced Ph.D. in clinical psychology who had extensive Rorschach training and had established acceptable levels of reliability in scoring these dimensions in a prior sample. The judge who scored the concept of the object scale was an undergraduate who had been especially trained in this procedure in a prior project and had established acceptable reliability in this prior study.

Both judges scored the 180 Rorschach protocols in random order and were uninformed about any aspects of the 90 patients (such as age and sex) and whether the Rorschach was from Time 1 or Time 2. In addition, each judge scored the various scoring systems without knowledge of the results of the other ratings and without information about any details of the clinical records. Reliability estimates for these various Rorschach scores (conventional scores, concept of the object, MOA, and thought disorder) were all at acceptable levels (Item Alpha $>.70$).

A number of Rorschach variables are summation scores that reflect the frequency with which a particular type of response occurs in a Rorschach protocol. To control statistically for response productivity, all summation scores were corrected by covariance for the total number of responses. Within a single sample, the covariance method is preferred to the more traditional ratio score, since a ratio score does not remove the effects of the denominator (Cohen & Cohen, 1975).

WECHSLER INTELLIGENCE TEST

Patients were also given an intelligence test as part of the initial assessment, usually the Wechsler Adult Intelligence Test (WAIS). To control for practice effect as much as possible, a different form of the Wechsler Intelligence Test was given at the second evaluation (usually either the Wechsler–Bellevue Form I or Form II). The Verbal IQ and the Performance IQ were used to elaborate the findings obtained with the Full Scale IQ in our data analyses.

HUMAN FIGURE DRAWINGS (HFDs)[2]

About one-third of 90 patients were asked to draw a person as part of the standard psychological assessment battery both at admission and again after at least 1 year of hospitalization and treatment. The patient was asked initially to "draw a picture of a whole person," and then, after the patient had drawn a whole person, he or she was requested to "now draw a picture of a whole person of the opposite sex." The drawings were executed on 8½ by 11 inch white paper with a freshly sharpened No. 2 lead pencil. To qualify for inclusion in the data analyses, both male and female figure drawings had to be more than primitive stick figures with little or no differentiation.

Thirty-two of the 90 patients in the study were given the HFD test at both Time 1 and Time 2 and produced drawings of a "whole person" that could be evaluated on the Goodenough–Harris (GH) (Harris, 1963) and Robins Balance-Tilt (RBT) (Robins, 1980) scoring procedures. Drawings were each given a code number and scored in random order. The HFDs were rated by judges blind to any identifying details of the patient. The judges also had no knowledge as to which drawings were from the same patient and whether the drawings were from early or late in the treatment process. The HFDs were evaluated by two scoring procedures: the Goodenough–Harris and the Robins Balance-Tilt.

Goodenough–Harris Scale

Goodenough (1926) developed a procedure for assessing the presence or absence of various items (parts of the human body and clothing) that could be expected to appear in the HFDs of children aged 1 to 15. Harris (1963) revised the Goodenough scale and concluded that the revised scale continued to measure developmental level and intelligence. Interrater reliability commonly exceeds .90 (Harris, 1963; McCarthy, 1944; Smith, 1937; Williams, 1935). Harris (1963) reported that after relatively brief training, judges can achieve high interrater reliability for this well-articulated, precisely specified rating procedure. As for validity, Harris (1963) and others (e.g., Ansbacher, 1952; Goodenough, 1926; Havighurst, 1946) found that the GH scale correlated positively with measures of intelligence and the individual's ability to form abstract concepts. Adler (1970) found that the scale also assessed the level of "cognitive maturity," or "maturity or sophistication of the body image representation" (p. 56).

Although the Goodenough (later the Goodenough–Harris) scale was developed particularly for children, Goodenough (1926) argued that the scale represents crucial developmental stages across the entire life span. Lowenfeld (1957) agreed that there was consistency between child and adult performance on HFDs and that the early stages lay the groundwork for the later stages. Chase (1941) used the Goodenough scale with adults and found significant differences between paranoids and normals, and between hebephrenics and normals. Darke and Geil (1948), Jones and Rich (1957), and Murphy (1956) found that the GH scale was an effective measure of personality dimensions with adults. Goodenough (1926) suggested that "personality traits can be found in the drawings" (p. 80), and DesLauriers and Halpern (1947) found that the Goodenough scale distinguished schizophrenic children from normals.

Witkin (Witkin–Marlens scale in Witkin et al. [1962]) developed a scale for assessing HFDs by systematically assessing the relative sophistication of body concept (degree of detailing and overall quality) expressed on the drawings. The Witkin–Marlens scale is essentially the same as the GH scale in that more "mature" or "differentiated" HFDs are those with more complete detailing and better quality. The GH scale, however, generally yields greater interrater reliability than the Witkin–Marlens scale because the Witkin–Marlens scale employs a procedure whereby judges arrive at an overall judgment of the figure drawing, whereas the GH is based on an objective, quantified scale.

Robins Balance-Tilt Scale

In contrast to the GH, the RBT scale is primarily a measure of psychopathology rather than intelligence and developmental maturity. Robins (1980) derived the concepts of "balance" and "tilt" from various sources.

Regarding "balance," Koppitz (1968) wrote that the "slant" of the figure is of critical importance, denoting the presence or absence of security, stability, or mental balance. Agreeing with Machover (1949), Koppitz related the toppling figure to "mental imbalance or a personality in flux" (p. 59). Hammer (1958) concurred with Wolff (1946) that imbalance indicates feelings of emotional inadequacy and insecurity. Hammer (1958) believed balance to be of utmost importance in determining the degree of pathology; for Hammer, an imbalanced HFD in adults denoted a preschizophrenic personality. Bridgman (1961) saw balance in the human figure as expressing "a sense of security," a "feeling or sense of balance" (p. 22). Koppitz (1968, p. 41) found a "slanting figure" occurring more frequently on HFDs of clinic patients as compared with those of well-adjusted students.

Robins (1980) based his operational definition of balance on Bridgman's (1961) definition of balance as "the center of gravity, from the pit of the neck, passing through the supporting foot or feet, or between the feet when they are supporting the weight equally" (p. 22). Most HFDs fit this category (i.e., standing straight, facing outward). In this case, a vertical line extended up from the midpoint of the stance of the feet should pass through the neck and the center of the head if the head is

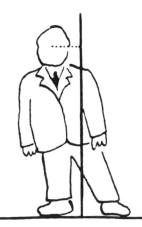

FIG. 3.1. Computation of balance of a Human Figure Drawing.

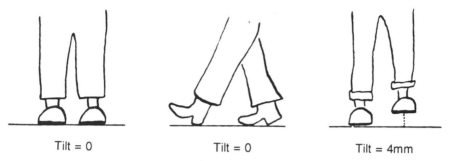

Tilt = 0   Tilt = 0   Tilt = 4mm

FIG. 3.2. Computations of tilt of a Human Figure Drawing.

drawn in the usual manner. The quantity of deviation from perfect balance is measured by the distance from the center of the head (arrived at by finding the center of the head as if it were a circle) to the extended vertical. As indicated in Figure 3.1, *balance* is defined as the deviation of the figure from the vertical axis.

The operational definition of *tilt* is the quantity by which one foot is "shorter" than the other (see Figure 3.2). The tilt scale is a variation of the balance scale but refers specifically to the feet of the figure. Although many authors do not distinguish between balance and tilt, there are instances when the balance can be strictly vertical but the tilt is not strictly horizontal. Tilt, therefore, measures a different dimension than balance.

The measurement of balance and tilt are corrected for the height of the figure (i.e., are divided by the height of the figure and multiplied by 100). In this way, a tiny figure with a 3-mm deviation from perfect balance is judged as "off balance" as a very large figure with 22 mm of deviation. The corrected scores of balance and tilt for the male and female drawings were converted to standardized (z) scores and summed to give the total RBT score. The same procedure was followed to obtain a total GH score.

Two independent raters (a graduate student in clinical psychology and an experienced clinical psychologist) established excellent interrater reliability ($r > .95$) in scoring both GH and RBT.

THEMATIC APPERCEPTION TEST (TAT)[3]

TAT protocols were assessed for three defense mechanisms (denial, projection, and identification) using a system developed by Cramer (1991). The TAT had been given to the 90 patients in a standard administration as part of the psychological assessment battery administered at admission and later in the treatment process. Patients' responses to three TAT cards (Cards 1, 14, and 13 MF) were assessed for three types of defenses—denial, projection, and identification. Responses to these three cards were selected for study because they were available for all the patients in the sample, the content of the pictures was realistic (i.e., not fantastic or surrealistic), and responses from two of the cards had been used in previous research on defenses as well as in the development of the scoring manual. These stories, with identifying data removed, were scored by an independent judge (an experienced doctorate-level clinical psychologist who had extensive prior experience with this scoring procedure) for the occurrence of different components of denial, projection, and identification.

Denial was scored for statements that included negation; denial of reality; reversal; misperception; omission of major characters or objects; overly maximizing the positive or minimizing the negative; and unexpected goodness, optimism, positiveness, or gentleness. Projection was scored for statements that included attribution of hostile feelings or intentions, or other normatively unusual feelings or intentions, to a character; additions of ominous people, animals, objects, or qualities; concern for protection from external threat; themes of pursuit, entrapment, and escape; apprehensiveness of death, injury, or assault; magical or autistic thinking; and bizarre story or theme. Identification was scored for statements that included themes of emulation of skills, characteristics, qualities, or attitudes; regulation of motives or behavior; self-esteem through affiliation; work and delay of gratification; role differentiation; and moralism. These criteria were derived from various theoretical discussions of each of the three defenses (e.g., Freud, 1946) as well as from the few previously published attempts to formulate a scoring system for defenses based on projective test data (e.g., Haworth, 1963). A more detailed presentation of these scoring procedures is available in Appendix 9.

The following story, told in response to TAT Card 1 (boy with violin) by one of the patients in the present study, illustrates the scoring system:

> There's something wrong with this boy physically and mentally. He's unhappy. He wants to play the violin, and he can't. Maybe he's deaf. Somebody else was in the room earlier and put it in front of him and left. He's not the kind of person who would pick it up and break it or anything. Is that enough? I don't know what the placemat's doing. It's obviously not something to eat.

Although the story begins with two examples of projection, the patient then resorts to using denial, which is unsuccessful in staving off the peculiar ideation at the conclusion of the story. Thus, this story would receive three scores for denial because of the use of negation: "He's not the kind of person who would . . . break it"; "I don't know what the placemat's doing"; and "It's . . . not something to eat." The story would also be scored twice for projection because of the addition of ominous qualities: "something wrong with this boy physically and mentally"; and "maybe he's deaf."

Previous work with this method indicated adequate interrater reliability (Cramer, 1991). A subsample of 47 stories from the present study were scored by a second doctorate-level clinical psychologist; the resulting interrater Pearson correlations were .80 for denial, .78 for projection, and .59 for identification. Judges' ratings were within 1 point of each other in 94% of the stories for ratings of denial and identification and in 83% of the stories for ratings of projection. Further evidence for the reliability in scoring this measure was provided by clinicians' judgments. Thirty-three scored stories—11 high on denial, 11 high on projection, and 11 high on identification—were presented in random order to two experienced doctorate-level clinical psychologists who were asked to indicate which of the three defenses was most prominent in each story. There was a high degree of agreement between the clinicians' judgments and the defense scores: The two judges each correctly identified 29 of the 33 stories.

Summary of Scoring of Test Protocols

In summary, as indicated in Table 3.3, the psychological test protocols were evaluated in a variety of ways to capture dimensions considered particularly relevant to an assessment of psychopathology and the process of therapeutic change.

1. The Rorschach protocols were evaluated for the following variables:
   a. Composite thought disorder (the weighted sum of responses indicating boundary disturbances—contamination, confabulation, and fabulized combination, controlling by covariance overall response productivity).
   b. The concept of the human object (OR) for accurately perceived (OR+) responses and inaccurately perceived (OR−) responses. Both the weighted sum (controlling for overall number of Rorschach responses) and the developmental mean were used to measure OR+ and OR−.
   c. The mutuality of autonomy—the average score of responses

TABLE 3.3
Overview of Research Design:
Evaluations at Admission and Later in Treatment

A. Manifest clinical and social behavior in clinical case records
    1. Clinical symptoms (Strauss–Harder Rating Scales)
        a. Neurotic
        b. Psychotic
        c. Labile Affect (Bizarre-Disorganized)
        d. Flattened Affect (Bizarre-Retarded)
    2. Social Behavior Fairweather Rating Scale of Ward Behavior
        a. Interpersonal communication
    3. Interpersonal relations (Menninger Scales)
        a. Motivation for treatment
        b. Sublimatory effectiveness
        c. Impulsivity
        d. Superego integration
        e. Object relations
B. Psychological test variables
    1. Rorschach
        a. Accurate Object Representation (OR+)
            (capacity for interpersonal relations)
        b. Inaccurate Object Representation (OR−)
            (investment in inappropriate, possibly autistic relationships)
        c. Capacity for Affect Modulation (Sum C)
            (color responses on the Rorschach)
        d. Thought disorder
            (impairment in differentiation and integration)
        e. Capacity for reality testing
            (F+% on Rorschach)
        f. Mutuality of Autonomy (Urist Scale)
        g. Adaptive Fantasy (M+)
            (accurately perceived human movement)
        h. Maladaptive Fantasy (M−)
            (inaccurately perceived human movement)
    2. Wechsler Intelligence Test (WAIS, WBI, WBII)
    3. Human Figure Drawings
    4. Thematic Apperception Test (TAT)
        (defenses of denial, projection, and identification)

on the continuum of themes from mutual empathic relatedness to malevolent engulfment and destruction. This measure was supplemented by also considering the level of each
patient's single most malevolent and single most benevolent
responses.

    d. Traditional Rorschach scores of degree of reality testing

(F+%), the number of accurately perceived and inaccurately perceived human movement responses (M+, M−), and the weighted sum of color responses.

2. Intelligence as assessed by one of the Wechsler intelligence tests (Full Scale, Verbal, and Performance IQ).
3. Assessment of the degree of articulation and differentiation (Goodenough–Harris scale) and the degree of organization (balance-tilt) in HFDs.
4. TAT protocols were assessed for the total indication of three types of defense: denial, projection, and identification.

Thus, in addition to the 7 ratings made on the clinical case records (4 symptoms scales and 3 measures of interpersonal relatedness), 10 basic psychological test variables were derived from the psychological test protocols: Four variables were derived from the concept of the human object in accurately and inaccurately perceived Rorschach responses, composite thought disorder, the average degree of benevolence and mutuality in the MOA scale, Full Scale IQ, the extent of total defenses appearing in TAT stories, and the degree of differentiation (GH) and organization (RBT) in human figure drawings. These 10 test variables were relatively independent at initial assessment. The various test variables are relatively uncorrelated at Time 1; almost all the correlations between the various test variables are less than .35. Exceptions occurred on the Rorschach, in which thought disorder had a substantial correlation with degree of reality testing (F+%) ($r = -.47$), the MOA mean score ($r = .49$), and the weighted sum of inaccurately perceived object representations (OR−) ($r - .67$). Degree of reality testing also correlated significantly with the MOA mean ($r = -.41$). Also, the two measures of accurately perceived object representation (OR +) (developmental mean and weighted sum) are highly correlated ($r = .51$), whereas this relationship for inaccurately perceived object representation (OR−) is not as substantial ($r = .36$). The number of accurately perceived human movement responses (M+) correlated significantly with the number of inaccurately perceived human movement responses (M−) ($r = .54$), and with the weighted sum and developmental mean of accurately perceived object representation (OR+) ($r = .72$ and .54, respectively). Correlations of the various test measures with Full Scale IQ were insubstantial ($r < .15$), except for the developmental mean of inaccurately perceived human forms (OR−) ($r = .36$). Overall, the various measures derived from the psychological test protocols (the Rorschach, TAT, Wechsler Intelligence Test, and HFDs) are relatively independent at the initial testing.

MEDIATOR CONTROL VARIABLES

A number of variables external to the treatment process itself can influence the direction and rate of therapeutic change, including the severity of the patient's pathology at admission to the hospital, the level of premorbid adjustment prior to hospitalization, the sex of the patient, the use of medication as part of the treatment process, and the level of the therapist's experience. We examined the effects of each of these potentially confounding variables on the basic results.

To control for level of premorbid adjustment, the initial case records of all 90 subjects were rated on two scales, one developed by Zigler and Phillips (1962) and the other by Goldstein (1978) and his colleagues (Goldstein, Held, & Cromwell, 1968; Goldstein, Rodnick, Evans, & May, 1975), designed to assess level of premorbid adjustment. Interrater reliability was at an acceptable level (Item Alpha >.80) for both these scales. (The Zigler–Phillips and the Goldstein scales of premorbid social adjustment are presented in Appendix 7.) We also noted the years of experience of the primary therapist and whether the patient was receiving psychoactive medication. Also, two experienced clinical psychologists reviewed the clinical case records at Time 1 and rated the severity of psychopathology into three categories (psychotic, severe personality disorder including borderline and narcissistic pathology, and severe neurotic disturbances, primarily depression). The judges had an acceptable level of reliability (78% agreement) in making this distinction. Differences between the two judges were resolved by consultation. We evaluated the impact of these various mediator variables on the assessment of change as measured by the variables derived from the psychological tests and the ratings of the clinical case records.

DIFFERENTIATION AMONG TYPES OF PATIENTS

Rather than expecting all patients to change in the same way, we thought it seemed more likely that different types of patients might change in different ways. As discussed earlier, we used the conceptualization developed by Blatt and Shichman (1983) to distinguish between two broad configurations of psychopathology: "anaclitic" and "introjective" psychopathologies. These two basic configurations of psychoology, as described in detail on pages 14 to 18, and a synopsis of the characteristics of the anaclitic and introjective diagnostic configurations are presented in Appendix 8.

Based on the initial case records, two judges rated the patient's pathology was primarily anaclitic or introjective. They rated each patient on a 100-point scale indicating the extent to which the patient was predominantly anaclitic or introjective. Judges were able to make this discrimination with a high degree of reliability. Of the 18 cases they jointly rated, the two judges agreed on 17 in terms of whether the patient was rated as predominantly anaclitic or introjective. The Item Alpha for their rankings using the 100-point scale was .93.

Each judge rated one-half of the sample for the anaclitic–introjective distinction. Forty-two of the subjects were considered to be primarily anaclitic, and 48 were considered as primarily introjective. Approximately 67% of the anaclitic patients were women, and 67% of the introjective patients were men. Analyses of change, using ratings derived from the clinical case records and the psychological test protocols, were conducted both for the entire sample of 90 patients and for 42 anaclitic and 48 introjective patients separately. Because the anaclitic–introjective distinction is sex-linked, the data were also evaluated for the extent to which the assessment of change was influenced by sex rather than the clinical distinction of anaclitic and introjective types of patients.

Statistical Analyses

The data were approached in several ways to answer a number of different questions.

First, we were interested in the general impact of hospitalization and treatment on the total sample. Thus, variables from the clinical case records and the psychological protocols at Time 1 and Time 2 were examined using a two-factor repeated measures analysis of variance design to compare change in the patients with anaclitic and introjective psychopathology. Matched t tests were also used to examine differences in degree of change in the two types of patients when there was a significant interaction between degree of change and type of patient. These results are presented in the first section of the next chapter.

We also evaluated the effect size (Cohen, 1984) of changes noted in clinical case record ratings and psychological test protocols over the course of treatment. Although there are no established procedures or computer programs for assessing effect size in a repeated measures design, effect size was estimated in this research by evaluating the mean change in terms of the basic variability of the measure (i.e., difference between means at Time 1 and Time 2, divided by the average of the standard deviations at Time 1 and Time 2). This is a conservative estimate of effect size because it is uncorrected for internal correlations. An effect size of .20 was considered as minimally acceptable, .30 to .50 as moderate, and greater than .50 as substantial.[4]

Second, we were interested in the effects of mediator variables, such as the use of psychoactive medication, the level of the therapist's experience, the sex of the patient, the severity of the patient's pathology, and the level of the patient's premorbid social adjustment, on the treatment process. Using two-way analyses of covariance, we examined the effects of each of these possible mediator variables on the change as measured by the various clinical case record ratings and psychological test variables. We compared the level of the clinical case record ratings and the psychological test variables at Time 2, covaried on Time 1, for anaclitic and introjective patients with high and low premorbid adjustment; patients independently considered to be psychotic, with severe character pathology or severe neurotic disturbance (e.g., depression); patients receiving or not receiving medication during treatment; and patients with more experienced (with at least 6 years postdoctoral experience) or less experienced (2 to 6 years of postdoctoral experience) therapists. These findings are presented in the second section of the next chapter.

Third, we were interested in the configuration of change. We based these analyses on the assumption that even though the total group of patients might exhibit significant change in a constructive direction, individual patients could change to various degrees, including some patients who might even regress in treatment. Thus, we sought to examine if there were clusters of variables that changed over time as indicated by correlations among various measures of change within individuals. We correlated change scores on the various case record ratings with change scores on the psychological test variables, for anaclitic and introjective patients, to see if there were particular configurations of change that characterized these two groups of patients.

Fourth, we attempted to evaluate the strength and nature of the relationship between the assessment of psychological test records at admission (Time 1) and clinical status at Time 2 in terms of symptoms and social adjustment as rated from the clinical case records. In this analysis, we sought to identify possible psychological characteristics at Time 1 that would be predictive of clinical status at Time 2. Beyond the predictive models that can be developed through multiple regression and canonical correlation analyses, causal processes can be inferred from analytic techniques such as cross-lagged correlation and path analysis, especially in longitudinal designs in which there is assessment of both predictor and criterion variables at Time 1 and Time 2. In this study, we used a path analytic model to examine our data for possible psychological test variables at Time 1 that would be prognostic of the extent of clinical change.

The path analytic technique requires a specification of unidirectional relationships (paths) among variables and the computation of indicators of the magnitude of effects (path coefficients). Mathematically, a multiple regression equation is fitted to the variables in the path model and the standardized regression weights (b_i^*) become the path coefficients. Although the scale and the interpretation of path coefficients are similar to correlations, they differ from correlations in two important ways: a path coefficient describes a one-directional effect rather than a nondirectional relationship, and a path coefficient is more like a partial correlation in that the effect that it describes statistically controls for the effect of all other variables on the criterion specified within the model. The statistical procedures of path analysis facilitate the examination of the relationships between estimates of change in variables from independent sources—from the social behavior reported in the clinical case records and from variables of psychological organization and functioning derived from the psychological test records. The details of this technique, the specific model we used, and the results are presented in Chapter 8.

Thus the results are organized to address four basic questions:

1. Are there consistent and systematic behavioral and psychological changes in the patients of the present sample during the period in which they were in treatment?
2. Are there possible confoundings of any results by variables external to the treatment process?
3. Are there consistent configurations of change? Do clusters of variables systematically change within subjects as various types of patients process or regress in the treatment process?
4. What is the progress of change? Is it possible to predict change and, if so, what dimensions serve as possible predispositional variables leading to change in the treatment process?

Notes

1. As noted by Blatt, Tuber, and Auerbach (1990), there are substantial differences between this system for scoring thought disorder and the one proposed by Exner (1978; Exner, Weiner, & Schuyler, 1976; Weiner & Exner, 1978). In particular, the distinction between a fabulized combination-regular and a fabulized combination-serious, a thought disorder score not found in the

Exner system, is an extension of Holt's (1963) differentiation between (1) the combination of two independent and clearly separate objects in an incongruous relationship (e.g., a bear standing on a butterfly), and (2) a combination in which two parts are placed together in an incongruous relationship within a single object (e.g., a bear with a man's head), such that each of the parts tends to lose its separate definition and integrity. The latter response, the fabulized combination-serious, is more akin to a contamination, in which the two objects or parts lose their separate identities and merge together to create an incongruous, illogical entity. In this sense, it indicates a more serious type of thought disorder than does the fabulized combination-regular, in which the separate definition and identity of the two objects or parts are maintained. Research (Blatt & Berman, 1984; Lerner, Sugarman, & Barbour, 1985; Wilson, 1982, 1985) supports the formulation that these two types of fabulized combinations indicate very different levels of pathological thinking.

Exner (1978; Exner et al., 1976) scores the fabulized combination-serious response as an incongruous combination (INCOM). In contrast to Holt (1962) and Blatt & Berman (1984), Exner considered this type of response less disturbed than the fabulized combination-regular, primarily because he found that the incongruous combination score is more frequent in a normal sample than is the fabulized combination-regular (Exner's FABCOM score). The relatively higher frequency of Exner's incongruous combination response as compared to his FABCOM score is probably an artifact of Exner's placing several different types of responses within the INCOM category. He included not only the fabulized combination-serious response, as defined by Holt (1963) and Blatt and Berman (1984), but also responses in which form and color are arbitrarily and unrealistically combined (e.g., pink bears). Exner's inclusion of FCarb responses (Allison, Blatt, & Zimet, 1968; Rapaport, Gill, & Schafer, 1945), along with the fabulized combination-serious, in his incongruous combination category, may be the reason why he found that this category occurs with a greater frequency in normals than does the fabulized combination-regular. Exner provided no theoretical or empirical justification, however, for combining the fabulized combination-serious response and the arbitrary color response (FCarb) into a single scoring category, INCOM. The FCarb score reflects an individual's difficulty integrating affective experiences with logical thought (cf. Rapaport et al., 1945), whereas the fabulized combination-serious score reflects difficulty maintaining a boundary between independent and separate ideas and concepts (Blatt & Wild, 1976). Thus, until there is more substantial theoretical rationale or empirical support for Exner's decision to merge fabulized combination-serious and arbitrary color responses into the INCOM category, it seems judicious to maintain the distinction between the two very different types of thought disorder expressed in fabulized combination-serious and fabulized combination-regular responses. Empirical findings (Lerner et al., 1985; Wilson, 1982, 1985) suggest that it seems appropriate to view the fabulized combination-serious responses as a more severe form of pathological thought.

2. Material in this section is derived from an article (Robins, Blatt, & Ford, 1991) published in the *Journal of Personality Assessment*.
3. Material in this section is derived from an article (Cramer, Blatt, & Ford, 1988) published in the *Journal of Personality Assessment*.
4. We are indebted to Professors Robert Manuck and Donald M. Quinlan at Yale University and Professor Patrick Shrout at New York University for their consultation and advice on this matter.

CHAPTER 4

Therapeutic Change in Clinical Case Reports and on the Rorschach

This chapter will consider the evaluation of therapeutic change as expressed in ratings of clinical behavior described in the clinical case reports prepared on each patient after the first 6 weeks of hospitalization and then again, on average, after 15 months of intensive treatment including psychoanalytically oriented individual psychotherapy four times weekly. The case records were rated for manifest clinical symptoms of psychosis, neurosis, and labile and flattened affect, as well as for the quality of social interactions with other patients and members of the clinical staff. In addition, Rorschach protocols administered at these same two times in the treatment process were independently evaluated for a variety of dimensions including thought disorder and the quality of the representation of the human figure and the nature of its interactions.

In data analyses to follow, we will assess therapeutic change for the total sample of patients as well as for patients with predominantly anaclitic disorders and those with predominantly introjective disorders. Initially we will consider change in clinical symptoms and social behavior as assessed from the clinical case reports, followed by analyses of variables from the Rorschach protocols.

PSYCHOLOGICAL AND BEHAVIORAL CHANGE

Changes in Social Behavior and Clinical Systems

Table 4.1 presents a two-way analysis of variance (ANOVA) for a repeated measures design comparing anaclitic and introjective patients

TABLE 4.1

Two-Way Analysis of Variance of Case Record Ratings of Social Behavior
for Anaclitic and Introjective Patients at Time 1 and Time 2

| | Means | | | | ANOVA (df = 1.88) F values (repeated measures) | | |
| | Anaclitic | | Introjective | | | | |
	T1	T2	T1	T2	A/I	T1/T2	A×B
Menninger Scales							
Factor I (Interpersonal relatedness)	−1.08	.18	−.94	1.72	2.40	26.57****	3.18†
Motivation for treatment	33.29	39.62	32.58	44.77	1.13	35.31****	3.37†
Sublimatory effectiveness	34.29	42.55	39.19	47.19	5.21*	29.08****	.01
Superego integration	36.14	36.00	34.92	39.02	.41	3.69*	3.68*
Object relations	29.98	31.31	29.69	34.73	1.55	11.38***	3.55†
Factor II (Impulsivity)	49.79	51.90	46.29	46.21	3.32†	.23	.31
Fairweather							
Interpersonal communication	1.31	1.32	1.34	1.26	.11	1.67	2.14

†p<.10   *p<.05   ***p<.001   ****p<.0001

at Time 1 and Time 2 on measures of social behavior as assessed from the clinical case records (the Menninger Factors of Interpersonal Relations and the Fairweather Scale of Interpersonal Communication).[1] The data clearly and consistently indicate that after an average of 15 months of treatment there are substantial constructive changes in social behavior and interpersonal relations in the total group of patients. As indicated in Table 4.1, significant and constructive change was found on Menninger Factor I (p<.0001) for the total sample. Matched t tests (Table 4.2) comparing change in both anaclitic and introjective patients at Time 1 and Time 2 indicate that both groups demonstrated significant change on this factor (t = −2.15, p<.05; t = −5.14, p<.001, respectively.) Effect size of these differences is substantial for the total sample (.64), especially for introjective (.79) as compared with anaclitic patients (.45).

Significant (p<.05) and constructive change was found for the total group of patients on each of the four scales that make up Menninger Factor I: Motivation for Treatment, Social and Sublimatory Effectiveness, Superego Integration, and Object Relations (effect size on these four scales for the total sample ranged from .25 to .78, with an average effect size of .53). There was no significant change on Menninger Factor II, Impulsivity.

While the primary findings are the main effects across time for the

TABLE 4.2

Matched *t* Tests and Effect Size of Changes in Case Record Ratings of Social Behavior for Anaclitic and Introjective Patients at Time 1 and Time 2

	Matched *t* tests			Effect size		
Case record variables	Total sample (N = 90)	Anaclitic patients (N = 42)	Introjective patients (N = 48)	Total sample (N = 90)	Anaclitic patients (N = 42)	Introjective patients (N = 48)
Menninger Scales						
Factor I (Interpersonal relatedness)	−5.09****	−2.15*	−5.14***	.64	.45	.79
Motivation for treatment	−5.86****	−2.72**	−5.59****	.78	.54	.98
Sublimatory capacity	−5.42****	−3.70***	−3.92***	.66	.70	.65
Superego integration	−1.83†	.09	−2.74**	.25	.02	.46
Object relations	−3.33***	−.90	−3.84***	.44	.20	.59
Factor II (Impulsivity)	.48	−.75	.03	.06	.14	.01
Fairweather						
Interpersonal communication	1.28	−.17	2.05*	.14	.06	.35

†*p* < .10 **p* < .05 **p < .01 ***p < .001 ****p < .0001

entire sample, there are trends ($p<.10$) toward significant interactions with the anaclitic–introjective distinction on three of the Menninger Scales: Motivation for Treatment, Superego Integration, and Object Relations. Matched t tests indicate that while anaclitic patients improved significantly on one of these three scales (Motivation for Treatment, $t = -2.72$; $p<.01$), the primary effects over time are a consequence of a significantly greater improvement in the introjective patients. Introjective patients improved on Motivation for Treatment and Object Relations to a highly significant degree ($t = -5.59$ and -3.84, respectively; $p<.0001$). Introjective patients also had a significant increase ($t = 2.74$; $p<.01$) in Superego Integration, while anaclitic patients had a slight, nonsignificant decline on this variable. The difference between changes of anaclitic and introjective patients on Superego Integration is the only significant ($p<.05$) interaction. This significant difference between the two groups on degree of improvement in Superego Integration is consistent with theoretical formulations that superego concerns are primary for introjective rather than anaclitic patients (Blatt, 1974, in press; Blatt & Shichman, 1983). Introjective patients generally seem somewhat more treatment responsive, however, at least in terms of improvement in social behavior.

While there was no indication of significant change for the entire sample, nor a significant interaction term, for the Fairweather Scale of Interpersonal Communication, matched t tests indicate significant improvement on this scale for introjective patients ($t = 2.05$; $p<.05$) (effect size $= .35$).

Table 4.3 presents the analysis of the four Strauss–Harder scales for

TABLE 4.3
Two-Way Analysis of Variance of Case Record Ratings of Clinical Symptoms for Anaclitic and Introjective Patients at Time 1 and Time 2

| | Natural means | | | | ANOVA ($df = 1.88$) F values (repeated measures) | | |
| | Anaclitic | | Introjective | | | | |
	T1	T2	T1	T2	A/I	T1/T2	A×B
Strauss–Harder symptoms							
Neurotic	6.98	6.79	7.21	5.75	.99	4.25*	2.27
Psychotic	2.26	2.55	3.12	2.31	1.17	1.53	5.10*
Labile Affect	1.31	1.64	1.19	.90	4.49*	0	3.90*
Flattened Affect	.60	.38	.56	.15	1.13	8.33**	.82

*$p<.05$ **$p<.01$

different clusters of clinical symptoms. Significant decreases ($p<.05$) in symptoms were noted for the total sample on the Neurotic and Flattened Affect scales (effect size of these differences are .31 and .42, respectively). These changes in neurotic symptoms and Flattened Affect, however, are primarily the consequence of significant changes in these symptoms in the introjective patients ($t = 2.88$ and 2.99, respectively; $p<.01$) (effect size of .54 and .55, respectively) but not in the anaclitic patients ($t = .28$ and 1.20, respectively). A significant interaction term, however, was also noted on the Psychotic and Labile Affect scales. Matched t tests (see Table 4.4) indicate that while introjective patients had a significant decrease ($t = 2.23$; $p<.05$) (effect size = .41) of psychotic symptoms, anaclitic patients had a nonsignificant increase in psychotic symptoms ($t = -0.92$; n.s.). Anaclitic patients also had a nonsignificant increase in Labile Affect($t = -1.28$; n.s.), while introjective patients had a nonsignificant decrease on this scale ($t = 1.55$; n.s.).

Thus, the analysis of data gained from the clinical case records—the assessment of change in social behavior, interpersonal relations, and several types of clinical symptoms—indicates significant improvement in the total sample during the treatment process, but especially for patients with an introjective type of psychopathology. Generally, the effect size of these changes in introjective patients is substantial. Introjective patients seem to improve more rapidly and in more manifest form. Improvement in anaclitic patients seems to occur more slowly and subtly and to a much less substantial degree than change in patients with an introjective type of pathology. Change in anaclitic patients is noted particularly in changes in the quality of their interpersonal relations but not in manifest clinical systems.

It should be stressed that careful methodological controls were established for the rating of the clinical case records. Case records of each patient were scored by a different judge at Time 1 and at Time 2 without knowledge of the other ratings. Two judges each scored half the cases at Time 1 and then the other half at Time 2. In addition, these ratings of the various case record variables are relatively independent of each other (see Chapter 9, Footnote 3, p. 195).

Even though judges making the ratings at Time 2 were uninformed about the case ratings at Time 1, and each judge scored the other half of the records at Time 2, it was not possible to disguise whether a case record was from Time 1 or Time 2. Therefore, it is possible that both judges could have been influenced by a general halo effect and were biased toward seeing better functioning at Time 2. Thus, it is important to note that on several of the scales anaclitic and introjective patients changed differentially, and, even further, on a few scales patients with

TABLE 4.4

Matched *t* Tests and Effect Size of Changes in Case Record Ratings of Clinical Symptoms for Anaclitic and Introjective Patients at Time 1 and Time 2

	Matched *t* tests			Effect size		
	Total sample (N = 90)	Anaclitic patients (N = 42)	Introjective patients (N = 48)	Total sample (N = 90)	Anaclitic patients (N = 42)	Introjective patients (N = 48)
Strauss–Harder symptoms						
Neurotic	2.05*	0.03	2.80**	.31	.07	.54
Psychotic	1.21	−0.92	2.23*	.17	.22	.41
Labile Affect	0	−1.28	1.55	.00	.25	.26
Flattened Affect	2.89*	1.20	2.99**	.42	.12	.55

*p<.05   **p<.01

an anaclitic type of psychopathology changed in a negative direction. It seems unlikely, therefore, that a simple positive halo effect distorted the ratings of the clinical case records and accounted for the significant positive changes noted in these ratings. Rather, it seems that the judges were providing consistent and reliable differentiation of the clinical case records and that the results accurately reflect significant and constructive therapeutic changes in a substantial number of the patients during the time interval assessed in this study. This conclusion is supported even further by the results of psychological test protocols. Significant and constructive changes were noted on several key psychological test variables, and the judges who scored these protocols were completely uninformed about the patient. They had no way of knowing anything about the case record ratings, not even the patient's sex, age, or diagnosis, nor any way of identifying whether a test protocol was from Time 1 or Time 2.

Changes on Psychological Test Protocols

Tables 4.5 to 4.12 present a detailed analysis of variables derived from the scoring of the Rorschach protocols. Tables 4.5 and 4.6 indicate a

TABLE 4.5
Two-Way Analysis of Variance for Thought Disorder on the Rorschach
for Anaclitic and Introjective Patients at Time 1 and Time 2

| | Natural means | | | | ANOVA (df = 1.88) F values (repeated measures) | | |
| | Anaclitic | | Introjective | | | | |
	T1	T2	T1	T2	A/I	T1/T2	A×B
Composite Thought Disorder Index	24.95	21.02	26.19	23.79	.05	5.52*	.44
Types of thought disorder							
Contamination	.12	.05	.06	.10	.15	.39	1.98
Contamination tendency	.48	.21	.40	.38	0	3.04†	1.81
Fabulized combination (serious)	1.26	1.26	1.56	1.69	.27	.28	.33
Confabulation	1.71	1.19	1.17	.71	2.12	5.44*	.11
Confabulation tendency	.31	.50	.54	.58	.79	.50	.27
Fabulized to confabulation	1.81	1.52	1.90	1.60	.06	5.92**	.06
Fabulized combination (regular)	.74	.64	.94	.85	.27	1.71	.06

†p<.10   *p<.05   **p<.01

TABLE 4.6

Matched *t* Tests and Effect Size of Changes in Thought Disorder on the Rorschach of Anaclitic and Introjective Patients at Time 1 and Time 2

	Matched *t* tests			Effect size		
	Total sample ($N = 90$)	Anaclitic patients ($N = 42$)	Introjective patients ($N = 48$)	Total sample ($N = 90$)	Anaclitic patients ($N = 42$)	Introjective patients ($N = 48$)
Composite Thought Disorder Index	2.36*	2.04*	1.29	.23	.31	.17
Types of thought disorder						
Contamination	.62	1.34	−.55	.09	.31	.10
Contamination tendency	1.74†	2.23*	.35	.24	.45	.07
Fabulized combination (serious)	.53	.91	0	.06	.14	0
Confabulation	2.34*	1.56	1.82†	.25	.27	.23
Confabulation tendency	−.71	−.94	−.15	.10	.20	.03
Fabulized to confabulation	2.45*	1.88†	1.58	.25	.28	.23
Fabulized combination (regular)	1.31	1.16	.74	.15	.18	.12

†*p*<.10   *p*<.05

significant ($F = 5.52$; $p<.05$) decline in thought disorder for the entire sample from initial to subsequent testing (effect size $= .23$). Not only was there a significant decline in total thought disorder for the entire sample, but there was also a significant decline in several component types of thought disorder that contribute to the composite thought-disorder score—especially in the more serious forms of thought disorder for which there were more substantial base rates—contamination tendencies, confabulations, and confabulation tendencies (fabulized to confabulation). In addition to a significant decrease in thought disorder, Tables 4.7 and 4.8 indicate that there was also a significant increase ($p<.05$) in the amount of adaptive fantasy (M+ responses) on the Rorschach from Time 1 to Time 2 for the total sample (effect size $= .20$).

Tables 4.9 and 4.10 present analyses of the concept of the object on the Rorschach. As discussed earlier, human responses in the Rorschach protocols were evaluated for the degree of differentiation, articulation, and integration. Two different measures were used to assess these dimensions: the mean developmental level and a developmental index (the total weighted sum) for the differentiation, articulation, and integration (motivation of action, integration of action, and the content and nature of interactions) of human responses. Consistent with prior research (Blatt et al., 1976b), analyses of these variables were conducted separately for accurately (F+) and inaccurately perceived (F−) human figures.

Tables 4.9 and 4.10 present an analysis of the mean developmental level and the weighted sum (the developmental index) for differentia-

TABLE 4.7

Two-Way Analysis of Variance of Several Traditional Rorschach Variables for Anaclitic and Introjective Patients at Time 1 and Time 2

| | Natural means | | | | ANOVA ($df = 1.88$) F values (repeated measures) | | |
| | Anaclitic | | Introjective | | | | |
	T1	T2	T1	T2	A/I	T1/T2	A×B
Rorschach Variables							
Adherence to Reality (F+%)	71.02	69.57	70.96	71.36	.11	.05	.21
Affective Lability (Sum C)	3.61	3.92	3.69	3.42	.60	.36	.66
Adaptive Fantasy (M+)	2.43	2.83	2.33	2.85	.13	3.68*	.18
Maladaptive Fantasy (M−)	.33	.19	.27	.29	.28	1.86	1.43
Number of Responses (R)	32.43	36.95	37.35	39.69	1.67	3.34†	.35

†$p<.10$ *$p<.05$

TABLE 4.8

Matched *t* Tests and Effect Size of Changes in Traditional Rorschach Variables for Anaclitic and Introjective Patients at Time 1 and Time 2

	Matched *t* tests			Effect size		
	Total sample (N = 90)	Anaclitic patients (N = 42)	Introjective patients (N = 48)	Total sample (N = 90)	Anaclitic patients (N = 42)	Introjective patients (N = 48)
F+% (Adherence to reality)	.23	0.45	−.16	.03	.09	.03
Sum Color (Affective Lability)	.60	−.15	1.25	.06	.03	.15
Human Movement + (Adaptive Fantasy)	−1.93†	−.96	−1.76†	.20	.15	.23
Human Movement − (Maladaptive Fantasy)	1.36†	2.17*	−.16	.19	.41	.04
Number of Rorschach responses	−1.83†	−2.23*	−.79	.20	.31	.13

†*p*<.10   **p*<.05

TABLE 4.9

Two-Way Analysis of Variance of Concept of the Object and Mutuality
of Autonomy on the Rorschach for Anaclitic and Introjective Patients
at Time 1 and Time 2

| | Natural means | | | | ANOVA ($df = 1.88$) F values (repeated measures) | | |
| | Anaclitic | | Introjective | | | | |
	T1	T2	T1	T2	A/I	T1/T2	A×B
Concept of the Object							
Appropriate Object Relations (OR+)							
Mean developmental level	.19	.21	−.03	−.32	.26	.08	.09
Developmental index	−.06	−.07	−.12	.23	.02	.11	.11
Inappropriate Object Relations (OR−)							
Mean developmental level	−.97	−1.66	.92	1.39	9.40**	.02	1.22
Developmental index	−.52	−1.22	.96	.56	2.90+	.86	.07
Mutuality of Autonomy (MOA)							
Mean score	3.02	3.05	2.97	2.72	.96	.66	1.15
Most malevolent score	4.64	4.43	4.60	4.08	.36	3.34+	.58
Most benevolent score	1.62	1.67	1.54	1.65	.13	.32	.04

+$p<.10$ **$p<.01$

tion, articulation, and integration of accurately (OR+) and inaccurately
(OR−) perceived responses with human content. The results indicate
that these variables do not change for the total sample from initial to
second testing, but they do significantly distinguish anaclitic and introjective patients. Anaclitic patients have significantly less investment in
the elaboration of inaccurately perceived human forms (OR−) than do
introjective patients. Anaclitic and introjective patients, however, do not
change significantly over the course of treatment on these measures of
the concept of the object on the Rorschach. There was a tendency
($p<.10$), however, for both anaclitic and introjective patients to have
Rorschach responses that portrayed a less malevolent type of interaction
(lower most malevolent score on the Mutuality of Autonomy) at Time 2
in comparison with Time 1 (effect size for total sample on this variable =
.21).

Tables 4.11 and 4.12 present the assessment of change in intelligence test scores from Time 1 to Time 2. Both Full Scale and Performance IQ scores increased significantly ($p<.05$) during treatment (effect
size = .18 and .34, respectively). There was a trend toward a significant
interaction ($p<.10$) on the Performance IQ. While the Performance IQ of

TABLE 4.10

Matched *t* Tests and Effect Size of Changes in the Concept of the Object and Mutuality of Autonomy on the Rorschach for Anaclitic and Introjective Patients at Time 1 and Time 2

	Matched *t* tests			Effect size		
	Total sample (N = 90)	Anaclitic patients (N = 42)	Introjective patients (N = 48)	Total sample (N = 90)	Anaclitic patients (N = 42)	Introjective patients (N = 48)
Concept of the Object						
Appropriate Object Relations (OR+)						
Mean developmental level	.28	−.02	.41	.03	.00	.07
Developmental index	−.34	.01	−.48	.04	.00	.02
Inappropriate Object Relations (OR−)						
Mean developmental level	.14	.90	−.65	.02	.16	.10
Developmental index	.93	1.64+	.39	.10	.28	.06
Mutuality of Autonomy (MOA)						
Mean Score	.88	−.15	1.65+	.11	.03	.24
Most malevolent source	1.89+	.71	1.94+	.21	.12	.29
Most benevolent source	−.58	−.21	−.68	.09	.05	.13

+*p*<.10

Table 4.11

Two-Way Analysis of Variance of Intelligence Test Scores for Anaclitic
and Introjective Patients at Time 1 and Time 2

| | Natural means | | | | ANOVA ($df = 1.88$) F values (repeated measures) | | |
| | Anaclitic | | Introjective | | | | |
	T1	T2	T1	T2	A/I	T1/T2	A×B
Intelligence test							
Full Scale IQ	116.9	118.2	120.7	122.5	4.14*	4.31˙	.15
Verbal IQ	120.2	120.0	124.6	123.5	3.40⁺	.61	.36
Performance IQ	110.0	112.0	111.8	116.9	2.39	17.10****	3.21⁺

⁺$p<.10$ *$p<.05$ ****$p<.0001$

anaclitic patients tended to increase during treatment ($t = -1.79$; $p<.10$), the primary effect is with introjective patients whose Performance IQ increased to a highly significant degree ($t = -3.82$; $p<.001$) (effect size = .43). It is important to stress that the assessment of intelligence at Time 1 and Time 2 was conducted with different forms of the Wechsler Intelligence Test (the WAIS and the Wechsler–Bellevue Forms I and II), which controlled, as much as possible, for practice effects.

In summary, the total group of 90 patients in this study demonstrated significant and consistent positive changes in both independently assessed clinical case records and psychological test protocols during the course of long-term, intensive treatment. The data indicate significant overall improvement in the quality of interpersonal behavior and a reduction of clinical symptoms. While interpersonal relations improved significantly in both groups, symptom reduction occurred primarily in introjective patients. Independently administered and scored psychological tests support these findings and indicate improvement in a number of crucial test variables for the total sample. The improved social behavior and decrease in symptoms observed in the clinical case reports are paralleled by a significant increase in the number of accurately perceived human movement responses (M+ responses) and a significant reduction in thought disorder on the Rorschach. The positive and constructive changes noted in social behavior and clinical symptoms in the case reports are also paralleled by a significant increase in intelligence test scores, particularly the Performance IQ. The significant increase in Performance IQ in introjective patients suggests that one of the consequences of treatment was a substantial reduction in the level of

TABLE 4.12

Matched *t* Tests and Effect Size of Changes in Intelligence Test Scores
for Anaclitic and Introjective Patients at Time 1 and Time 2

Intelligence test	Matched *t* tests			Effect size		
	Total sample (*N* = 90)	Anaclitic patients (*N* = 42)	Introjective patients (*N* = 48)	Total sample (*N* = 90)	Anaclitic patients (*N* = 42)	Introjective patients (*N* = 48)
Full Scale IQ	−2.09*	−1.36	−1.58	.18	.14	.23
Verbal IQ	.78	.11	.92	.04	.02	.05
Performance IQ	−4.08****	−1.79†	−3.82***	.34	.23	.43

*$p<.05$ ***$p<.001$ ****$p<.0001$

depression (Allison, Blatt, & Zimet, 1968/1988). Psychological test measures of object relations such as the developmental index and the mean developmental level of the concept of the object as well as the Mutuality of Autonomy on the Rorschach, however, failed to reflect the significant changes observed on these other variables.

POTENTIALLY CONFOUNDING VARIABLES AFFECTING THERAPEUTIC CHANGE

A number of variables such as the level of the therapist's experience, the use of medication, the level of the patient's premorbid social adjustment, and the initial severity of the patient's pathology could potentially account for the findings of significant therapeutic change. We examined the relationship of these mediator variables to the patient's initial level of functioning (as reported in the clinical case records and as assessed on psychological tests) as well as to estimates of therapeutic change.

Effects of Therapist's Experience

Correlations between years of therapist experience and aspects of the clinical case record and psychological test protocols at Time 1 indicate that more experienced therapists were assigned patients who had significantly ($p<.05$) more clinical symptoms, especially labile affect, at Time 1.

Therapists were classified into more- and less-experienced groups based on a median split of the number of years of experience. More-experienced therapists had 6 to 34 years of postdoctoral training and/or experience, while less-experienced therapists had less than 6 years of postdoctoral experience. Using a two-way analysis of covariance, we examined the effects of the level of therapist's experience for anaclitic and introjective patients on ratings of the clinical case records and on psychological test variables at Time 2, controlling for the initial level of these variables at Time 1. As indicated in Table 4.13, the level of the therapist's experience had no significant relationship to changes in clinical case record ratings of social behavior or clinical symptoms at Time 2 except for a trend ($p<.10$) for the patients of less-experienced therapists to have higher scores on Sublimatory Effectiveness at Time 2, controlling for the level of this variable at Time 1. Table 4.14 presents the impact of the level of therapist experience on changes in the psychological test

TABLE 4.13

Two-Way Analysis of Covariance for the Effect of the Level of Therapist Experience on Case Record Ratings (Time 2/Time 1) of Anaclitic and Introjective Patients

| | Covariate means | | | | F values ($df = 1.85$) | | |
| | Anaclitic | | Introjective | | | | |
Case record variables	More experience (>6 yr)	Less experience (<6 yr)	More experience (>6 yr)	Less experience (<6 yr)	A/I	Experience	A×B
Menninger Scales							
Factor I (Interpersonal relatedness)	.04	.35	1.40	2.07	4.39*	.45	.06
Motivation for treatment	−.02	.25	.46	.66	3.65†	1.04	.02
Sublimatory effectiveness	−.26	.05	.09	.58	4.05*	3.21†	.18
Superego integration	.33	.11	.47	.33	.70	.75	.04
Object relations	.06	−.04	.39	.47	4.92*	.11	.01
Factor II (Impulsivity)	.02	.34	−.07	−.19	2.22	.25	1.20
Fairweather							
Interpersonal communication	1.31	1.33	1.25	1.26	1.60	.09	0
Strauss–Harder symptoms							
Neurotic	.04	.04	−.24	−.44	3.83*	.27	.24
Psychotic	2.38	2.80	2.10	2.45	.90	1.35	.01
Labile Affect	.14	.44	−.21	−.34	8.78**	.21	1.26
Flattened Affect	.39	.37	.22	.06	3.84*	.53	.33

†$p<.10$ *$p<.05$ **$p<.01$

TABLE 4.14

Two-Way Analysis of Covariance for the Effect of the Level of Therapist Experience on Psychological Test Variables (Time 2/Time 1) of Anaclitic and Introjective Patients

| | Covariate means | | | | F values (df = 1.85) | | |
| | Anaclitic | | Introjective | | | | |
Test record variables	More experience (>6 yr)	Less experience (<6 yr)	More experience (>6 yr)	Less experience (<6 yr)	A/I	Experience	A×B
Rorschach							
Concept of the Object							
Appropriate Object Relations (OR+)							
Mean developmental level	.94	-.41	.20	-.89	.49	1.95	.02
Developmental index	.22	-.32	.30	.18	.08	.10	.04
Inappropriate Object Relations (OR−)							
Mean developmental level	-2.19	-.56	.32	1.95	7.87**	3.45†	.00
Developmental index	-1.08	-.93	-.38	1.31	4.82*	1.91	1.34
Mutuality of Autonomy (MOA)							
Mean score	3.36	2.80	2.86	2.57	3.08†	3.98*	.41
Most malevolent score	4.76	4.17	4.20	3.94	1.31	1.56	.24
Most benevolent score	2.00	1.42	1.89	1.33	.27	8.97**	.00
Composite thought disorder	.30	-7.09	-1.59	-2.59	.10	1.08	.62
Traditional measures							
Adherence to reality (F+%)	66.16	72.11	70.28	72.77	.53	1.65	.28
Adaptive Fantasy (M+)	.31	.01	.38	.05	.02	.66	.00
Maladaptive Fantasy (M−)	.05	-.20	.02	-.09	.10	2.12	.35
Affective Lability (Sum Color)	-.11	.45	-.56	-.06	.88	1.11	.00
Number of responses (R)	34.56	40.71	39.43	37.77	.10	.53	1.59
Intelligence test							
Full Scale IQ	119.10	120.00	122.10	120.10	1.03	.14	.99
Verbal IQ	122.60	121.50	122.20	121.00	.07	.41	0
Performance IQ	111.30	113.50	117.42	114.95	5.63*	.01	2.10

†p<.10 *p<.05 **p<.01

variables. Patients with less-experienced therapists had significantly ($p<.05$) lower malevolent scores on the Mutuality of Autonomy (MOA) scale at Time 2, but they also tended ($p<.10$) to have greater investment in inaccurately perceived human representations (OR−). Given the large number of variables evaluated, however, the differences on these two variables are likely to be due to chance. Generally, the level of the therapist's experience seemed to have little influence on the degree to which patients changed over the treatment process as assessed for both clinical case records and Rorschach protocols.

Effects of Medication

Twelve patients received psychoactive medication during the first 6 weeks of hospitalization, and these 12 patients at admission had significantly ($p<.05$) poorer premorbid social adjustment as rated on both the Zigler–Phillips scale and the Goldstein scale. They also had significantly ($p<.05$) more clinical symptoms, especially neurotic symptoms and labile affect, lower Performance IQ, and a tendency ($p<.10$) toward poorer social adjustment as assessed on Factor I of the Menninger scales at admission to the hospital. Based on two-way analyses of covariance, there were no significant relationships, however, between the use of medication and changes from Time 1 to Time 2 in the level of social behavior or the severity of clinical symptoms as rated from the clinical case records (see Table 4.15). But as indicated in Table 4.16, patients who received medication had a significantly ($p<.05$) greater decrease in the amount of maladaptive fantasy on the Rorschach and a significantly ($p<.01$) greater increase in Verbal and Full Scale IQ from Time 1 to Time 2. Although only 2 of the 12 patients receiving psychoactive medication early in treatment were still receiving medication at Time 2, there were some indications that medication facilitated therapeutic change to some degree as assessed on psychological tests (decreased number of M− responses on the Rorschach and an increase in IQ).

Effects of Premorbid Social Adjustment

Premorbid social adjustment, as assessed by the mean score of the Goldstein and Zigler–Phillips measures of premorbid social adjustment, correlated significantly with a number of measures at the initial evaluation.[2] More disruptive premorbid social adjustment prior to hospitalization was associated with indications of greater disturbance in both the initial clinical case record and psychological tests obtained at admission

TABLE 4.15

Two-Way Analysis of Covariance for the Effect of Medication on Case Record Ratings
(Time 2/Time 1) of Anaclitic and Introjective Patients

| | Covariate means | | | | F values (df = 1.85) | | |
| | Anaclitic | | Introjective | | | | |
Case record variables	Medication	No medication	Medication	No medication	A/I	Medication	A×B
Menninger Scales							
Factor I (Interpersonal relatedness)	-1.28	.43	2.01	1.65	4.06*	.28	.76
Motivation for treatment	-.15	.18	.86	.50	3.82*	0	1.01
Sublimatory effectiveness	-.53	-.01	-.01	.35	1.84	1.82	.06
Superego integration	-.05	.24	.48	.40	1.22	.12	.35
Object relations	-.38	.03	.44	.42	4.00*	.42	.50
Factor II (Impulsivity)	.53	.15	-.48	-.07	4.33*	0	1.81
Fairweather							
Interpersonal communication	1.21	1.34	1.24	1.26	.14	1.20	.63
Strauss–Harder symptoms							
Neurotic	.21	.01	-.06	-.36	1.31	.73	.03
Psychotic	2.76	2.58	2.64	2.20	.25	.42	.07
Labile Affect	.38	.30	-.44	-.25	5.96**	.04	.25
Flattened Affect	.32	.39	.44	.10	.20	.50	1.23

*p<.05 **p<.01

TABLE 4.16

Two-Way Analysis of Covariance for the Effect of Medication on Psychological Test Variables
(Time 2/Time 1) of Anaclitic and Introjective Patients

| | Covariate means | | | | F values ($df = 1.85$) | | |
| | Anaclitic | | Introjective | | | | |
Test record variables	Medication	No medication	Medication	No medication	A/I	Medication	A×B
Rorschach							
Concept of the Object							
Appropriate Object Relations (OR+)							
Mean developmental level	.40	.12	2.41	-.66	.24	1.76	1.19
Developmental index	2.50	-.52	-.54	.36	.51	.48	1.67
Inappropriate Object Relations (OR-)							
Mean developmental level	-1.26	-1.26	1.62	.96	3.63†	.06	.06
Developmental index	-2.05	-.81	-.54	.47	2.02	1.35	.01
Mutuality of Autonomy (MOA)							
Mean score	3.32	3.00	2.64	2.75	2.19	.12	.46
Most malevolent score	5.14	4.30	4.26	4.07	1.23	1.08	.40
Most benevolent score	1.82	1.64	1.33	1.69	.59	.10	.90
Composite thought disorder	-8.64	-3.12	-4.72	-1.64	.21	.52	.04
Traditional measures							
Adherence to reality (F+%)	65.42	70.25	70.02	71.56	.38	.44	.12
Adaptive Fantasy (M+)	.07	.15	-.06	.28	0	.14	.05
Maladaptive Fantasy (M-)	-.42	-.03	-.28	.01	.27	3.81*	.08
Affective Lability (Sum Color)	1.72	-.05	-.36	-.34	2.57	1.41	1.41
Number of responses (R)	47.42	36.52	37.22	38.92	.75	1.06	1.99
Intelligence test							
Full Scale IQ	125.70	118.70	124.80	120.50	.05	8.19**	.54
Verbal IQ	129.60	120.60	125.60	121.00	.61	9.22**	.96
Performance IQ	117.20	111.90	117.90	116.10	1.20	2.38	.64

†$p<.10$ *$p<.05$ **$p<.01$

to the hospital. Both the mean Goldstein score and the mean Zigler–Phillips score correlated significantly ($p<.05$) with several Menninger scales (Motivation for Treatment, Superego Integration, and Object Relations), the Fairweather Scale of Interpersonal Communication, and the Neurotic symptom scale from the Strauss–Harder. In addition, the better the premorbid adjustment as measured on the Goldstein scale, the greater ($p<.05$) the number of accurately perceived, well-differentiated, articulated, and integrated human figures (OR+) on the Rorschach at Time 1. Also, there was a trend ($p<.10$) for good premorbid social adjustment, as assessed on both the Goldstein and the Zigler–Phillips scales, to correlate with responses to the Rorschach that conveyed more benevolent and reciprocal interactions at Time 1 as rated on the MOA scale.

Despite the fact that the two measures of premorbid social adjustment were significantly related to a number of important dimensions of clinical functioning at Time 1, premorbid adjustment was essentially unrelated to any measures of change in the treatment process. Using a two-way analysis of covariance, we examined the effects of premorbid adjustment for anaclitic and introjective patients on ratings of the clinical case records and on psychological test variables at Time 2, controlling for the initial level of these variables at Time 1. As indicated in Tables 4.17 and 4.18, the level of premorbid social adjustment as assessed by the mean score on the Goldstein scale had no significant relationship to change in social behavior or clinical symptoms, nor to change on any of the major psychological test variables. As indicated in Tables 4.19 and 4.20, however, premorbid social adjustment as assessed by the mean Zigler–Phillips score was significantly related ($p<.05$) only to change in maladaptive fantasy on the Rorschach (M−). Poor premorbid patients had a significantly greater decrease in maladaptive fantasy at Time 2 than did good premorbid patients. This finding, however, is likely due to chance variation because it was the only significant finding that emerged from among the large number of comparisons that were made with the two measures of premorbid adjustment.

Effects of Initial Severity of Psychopathology

Two experienced clinicians reviewed the 90 clinical case records prepared at admission for patients in this study, and they classified the patients as either psychotic, severe character pathology (i.e., borderline or narcissistic) or neurotic character pathology (i.e., depressed). The judges agreed on 78% of the cases and resolved their differences on the remaining cases through consultation. In this sample, 20% ($n = 29$) of

TABLE 4.17

Two-Way Analysis of Covariance for the Effect of Premorbid Level (Mean Goldstein) on Case Record Ratings (Time 2/Time 1) of Anaclitic and Introjective Patients

Case record variables	Covariate means				F values ($df = 1.85$)		
	Anaclitic		Introjective				
	Good premorbid	Poor premorbid	Good premorbid	Poor premorbid	A/I	Premorbid	A×B
Menninger Scales							
Factor I (Interpersonal relatedness)	.67	-.33	1.29	2.01	4.12*	.03	1.36
Motivation for treatment	.28	-.04	.40	.66	3.16†	.01	1.57
Sublimatory effectiveness	.02	-.21	.22	.38	3.08†	.02	.71
Superego integration	.16	.24	.26	.54	.88	.74	.22
Object relations	.18	-.28	.28	.53	5.04*	.24	3.01†
Factor II (Impulsivity)	.26	.13	-.19	-.06	2.50	0	.43
Fairweather							
Interpersonal communication	1.29	1.35	1.29	1.22	1.72	0	1.69
Strauss–Harder symptoms							
Neurotic	-.13	.25	-.27	-.37	3.90*	.47	1.51
Psychotic	2.51	2.72	2.67	1.94	.87	.66	2.09
Labile Affect	.23	.40	-.38	-.18	9.87**	.90	.01
Flattened Affect	.27	.51	.08	.20	4.17*	2.17	.26

†$p<.10$ *$p<.05$ **$p<.01$

TABLE 4.18

Two-Way Analysis of Covariance for the Effect of Premorbid Level (Mean Goldstein) on Psychological Test Variables (Time 2/Time 1) of Anaclitic and Introjective Patients

	Covariate means				F values (df = 1.85)		
	Anaclitic		Introjective				
Test record variables	Good premorbid	Poor premorbid	Good premorbid	Poor premorbid	A/I	Premorbid	A×B
Rorschach							
Concept of the Object							
Appropriate Object Relations (OR+)							
Mean developmental level	.16	.55	.61	−.96	.19	.25	1.68
Developmental index	.65	−.98	.14	.33	.15	.47	.76
Inappropriate Object Relations (OR−)							
Mean developmental level	−1.70	−.70	2.26	.06	7.05*	.47	3.32†
Developmental index	−1.20	−.71	.70	.08	3.97*	.01	.69
Mutuality of Autonomy (MOA)							
Mean score	3.09	2.99	2.74	2.73	2.03	.06	.03
Most malevolent score	4.47	4.36	4.30	3.93	.78	.47	.15
Most benevolent score	1.82	1.48	1.57	1.70	.00	.29	1.50
Composite thought disorder	−5.08	2.52	−4.65	.04	.14	.80	.07
Traditional measures							
Adherence to reality (F+%)	68.88	70.39	71.12	71.53	.27	.08	.03
Adaptive Fantasy (M+)	.30	−.07	.13	.33	.08	.05	.54
Maladaptive Fantasy (M−)	−.16	−.01	−.12	.04	.14	1.72	.00
Affective Lability (Sum Color)	.49	−.13	−.51	−.22	1.14	.10	.78
Number of responses (R)	36.27	40.30	40.13	37.57	.03	.06	1.10
Intelligence test							
Full Scale IQ	119.79	119.46	121.54	120.88	1.14	.12	.01
Verbal IQ	121.72	122.26	122.28	121.19	.02	.03	.24
Performance IQ	113.46	111.51	116.35	116.37	5.83**	.36	.38

†$p<.10$ *$p<.05$ **$p<.01$

TABLE 4.19

Two-Way Analysis of Covariance for the Effect of Premorbid Level (Mean Zigler–Phillips) on Case Record Ratings (Time 2/Time 1) of Anaclitic and Introjective Patients

| | Covariate means | | | | F values ($df = 1.85$) | | |
| | Anaclitic | | Introjective | | | | |
Case record variables	Good premorbid	Poor premorbid	Good premorbid	Poor premorbid	A/I	Premorbid	A×B
Menninger Scales							
Factor I (Interpersonal re-latedness)	.15	.26	1.74	1.65	4.07*	.00	.02
Motivation for treatment	–.00	.23	.48	.60	3.38†	.55	.05
Sublimatory effectiveness	.03	–.17	.36	.26	2.81†	.43	.05
Superego integration	.34	.10	.52	.32	.86	1.09	0
Object relations	–.18	.08	.52	.34	5.46*	.05	1.10
Factor II (Impulsivity)	.13	.25	.14	–.34	2.04	.83	2.15
Fairweather							
Interpersonal communication	1.39	1.27	1.26	1.25	2.32	1.44	1.09
Strauss–Harder symptoms							
Neurotic	.15	–.03	–.39	–.27	4.02*	.03	.63
Psychotic	2.73	2.50	1.74	2.72	1.41	1.36	3.47†
Labile Affect	.53	.16	–.35	–.20	10.58***	.32	1.83
Flattened Affect	.34	.40	.16	.13	3.22†	.02	.12

†$p<.10$ *$p<.05$ ***$p<.001$

TABLE 4.20

Two-Way Analysis of Covariance for the Effect of Premorbid Level (Mean Zigler–Phillips) on Psychological Test Variables (Time 2/Time 1) of Anaclitic and Introjective Patients

| | Covariate means | | | | F values (df = 1.85) | | |
| | Anaclitic | | Introjective | | | | |
Test record variables	Good premorbid	Poor premorbid	Good premorbid	Poor premorbid	A/I	Premorbid	A×B
Rorschach							
Concept of the Object							
Appropriate Object Relations (OR+)							
Mean developmental level	.50	−.06	−1.24	.54	.43	.48	1.82
Developmental index	.38	−.41	.43	.10	.07	.27	.05
Inappropriate Object Relations (OR−)							
Mean developmental level	−1.32	−1.23	.67	1.35	6.27**	.19	.11
Developmental index	−.95	−1.01	.57	.18	3.91*	.11	.06
Mutuality of Autonomy (MOA)							
Mean score	3.18	2.95	2.80	2.67	2.32	.71	.06
Most malevolent score	4.70	4.23	4.21	3.99	1.14	1.02	.12
Most benevolent score	1.47	1.79	1.73	1.58	.01	.19	1.44
Composite thought disorder	−3.58	−4.14	2.28	−5.66	.29	1.10	.83
Traditional measures							
Adherence to reality (F+%)	70.14	69.17	75.27	68.07	.38	1.55	.90
Adaptive Fantasy (M+)	.21	.08	.10	.36	.04	.03	.23
Maladaptive Fantasy (M−)	.09	−.21	.06	−.11	.09	3.77*	.30
Affective Lability (Sum Color)	−.27	.53	.02	−.65	.78	.02	2.13
Number of responses (R)	37.89	38.22	34.22	42.48	.01	1.97	1.66
Intelligence test							
Full scale IQ	118.26	120.50	120.51	121.76	1.39	1.35	.12
Verbal IQ	120.78	122.63	120.23	122.88	.01	1.68	.06
Performance IQ	111.54	115.33	116.19	116.49	5.80**	.42	.22

*p<.05   **p<.01

the patients were considered psychotic, 70% (n = 50) as having severe character pathology, and 10% (n = 11) as neurotic. Level of severity of psychopathology was significantly ($p<.05$) related to a number of clinical dimensions at the initial assessment. Psychotic patients had significantly more disturbed premorbid histories than the patients with neurotic character pathology and tended ($p<.10$) to be somewhat older. There was also a tendency for there to be more males in the psychotic group and more females in the severe character disorder group. No significant differences were found among the three diagnostic groups, however, in the level of experience of their therapists or in patients that received psychoactive medication.

Patients in the psychotic group had significantly ($p<.0001$) lower ratings at admission on each of the four Menninger scales (Motivation for Treatment, Sublimatory Capacity, Superego Integration and Object Relations) that make up the first Menninger factor (Interpersonal Relations). The three diagnostic groups did not differ significantly, however, on the second Menninger factor, Impulsivity. The three diagnostic groups also differed significantly ($p<.005$) on the Fairweather Scale of Interpersonal Communication, with significantly greater interpersonal disruption noted primarily in the psychotic group. In terms of clinical symptoms, the three groups differed significantly ($p<.01$) on the Neurotic, Psychotic, and Flattened Affect scales of the Strauss–Harder, with the psychotic group displaying more frequent and/or severe symptoms on all three scales. No significant differences were found, however, between the three groups on the Labile Affect scale.

In terms of variables derived from psychological tests, the psychotic group had significantly ($p<.001$) more impaired reality testing (lower F+%) and greater thought disorder on the Rorschach than the other two groups. The psychotic group also tended ($p<.07$) to attribute more malevolent interactions on the Rorschach as assessed by the MOA scale.

Most of these differences noted among the three diagnostic groups at the initial evaluation diminished substantially at the second evaluation. At the second evaluation, the psychotic group continued to show somewhat greater impairment on the Rorschach, including lower reality testing (F+%) ($p<.03$) and somewhat greater ($p<.09$) thought disorder, but there were no significant differences among the three groups on any of the behavioral assessments on the Menninger or Strauss–Harder scales. The only difference among the three groups in variables derived from the clinical case records that approached significance ($p<.06$) was the tendency for the psychotic group to have more impaired interpersonal communication as assessed on the Fairweather Scale of Interpersonal Communication than the group with neurotic character pathology.

TABLE 4.21

Two-Way Analysis of Covariance for the Effect of Severity of Pathology on Change in Case Record Ratings (Time 2/Time 1) of Anaclitic and Introjective Patients

| | Covariate means | | | | | | F values (df = 1.83) | | |
| | Anaclitic | | | Introjective | | | | | |
Case record variables	Psychosis (N = 13)	Character disorder (N = 24)	Neuros.s (N = 5)	Psychosis (N = 16)	Character disorder (N = 26)	Neurosis (N = 6)	A/I	Premorbid	A×B
Menninger Scales									
Factor I (Interpersonal relatedness)	1.01	-.26	.45	-.63	2.55	.79	1.13	.15	2.19
Motivation for treatment	.52	-.10	.26	.36	.66	.55	1.16	.20	1.65
Sublimatory effectiveness	.38	.01	.60	-.03	.76	.10	.04	.46	4.32+
Superego integration	-.22	-.05	.19	-.16	.61	.16	.08	1.52	1.00
Object relations	.02	-.03	-.13	.08	.61	.50	3.27	.47	.88
Factor II (Impulsivity)	-.07	.32	.34	.02	-.23	.02	1.15	.18	1.03
Fairweather									
Interpersonal communication	1.38	1.30	1.26	1.29	1.26	1.14	1.74	1.21	.16
Strauss–Harder symptoms									
Neurotic	-.11	.23	-.45	-.23	-.38	-.36	3.67+	.53	1.09
Psychotic	3.30	2.37	1.71	2.69	2.09	2.06	1.19	2.62	.41
Labile Affect	.52	.12	.65	-.13	-.26	-.72	9.49*	.80	1.41
Flattened Affect	.44	.38	.21	.36	.05	.01	3.55	1.16	.40

+$p < .10$ *$p < .05$

TABLE 4.22

Two-Way Analysis of Covariance for the Effect of Severity of Pathology on Change in Psychological Test Variables (Time 2/Time 1) of Anaclitic and Introjective Patients

| | Covariate means | | | | | | F values (df = 1,83) | | |
| | Anaclitic | | | Introjective | | | | | |
Test record variables	Psychosis (N = 13)	Character disorder (N = 24)	Neurosis (N = 5)	Psychosis (N = 16)	Character disorder (N = 26)	Neurosis (N = 6)	A/I	Pathology	A×B
Rorschach									
Concept of the Object									
Appropriate Object Relations (OR+)									
Mean developmental level	.22	.81	−3.05	−.53	−.50	1.32	.55	.29	2.20
Developmental index	.90	−.38	−1.28	.03	.27	.76	.22	.13	.39
Inappropriate Object Relations (OR−)									
Mean developmental level	−1.39	−1.36	−.32	.33	1.29	1.74	3.75*	.34	.11
Developmental index	−.97	−.93	−1.19	−.28	.61	.88	3.06	.20	.24
Mutuality of Autonomy (MOA)									
Mean score	3.00	3.12	2.77	2.85	2.67	2.66	.81	.18	.26
Most malevolent score	4.63	4.37	4.13	4.30	4.02	3.85	.06	.41	.00
Most benevolent score	1.69	1.66	1.60	1.81	1.54	1.67	.01	.23	.16
Composite thought disorder	.14	−5.22	−8.14	−3.55	−2.56	4.35	.61	.13	.72
Traditional measures									
Adherence to reality (F+%)	64.70	71.04	75.17	67.44	72.50	76.89	.25	1.78	.02
Adaptive Fantasy (M+)	1.35	−.35	−.67	.13	.26	.43	.13	1.96	2.80
Maladaptive Fantasy (M−)	−.05	−.07	−.33	−.08	−.08	.35	2.17	.09	1.89
Affective Lability (Sum Color)	−1.05	.83	.44	−.43	−.63	1.14	.01	2.05	2.28
Number of responses (R)	36.11	38.47	41.31	38.43	39.30	36.83	.01	.12	.21
Intelligence test									
Full Scale IQ	121.37	118.94	119.40	123.94	120.22	116.95	.07	2.55†	.55
Verbal IQ	123.95	120.76	122.73	123.76	121.23	117.52	.65	1.50	.59
Performance IQ	112.19	112.96	112.39	118.46	115.67	113.11	2.76	.45	.73

†p<.10   *p<.05

Despite the differences among the three diagnostic groups at the initial assessment, severity of psychopathology at admission did not have any significant effect on the extent of therapeutic change as assessed by changes in the ratings of the clinical case records and on changes in the variables derived from the psychological test protocols. In addition, severity of psychopathology did not interact significantly with the anaclitic–introjective distinction in influencing therapeutic change (see Tables 4.21 and 4.22). It is noteworthy that both severity of psychopathology at admission and the quality of premorbid adjustment as assessed on both the Goldstein and Zigler–Phillips scales were related to level of clinical functioning at Time 1 but unrelated to the extent of therapeutic change. These findings suggest that given the right therapeutic environment, patients apparently can change, on their own terms, to a comparable degree no matter how troubled they are initially.

Differences between Anaclitic and Introjective Patients

Patients in both the anaclitic and introjective groups were, on average, 21 years of age at time of admission. Six patients in both the anaclitic and introjective groups were receiving antipsychotic medications at the time of the first evaluation—after the first 6 weeks of hospitalization. There were no significant differences between anaclitic and introjective patients in their educational level and socioeconomic and occupational status or the socioeconomic and occupational status of their fathers. Mothers of anaclitic patients, however, were more often employed in higher-level (professional) positions than the mothers of introjective patients (28% as compared with 14%). There were no significant differences between anaclitic and introjective patients in level of premorbid adjustment as assessed by the Zigler–Phillips and Goldstein scales of premorbid adjustment.

The therapists of both groups had, on average, 7 to 8 years of postdoctoral training and/or experience. Patients in both groups were tested a second time, on average, approximately 15 months after entering the hospital. At the time of the second testing, virtually none of the patients was receiving antipsychotic medication (none of the anaclitic and only 2 of the 48 introjective patients were still receiving medication, and these 2 patients were each receiving the therapeutic equivalent of approximately 120 to 150 mg of thorazine per day).

In terms of psychological test and case record variables at the initial assessment, anaclitic and introjective patients were significantly different on only a few dimensions. In the ratings of the case records, introjective patients had significantly ($p<.05$) higher scores on the Strauss–

Harder psychotic scale, but they also had high ratings ($p<.04$) on the Menninger Scale for Sublimatory Effectiveness and somewhat higher ($p<.10$) Verbal IQ. Introjective patients also tended ($p<.10$) to describe human responses on the Rorschach in greater detail than did the anaclitic patients and to have greater investment in elaborating inaccurately perceived human forms.

Comparison of the degree of therapeutic change in anaclitic and introjective patients at Time 2 by one-way analyses of covariance, controlling for initial level at Time 1, indicates introjective patients had significantly greater improvement than anaclitic patients ($p<.04$) on the Menninger Factor I. In terms of the four individual Menninger scales that contribute to Factor I, introjective patients had a tendency for greater improvement than anaclitic patients on the Motivation for Treatment ($p<.08$), Sublimatory Capacity ($p<.08$), and Object Relations ($p<.03$) scales. As indicated in Table 4.23, introjective patients also had significantly greater improvement than anaclitic patients on three of the four Strauss–Harder scales (Neurotic [$p<.06$], Labile Affect [$p<.003$], and Flattened Affect [$p<.06$]). As indicated in Table 4.24, introjective patients

TABLE 4.23

One-Way Analysis of Covariance (Time 2/Time 1) Comparing
Anaclitic and Introjective Patients on Case Record Variables

	Covariate means		F values ($df = 1.87$)
	Anaclitic	Introjective	
Menninger Scales			
Factor I (Interpersonal re-latedness)	.22	1.69	4.17**
Motivation for treatment	.13	.55	3.24†
Sublimatory capacity	−.09	.31	3.18†
Superego integration	.20	.41	.97
Object relations	−.03	.42	4.92*
Factor II (Impulsivity)	.20	−.12	2.58
Fairweather			
Interpersonal communication	1.32	1.25	1.77
Strauss–Harder symptoms			
Neurotic	.04	−.33	3.70†
Psychotic	2.61	2.26	1.16
Labile Affect	.31	−.27	9.45**
Flattened Affect	.38	9.15	3.59†

†$p<.10$ *$p<.05$ **$p<.01$

Table 4.24

One-Way Analysis of Covariance (Time 2/Time 1) Comparing
Anaclitic and Introjective Patients on Psychological Test Variables

Test record variables	Covariate means		F values ($df = 1.87$)
	Anaclitic	Introjective	
Rorschach			
Concept of the Object			
Appropriate Object Relations (OR+)			
Mean developmental level	−.09	.25	.11
Developmental index	.16	−.28	.26
Inappropriate Object Relations (OR−)			
Mean developmental level	−.98	.35	4.00*
Developmental index	−1.26	1.04	6.60**
Mutuality of Autonomy (MOA)			
Mean score	3.04	2.73	2.16
Most malevolent score	4.42	4.09	.96
Most benevolent score	1.67	1.65	.01
Composite thought disorder	−3.92	−2.02	.23
Traditional measures			
Adherence to reality (F+%)	69.56	71.37	.31
Adaptive Fantasy (M+)	.13	.24	.07
Maladaptive Fantasy (M−)	.09	.03	.28
Affective Lability (Sum Color)	.21	−.34	1.20
Number of responses (R)	38.06	38.72	.05
Intelligence test			
Full Scale IQ	119.65	121.18	1.10
Verbal IQ	121.96	121.68	.03
Performance IQ	112.63	116.36	5.57*

*$p<.05$ **$p<.01$

also had a significantly greater increase ($p<.02$) of Performance IQ than anaclitic patients. It is important to note, however, that anaclitic patients showed significantly more therapeutic gain than introjective patients on the measures of object representation on the Rorschach. Anaclitic patients had a significantly greater decrease in Rorschach responses indicating fantasies about inappropriate, possibly autistic, interpersonal relationships as measured on the Rorschach concept of the object scale (OR−) by both the developmental index ($p<.05$) and the mean developmental level ($p<.01$) of inaccurately perceived human figures. Anaclitic patients had significantly greater reduction at Time 2 in the number of inaccurately perceived human figures on the Rorschach, in the degree to which they described them, and in the degree to which they attributed differentiated and complex activity to these figures. Thus, although introjective patients generally seemed to have made significantly greater therapeutic gain than anaclitic patients at the second evaluation in terms of behavior reported in the clinical case reports and Performance IQ, there were some indications in the psychological test protocols that therapeutic improvement in anaclitic patients was more evident in the representation of interpersonal relationships. Anaclitic, as compared to introjective, patients had a significantly greater reduction in the representation of unrealistic, possibly autistic, types of interpersonal relationships. (This important finding concerning the nature of clinical change in anaclitic patients is discussed in greater detail in Chapters 6 and 9.)

Effects of Sex

Because of significant differences between the number of men and women in the anaclitic and introjective groups (approximately 67% of the anaclitic patients were female, and 67% of the introjective patients were male), it was important to consider if the differences between

TABLE 4.25

Two-Way Analysis of Covariance for the Effect of Sex on Case Record Ratings (Time 2/Time 1) of Anaclitic and Introjective Patients

| | Covariate means | | | | F values ($df = 1.85$) | | |
| | Anaclitic | | Introjective | | | | |
Case record variables	Male	Female	Male	Female	A/I	Sex	A×B
Menninger Scales							
Factor I	.33	.16	1.21	2.57	4.66*	.60	1.01
Motivation for treatment	.37	.02	.43	.77	2.78†	0	2.09
Sublimatory effectiveness	−.05	−.10	.19	.53	3.44†	.39	.71
Superego integration	−.00	.30	.29	.63	1.98	2.12	.01
Object relations	.00	−.04	.28	.68	5.47*	.67	1.02
Factor II (Impulsivity)	.20	.20	−.18	−.02	1.97	.14	.13
Fairweather							
Interpersonal communication	1.23	1.36	1.24	1.28	.51	2.50	.92
Strauss–Harder symptoms							
Neurotic	−.21	.17	−.30	−.38	2.49	.52	1.34
Psychotic	2.48	2.67	2.64	1.56	1.97	1.84	3.65†
Labile Affect	.28	.32	−.40	−.03	6.84**	1.07	.73
Flattened Affect	.36	.39	.19	.07	3.50†	.10	.33

†$p<.10$ *$p<.05$ **$p<.01$

TABLE 4.26

Two-Way Analysis of Covariance for the Effect of Sex on Psychological Test Variables (Time 2/Time 1) of Anaclitic and Introjective Patients

| | Covariate means | | | | F values (df = 1,85) | | |
| | Anaclitic | | Introjective | | | | |
Test record variables	Male	Female	Male	Female	A/I	Sex	A×B
Rorschach							
Concept of the Object							
Appropriate Object Relations (OR+)							
Mean developmental level	.04	−.15	.94	−1.01	0	.96	.65
Developmental index	.10	.19	.28	−1.30	.51	.66	.82
Inappropriate Object Relations (OR−)							
Mean developmental level	−1.81	−.57	.46	.16	4.54*	.46	1.20
Developmental index	−1.52	−1.13	1.96	−.65	4.60*	1.47	2.67†
Mutuality of Autonomy (MOA)							
Mean score	3.18	2.97	2.81	2.59	2.82†	.86	.00
Most malevolent score	4.50	4.38	4.37	3.58	1.74	1.66	.91
Most benevolent score	1.85	1.57	1.61	1.71	.07	.19	.82
Composite thought disorder	−4.06	−3.83	−.49	−4.82	.09	.23	.29
Traditional measures							
Adherence to reality (F+%)	69.88	69.40	73.07	68.27	.09	.57	.39
Adaptive Fantasy (M+)	.11	.12	.68	−.55	.03	2.47	2.21
Maladaptive Fantasy (M−)	−.20	−.03	−.07	.04	.69	1.17	.05
Affective Lability (Sum Color)	−.43	.52	−.14	−.70	.80	.13	2.03
Number of responses (R)	40.95	36.54	40.10	36.32	.03	1.57	.01
Intelligence test							
Full IQ	121.09	115.75	122.29	119.03	.24	3.22†	.09
Verbal IQ	124.05	120.64	123.26	118.65	.65	5.06*	.12
Performance IQ	112.83	112.51	116.82	115.40	4.15*	.26	.10

†p<.10 *p<.05

changes that occurred in treatment of anaclitic and introjective patients were due primarily to sex differences. Based on analyses of covariance, we examined the effects of sex for anaclitic and introjective patients on the ratings of the clinical case records and psychological test variables at Time 2, controlling for the initial level of these variables at Time 1.

As indicated in Tables 4.25 and 4.26, there were no significant ($p<.05$) sex by group interactions on any of the variables from the clinical case records or the psychological test protocols. One interaction term did approach statistical significance ($p<.10$): At Time 2, anaclitic males tended to have fewer psychotic symptoms than did anaclitic females (2.48 versus 2.67; n.s.), while at Time 2 introjective males had more psychotic symptoms than did introjective females (2.64 versus 1.56; $p<.02$). There was also one significant ($p<.05$) main effect for sex at Time 2, controlling for initial level. Men had a significantly higher Verbal IQ ($p<.05$) than did women at Time 2. These few significant differences between men and women, however, do not seem to account for the large number of significant differences that were observed between the anaclitic and introjective patients. The clinical distinction between anaclitic and introjective forms of psychopathology seems much more central to understanding differences in treatment effects than differences based on sex.

SUMMARY

Patients who had more clinical symptoms and poorer premorbid social adjustment at Time 1 were more likely to receive antipsychotic medication and to be assigned to more experienced therapists, especially if the patients had greater affect lability. Anaclitic and introjective patients, however, seemed quite similar at Time 1, and there were no significant differences between the two groups in the number of patients in each group receiving medication or in the experience level of their therapists.

The level of the therapist's experience and the severity of the patient's pathology seemed unrelated to therapeutic change. There was some suggestion that the use of medication facilitated therapeutic improvement to some degree, particularly as measured by a decrease of maladaptive fantasy on the Rorschach (M−) and an increase in Verbal and Full Scale IQ. These effects of medication, however, did not seem substantial, and the degree of therapeutic change observed in the patients seemed far beyond the change accounted for by the effects of antipsychotic medication that had been administered initially to 12 of the patients.

We also investigated the possibility that the differences in changes noted in anaclitic and introjective patients were due to the significant disproportion of men and women in these two groups of patients. There were no significant group by sex interactions, however, on any of the variables derived from the Rorschach and the clinical case records.

In summary, the significant constructive changes noted over the course of the long-term, intensive treatment of seriously disturbed inpatients seemed to be consistent and systematic, and relatively uninfluenced by a wide range of potentially confounding variables that were external to the treatment process. The data generally indicate that substantial and constructive treatment effects occurred in the total group of patients and that some of these constructive effects were unique to anaclitic and introjective patients.[3]

Notes

1. Standard deviations of all measures derived from clinical case records and psychological test protocols at Time 1 and Time 2 are presented in Appendix 10.

2. Mean scores were used for the Goldstein and Zigler–Phillips measures of premorbid adjustment rather than the more usual sum scores because on occasion the case records lacked the information necessary to rate one of the variables included in these two measures of premorbid adjustment. Thus, mean scores were derived for both measures of premorbid adjustment to reflect the average premorbid level for those variables of the scales for which there was adequate information to make these ratings.

3. Data analyses of the stories told to the Thematic Apperception Test were not included in this chapter and are presented separately because prior research indicated that there are significant sex differences between females and males in their use of the three types of defense in TAT stories, thus requiring more detailed statistical analyses of the interaction between sex, anaclitic–introjective patients, and types of defenses. Data analyses of the human figure drawings are also reserved for a later chapter because the number of patients who had been given this procedure was substantially less than the data available from the Rorschach and the ratings of the clinical case records.

CHAPTER 5

Therapeutic Change on the Thematic Apperception Test[1]

Change over the course of long-term intensive treatment was also assessed from stories told to the cards of the Thematic Apperception Test (TAT). Cramer (1987, 1991) developed a method for systematically scoring different types of defenses on the TAT—denial, projection, and identification. This chapter examines the hypothesis that constructive change over the course of long-term treatment will be expressed both in the overall diminution of total defenses apparent in the TAT stories and by a shift in the TAT narratives to higher-level, developmentally more mature defenses over the course of treatment—from denial, to projection, to identification.

Denial is scored in a TAT story when there is evidence of the following: statements of negation, denial of reality, reversal, misperception, omission of major characters or objects, over-maximization of the positive or minimization of the negative, and unexpected goodness, optimism, positiveness, and gentleness.

Projection is scored when the TAT story contains attributions of hostile feelings or intentions to a character, or attribution of any other feelings or intentions that are normatively unusual for that card; additions of ominous people, animals, objects, or qualities; concern for protection against external threat; themes of pursuit, entrapment, and escape; apprehensiveness of death, injury, or assault; magical or autistic thinking; and a bizarre story or themes.

Identification is scored when there are themes of emulation of skills, characteristics, qualities, or attitudes, and themes of a regulation of motives or behavior, self-esteem through affiliation, work and delay of gratification, role differentiation, and moralism. (A more detailed description of this system for scoring defenses from responses to the TAT is presented in Appendix 9.)

According to theoretical formulations, the anaclitic and introjective personality configurations are each expected to be characterized by different types of defense mechanisms (Blatt & Shichman, 1983). Anaclitic defenses are expected to be primarily avoidant maneuvers—denial, repression, and displacement. The aim of these avoidant defenses, at least in part, is to maintain interpersonal relationships by minimizing and avoiding disruptive and conflictual feelings and impulses. Introjective defenses, on the other hand, are expected to be primarily counteractive and include projection, externalization, reaction formation, and overcompensation. The aim of these counteractive defenses is to protect and preserve the sense of self.

A comparison of the anaclitic and introjective patients in our study, however, indicates that initially these two groups do not differ significantly in the types of defenses they expressed in TAT stories ($t(88)$: denial $= -.73$; projection $= -1.24$; and identification $= 1.60$). Part of the reason why specific defenses were not found to be characteristic of anaclitic and introjective patients may be that the anaclitic and introjective distinction (Blatt, 1974, 1990b; Blatt & Shichman, 1983) as well as the use of particular defenses are sex-linked (Cramer, 1979). The failure to account for these sex differences may obscure the identification of particular defenses as characteristic of patients with anaclitic and introjective pathology.

Within our sample of 90 patients, the majority of anaclitic patients were women (28 women versus 14 men), whereas the majority of the introjective patients were men (31 men versus 17 women). These sex differences are consistent with sex-role stereotypes. Women are typically described as being more concerned with interpersonal relations and oriented toward affiliation, whereas men are described as being more concerned with personal autonomy and achievement (e.g., Blatt & Blass, 1990; Blatt & Shichman, 1983; Chevron, Quinlan, & Blatt, 1978; Gilligan, 1982; Horner, 1972; Josselson, 1973; McClelland, 1961). Developmental demands (Blatt & Shichman, 1983; Chodorow, 1978; Gilligan, 1982), cultural stereotypes, and perhaps biological predispositions all appear to contribute to an increased proclivity for women to focus more on anaclitic issues, whereas men more often focus on the introjective issues. Defense mechanisms also have been found to be sex related. Denial has consistently been found to be more often used by women, whereas projection is more characteristic of men (Cramer, 1979; Cramer & Carter, 1978; Gleser & Ihilevich, 1969; Gleser & Sacks, 1973; Gur & Gur, 1975; Sholz, 1973).

Research evidence indicates that cross-sex role orientation (or sexual identity) is related to cross-sex use of defenses. Cramer and Carter (1978) found a strong relationship between the use of sex-congruent defenses and sexual identity, whereas the use of sex-incongruent defenses was related to lower masculine identity in college men and lower feminine identity in college women. Also, Gleser and Ihilevich (1969) found that for men the use of male defenses correlated significantly with a masculine score on the Minnesota Multiphasic Personality Inventory (MMPI) Masculine–Feminine (MF) scale, whereas the use of female defenses in men correlated with a feminine MF score (see also LoPiccolo & Blatt, 1972). Likewise, Evans (1982), studying women only, found the use of male defenses to be related to high masculine scores on Bem's (1974) measure of sex-role orientation, whereas the use of female defenses was related to low masculine scores. Finally, Frank, McLaughlin, and Crusco (1984) found a positive relationship between a masculine sex-role orientation score on the Personality Research Form Androgyny Scale (Berzins, Welling, & Wetter, 1987) and the use of male defenses for men, whereas women showed a negative relationship between the use of male defenses and feminine sex-role orientation scores. Also, among women only, the use of male defenses was related to psychological distress, as was a feminine sex-role orientation in men.

These studies indicate that defense use is a function of sex and sexual orientation. Thus, it seems likely that sex would interact with a sex-linked personality configuration in determining defense use. In predicting that anaclitic patients will use more avoidant defenses such as denial, it may be important to account for the fact that denial is more typically a female defense. Anaclitic men may not use denial as fully as do anaclitic women or as do women more generally. Likewise, in predicting that introjective patients will be higher on counteractive defenses such as projection, it may be important to note that projection is predominantly a male defense. Thus, introjective women may not use projection as fully as do introjective men or as do men more generally. It is possible, then, that the lack of significant differences in defense use between patients characterized as anaclitic or introjective may be due to a confounding of defense use with sex. Moreover, one might expect different patterns of change in defense use following intensive treatment between those patients whose predominant developmental preoccupations are congruent with their sex and those patients whose predominant preoccupations are sex incongruent. One might also expect different patterns of correlations between TAT defenses and other measures of psychopathology and psychological functioning in males and females, and in those patients who use gender-congruent or incongruent defenses.

If, in fact, there is a congruence among the anaclitic/introjective configuration, defense use, and sex, it becomes important in evaluating therapeutic change to compare sex-congruent and sex-incongruent individuals. It is important to determine if defense use in sex-congruent patients (female anaclitic and male introjectives) and in sex-incongruent patients (male anaclitic and female introjective patients) is determined more by sex, by the anaclitic/introjective personality distinction, or by some interaction of the two. In addition to identifying the defense preferences of sex-incongruent patients, it is equally important to determine whether their defenses work as effectively or if they experience more conflict and thus manifest greater defensiveness than their sex-consistent counterparts (female anaclitics and male introjectives). Smith, O'Keeffe, and Jenkins (1988), for example, found that individuals with sex-incongruent personality characteristics (especially dependent men but also self-critical women) were more likely to experience depression in response to negative life experiences than were sex-congruent individuals (self-critical men and dependent women).

The TAT, administered at Time 1 and again at Time 2 as part of the psychodiagnostic test battery, provided the basis for the assessment of defense mechanisms. These test data were scored by a judge who had established acceptable levels of reliability in scoring these defenses on the TAT in prior studies. In this study, the judge scoring the TAT protocols had no knowledge of the case record, including the patient's sex and anaclitic/introjective designation. In addition, the judge had no way of identifying whether a TAT protocol was from Time 1 or Time 2.

The use of the defenses of denial, projection, and identification was assessed from the patient's responses to three TAT cards (1, 14, and 13 MF), according to a method developed by Cramer (1987, 1991). Each TAT story was scored for the occurrence of the three defenses. For each defense, there are seven categories that may be scored, each representing a different component of the defense. The categories for each defense are defined and explicit criteria (with numerous examples) are provided in Appendix 10. The frequency of use of each component of a defense in each TAT story determines the three defense scores for that story. The three scores are then summed across the three stories to determine an overall score for each defense. Adequate interrater reliability had been established for scoring each defense in the present sample (Item Alpha >.65) as well as with numerous other samples (Cramer, 1987, 1991; Cramer et al., 1988). For each patient, then, scores on the use of denial, projection, and identification, as well as total defense use (the sum of the three individual defenses), were available for Time 1 and again for Time 2.

CHANGE IN DEFENSES: DENIAL, PROJECTION, AND IDENTIFICATION

Table 5.1 presents two-way analyses of variance for a repeated measures design, assessing the change from Time 1 to Time 2 in total use of defenses and in the use of each of the three specific types of defense for anaclitic and introjective patients. As indicated in Table 5.1, there was a significant ($p<.05$) reduction of total defenses from Time 1 to Time 2. Although the interaction term was not significant, matched t tests (see Table 5.2) indicate that the significant reduction in total defenses used in TAT stories was primarily a function of a statistically significant ($p<.05$) reduction for introjective patients. The scores for anaclitic patients also diminished from Time 1 to Time 2, but this change did not reach statistical significance. As indicated in Table 5.2, the effect size was moderate for the significant reduction in the use of total defenses for the entire sample (effect size $= .30$), but especially for introjective patients (effect size $= .44$). Although the usage of each of the three types of defenses (denial, projection, and denial) diminished from Time 1 to Time 2 for both anaclitic and introjective patients, these differences were not significant.

TABLE 5.1
Analysis of Variance of TAT Ratings of Defense for Anaclitic
and Introjective Patients at Time 1 and Time 2

	Means				ANOVA ($df = 1.88$) F values (repeated measures)		
	Anaclitic		Introjective				
	T1	T2	T1	T2	A/I	T1/T2	A × B
Thematic Apperception Test defenses							
Total	6.28	5.59	6.60	5.21	.24	4.22*	.35
Denial	1.76	1.62	2.10	1.58	.29	1.46	.44
Projection	2.10	2.07	2.65	1.90	.29	2.42	1.88
Identification	2.43	1.90	1.85	1.73	1.82	2.54	1.04

*$p<.05$

TABLE 5.2

Matched *t* Tests and Effect Size for Comparison of Change in TAT Defenses
from Time 1 to Time 2 for Anaclitic and Introjective Patients

	Matched *t* tests			Effect size		
	Total sample ($n = 90$)	Anaclitic ($n = 42$)	Introjective ($n = 48$)	Total sample ($n = 90$)	Anaclitic ($n = 42$)	Introjective ($n = 48$)
Thematic Apperception Test defenses						
Total	2.25*	0.93	2.33*	.30	.15	.44
Denial	1.21	0.30	1.54	.18	.07	.29
Projection	1.51	0.07	1.92†	.20	.01	.39
Identification	1.59	1.50	0.62	.19	.28	.09

†$p < .10$ *$p < .05$

INTERACTIONS OF SEX WITH CHANGE IN DEFENSES

Examination of the effects of potentially confounding variables effecting the change in defense usage in TAT stories indicates, as expected, that there is a significant interaction between sex and types of defense use in anaclitic and introjective patients. To evaluate this interaction systematically, an analysis of variance (ANOVA) was performed to assess the use of defenses in anaclitic and introjective males and females at Time 1 and Time 2. At Time 1, the analysis yielded a significant anaclitic/introjective by sex interaction ($F(1, 86) = 8.73; p<.004$), indicating the importance of gender in determining defense use in anaclitic and introjective patients. Comparison of means, as presented in Table 5.3, indicates that at Time 1 anaclitic men had significantly higher total defense scores than both anaclitic women [$t(40) = 3.27; p<.002$] and introjective men [$t(43) = 1.93; p<.06$]. Furthermore, introjective women had significantly higher total defense scores than anaclitic women [$t(43) = 2.41; p<.02$]. Thus, as indicated in Table 5.3, at admission, gender-incongruent patients (anaclitic males and introjective females) had significantly higher total defense scores than gender-congruent patients.

TABLE 5.3
TAT Defense Scores at Time 1 and Time 2 for Male and Female
Anaclitic and Introjective Patients

Group	Denial		Projection		Identification		Total	
	M	SD	M	SD	M	SD	M	SD
Anaclitic men (n = 14)								
T1	2.64	3.88	3.14	2.41	3.21	2.61	9.00	5.79
T2	1.93	1.59	3.50	3.06	1.79	1.58	7.21	4.41
Introjective men (n = 31)								
T1	2.16	1.86	2.48	2.03	1.71	1.32	6.35	3.38
T2	1.16	1.39	1.87	1.33	1.84	1.66	4.87	2.32
Anaclitic women (n = 28)								
T1	1.32	1.22	1.57	1.50	2.04	1.55	4.93	2.31
T2	1.46	1.29	1.36	1.70	1.96	1.82	4.79	3.01
Introjective women (n = 17)								
T1	2.00	1.94	2.94	2.58	2.12	1.05	7.06	3.63
T2	2.35	2.15	1.94	2.11	1.53	0.87	5.82	3.64

Moreover, although the three-way interaction was not significant, planned comparisons indicated that the anaclitic men scored significantly higher on identification than introjective men [$t(43) = 2.58; p<.01$] and somewhat higher than anaclitic women [$t(40) = 1.84; p<.07$]. Also, anaclitic men scored somewhat higher on denial than did anaclitic women [$t(40) = 1.66; p<.10$]. Further, introjective women, introjective men, and anaclitic men all had higher projection scores than did anaclitic women [$t(43, 57,$ and $40) = 2.26, 1.94,$ and $2.60; p<.03, .06,$ and $.01$, respectively].

A similar ANOVA for the defense scores at Time 2 indicates a significant anaclitic/introjective by sex interaction [$F(1, 86) = 5.69; p<.02$]. Again, anaclitic men had higher total defense scores than anaclitic women [$t(40) = 2.10; p<.04$]. In addition, the anaclitic/introjective by sex by defense interaction was significant [$F(2, 172) = 3.84; p<.02$]. At Time 2, anaclitic men used significantly more of the male-type defense of projection than did anaclitic women [$t(40) = 2.93; p<.006$] or introjective men [$t(43) = 2.51; p<.02$]. Also at Time 2, introjective women used more of the female-type defense, denial, than did introjective men [$t(46) = 2.33; p<.02$] and somewhat more than did anaclitic women [$t(43) = 1.74; p<.09$].

Thus, the data indicate that there are significant differences in defense use between anaclitic and introjective patients, but primarily as a function of sex. Patients with gender-incongruent personality organization (introjective women and anaclitic men) had significantly higher total defense scores than did gender-congruent patients (anaclitic women and introjective men). This greater use of defenses in TAT stories suggests that gender-incongruent patients experience more conflict than gender-congruent patients. The importance of the issue of identity in gender-incongruent patients is indicated by the significant decrease in their use of identification in TAT stories from Time 1 to Time 2, suggesting that their greater level of conflict may be related to the unsatisfactory nature of their identification as it was experienced at the onset of the treatment.

The following story, told to TAT Card 1 at admission by an anaclitic male patient, illustrates this conflict around identification quite well.

> This little boy here—had an interest in music. He felt it in himself. He's been encouraged by his family to play the violin. He's still not sure if it's the thing for him to go into. Not sure whether the impetus, whether the idea of playing it was his or if it was imposed on him. A conflict whether to rebel or if it's his own desires. The violin is the symbol of who he is—an identity crisis over this thing. Through this conflict emerges a realization of who he is— emerges free of what they impose on him. He may go on to other things, but the violin is certainly an instrumental part of his development.

The findings also indicate that gender-incongruent patients use defenses at admission that are consistent with their opposite sex. Thus, anaclitic men showed a tendency to use more denial (a feminine defense) than did anaclitic women, and, likewise, introjective women used more projection (a masculine defense) than did anaclitic women. This finding regarding anaclitic men is consistent with Miller and Swanson (1960), who found that men with a feminine identity (both conscious and unconscious) scored higher on a measure of denial than other men. In terms of the impact of therapy on these gender-incongruent patients, it is important to note that at Time 2, after an average of 15 months of treatment, gender-incongruent patients used more gender-consistent defenses. At the second testing, anaclitic men used more projection than did anaclitic women or introjective men, and introjective women used more denial than did anaclitic women and introjective and anaclitic men. Thus, after 15 months of treatment, gender-incongruent patients shifted from gender-incongruent to gender-congruent defenses, consistent with the interpretation that the decrease from Time 1 to Time 2 in the use of the defense of identification in gender-incongruent patients reflects at least a partial discarding of a conflicted gender-incongruent identity. These findings indicate the importance of examining more systematically the interaction between sex and type of psychopathology in evaluating changes in the use of defenses over the course of long-term treatment.

To assess systematically changes in the use of defense mechanisms following 15 months of intensive psychotherapy, the defense scores were analyzed using a four-way ANOVA—a 2 (anaclitic/introjective) × 2 (gender) × 2 (time) × 3 (defense) design, with the last two variables as repeated measures.

As indicated in Table 5.3, total defense use decreased significantly from Time 1 to Time 2 [$F(1, 86) = 5.19$; $p<.02$]. Matched t tests comparing total defense use at Time 1 and Time 2 indicate that anaclitic patients had an insignificant decline in total defense use from Time 1 to Time 2 [$x = 6.28, 5.59$; $t = .93$, n.s.], but this change was statistically significant for introjective patients [$x = 6.60, 5.21$; $t = 2.33$; $p<.05$]. There was also a significant main effect for sex [$F(1, 86) - 4.62$; $p<.03$], which is best understood in terms of a highly significant anaclitic/introjective by sex interaction [$F(1, 86) = 13.09$; $p<.0005$]. Gender-incongruent patients, anaclitic men and introjective women, had higher total defense scores at both Time 1 and Time 2.

The time × defense × sex interaction approached significance [$F(2, 172) = 2.58$; $p<.08$], indicating that male patients showed a significant decrease in denial from Time 1 to Time 2 [$t(44) = 2.14$; $p<.04$]. Although the four-way interaction was not significant [$F(2, 172) = 2.03$; $p<.14$], planned comparisons for the gender-incongruent groups (anaclitic men and introjective women) indicated a significant decrease in identification scores from Time 1 to Time 2 [$t(13, 16) = 2.22$ and 2.42; $p<.05$, respectively].

In summary, overall analysis indicates significant decreases in defense use after 15 months of intensive treatment. Moreover, gender-incongruent males and females showed significant decreases in the use of identification, and male patients showed a significant decrease in the female-type defense of denial ($t(44) = 2.14$, $p<.04$). With treatment, gender-incongruent patients (anaclitic males and introjective females) have a substantial increase in their use of gender-congruent defenses. The four-way interaction also indicates that the significant decrease in the use of denial in male patients is primarily the consequence of the decrease, especially in male introjective patients ($t(30) = 3.70$, $p<.001$).

RELATION OF CHANGE IN DEFENSE SCORES TO OTHER MEASURES OF CHANGE

Changes in defense scores from Time 1 to Time 2, as rated on the TAT, were correlated with changes as rated from the clinical case records in terms of the Strauss–Harder scales of clinical symptoms (Psychotic, Neurotic, and Labile Affect) and in terms of interpersonal behavior (Menninger Factor I and the Fairweather Scale of Interpersonal Communication).

Changes in total defense use were positively correlated with changes on the Labile Affect scale for three of the four patient groups: anaclitic women ($r = .56$; $p<.001$), anaclitic men ($r = .55$; $p<.02$), and introjective men ($r = .36$; $p<.02$). This correlation was not significant for introjective women.

The correlations between the change scores (Time 2 minus Time 1) of the individual defenses (denial, projection, and identification) and the change scores for the Strauss–Harder Labile Affect scale are presented in Table 5.4. For anaclitic women, changes in denial were positively correlated with changes in labile affect ($r = .47$; $p<.006$). For introjective men, a decrease in projection was associated with a decrease in labile affect ($r = .32$; $p<.04$). Also, for anaclitic and introjective women, changes in identification were positively related to changes in labile affect scores ($r = .42$; $p<.01$ and .05, respectively).

The correlations between changes in individual defense scores (denial, projection, and identification) and changes on the ratings of interpersonal behavior from the clinical case records (Time 2 minus Time 1)

Table 5.4

Correlations of Changes in TAT Defense Scores with Changes in Labile Affect, Interpersonal Behavior, and Rorschach Measures

Defenses by group	Labile Affect	Fairweather Scale	Menninger Factor I	OR−	OR+	Mean MOA
Anaclitic men (n = 14)						
Denial	.43	−.10	−.46*	.53*	.03	.64**
Projection	.27	.41	.04	.15	.44	−.43
Identification	.22	.54*	.23	.21	.60**	−.29
Introjective men (n = 31)						
Denial	.23	−.16	−.01	.11	−.35*	.08
Projection	.32*	.47**	−.03	.34*	−.25	.33*
Identification	.18	−.06	.31*	−.01	.16	−.03
Anaclitic women (n = 28)						
Denial	.47**	.06	.03	−.30	−.49**	.51**
Projection	.26	−.13	−.20	−.05	.10	.18
Identification	.42**	−.33*	−.06	−.31	−.08	.19
Introjective women (n − 17)						
Denial	.33	.13	.10	−.04	−.26	−.14
Projection	−.23	−.16	.30	−.08	.21	−.29
Identification	.42*	.16	−.31	.24	.18	.23

*p<.05   **p<.01

are also presented in Table 5.4 for both gender-congruent and gender-incongruent patients. An increase in identification was associated with improvement in interpersonal relationships in these two groups of patients. For anaclitic women, an increase in identification was correlated with an improvement in the Fairweather Scale ($r = -.33$; $p<.04$). For introjective men, change in identification was significantly correlated with improvement on Menninger Factor I ($r = .31$; $p<.05$). Also, for male patients, decrease in the use of projection was related to increased capacity for interpersonal relations, as seen in the correlation with lower Fairweather scores (better interpersonal functioning) [introjective men ($r = .47$; $p<.004$) and anaclitic men ($r = .41$; $p<.07$)].

On the other hand, for gender-incongruent patients, a decrease in identification was associated with improvement in interpersonal relationships. For anaclitic men, a decrease in identification was correlated with a decrease in the Fairweather Scale (better interpersonal functioning; $r = .54$; $p<.02$). For introjective women, there was a tendency for a decrease in identification to be correlated with an increase in Menninger

Factor I ($r = -.31$; $p<.11$). Finally, for anaclitic men, a decrease in denial was associated with an increase on Menninger Factor I (better interpersonal functioning; $r = -.46$; $p<.05$).

Changes in defense scores on the TAT were also correlated with changes on Rorschach measures. We explored particularly the relationships of TAT defense scores with measure of object relations on the Rorschach as assessed by the Concept of the Object Scale (OR+ and OR−) (Blatt et al., 1976b) and the Mutuality of Autonomy Scale (MOA) (Urist, 1977). A decrease in the use of denial was associated with a significant increase in OR+ scores for gender-congruent patients (anaclitic women, $r = -.49$; $p<.004$; introjective men, $r = -.35$; $p<.03$). For anaclitic men, a decrease in denial was associated with a decreased investment in inappropriate, possibly autistic representations of interpersonal interactions (OR−) ($r = .53$; $p<.03$). For both anaclitic males and females, a decrease in denial was associated with less malevolence in mean MOA scores (anaclitic men, $r = .64$; $p<.007$; anaclitic women, $r = .51$; $p<.003$).

Also, for both anaclitic females and males, a decrease in the use of identification was associated with changes in the object-relations measures. For anaclitic women, a decrease in the use of identification was associated with an increase in OR− scores ($r = -.31$; $p<.06$), whereas for anaclitic men, it was associated with a decreased investment in representations of appropriate interpersonal interactions (OR+) ($r = .60$; $p<.01$).

Finally, for anaclitic men, an increase in the use of projection was associated with an increase on OR+ scores ($r = .44$; $p<.06$), whereas for introjective men, a decrease in the use of projection was associated with a decrease in OR− scores ($r = .34$; $p<.03$) and a decrease in the level of malevolent interactions as measured by the mean MOA ($r = .33$; $p<.04$).

SUMMARY

In summary, the results demonstrate the efficacy of the assessment of defenses on the TAT as a measure of therapeutic change. Following approximately 15 months of treatment, the total group of patients decreased significantly in their overall use of defense, and this decrease was significantly correlated, in three of four patient groups (anaclitic and introjective men and anaclitic women), with a decrease in the independent rating of labile affect from the clinical case records. Significant changes in level of defense use were also related to changes in clinical symptomatology, interpersonal relations, and investment in object relationships, but these relationships differed as a function of the interaction between sex, defense use, and anaclitic/introjective personality organization. For gender-incongruent (anaclitic) men, significant decrease in the use of identification was significantly associated with less investment in the representation of satisfying interpersonal relationships (OR+) but improved interpersonal behavior (Fairweather Scale). The significant increase among anaclitic men in the gender-congruent defense of projection was significantly associated with greater investment in Rorschach responses reflecting satisfying interpersonal relationships (OR+, MOA) but with poorer interpersonal behavior (Fairweather scale). Although the decrease from Time 1 to Time 2 in the anaclitic men's use of denial was not statistically significant, it was related significantly to a decreased investment in unsatisfying, possibly malignant interpersonal relationships on the fantasy level (OR−, MOA) and improved interpersonal functioning (Menninger Factor I).

For gender-congruent (introjective) men, the significant decrease in the use of denial from Time 1 to Time 2 was significantly associated with an increased investment in the representations of appropriate interpersonal relationships (OR+). Also, a decrease in the use of projection was related to decreases in clinical symptoms, better interpersonal communications (Fairweather Scale), and less investment in the representation of unsatisfying, malignant interpersonal relationships on the fantasy level (OR−, MOA). Also, an increase in the use of identification in this sex-congruent patient group was associated with improvement in interpersonal relationships (Menninger Factor I).

Among the gender-congruent (anaclitic) women, decreased use of denial was related to decreased labile affect and increased investment in the representation of satisfying interpersonal relations (OR+) that are benign and mutually facilitating (MOA). Again, as with males, in this gender-congruent group, increased use of identification was associated with improved interpersonal relationships (Fairweather Scale) and less investment in the representation of unsatisfying relationships (OR−), but also with an increase in clinical symptoms (labile affect).

Finally, among gender-incongruent (introjective) women, a significant decrease in the use of identification was related to a decrease in clinical symptoms and improved interpersonal relationships (Menninger Factor I). The significant increase in the use of denial, however, was not associated with changes in other variables.

These findings in males and females indicate that an increase in identification among gender-congruent patients and a decrease in identification among gender-incongruent patients were generally related to improved psychological functioning. Moreover, an increase in gender-congruent defenses among gender-incongruent patients was related to psychological improvement, whereas a decrease in gender-congruent defenses among gender-congruent patients was related to psychological improvement. Finally, for male patients, a decrease in the gender-incongruent defense of denial was related to improved functioning.

These findings indicate that investigations of defense mechanisms must consider whether the defenses are gender congruent or gender incongruent, which in this study produced opposite effects. Second, the measure of the defense of identification should be interpreted cautiously with more seriously disturbed patients. High scores on identification may be indicative of a primitive, pathological identification that interferes with normal development, rather than being an indication of psychological strength. But overall the TAT data demonstrate significant and substantial constructive change over the 15 months that the patients participated in the therapeutic program.

NOTES

1. Material for this chapter was drawn from articles (Cramer & Blatt, 1990; Cramer, Blatt & Ford, 1988) published in *The Journal of Personality Assessment* and *The Journal of Consulting and Clinical Psychology.*

CHAPTER 6

Therapeutic Change on Human Figure Drawings[1]

There is considerable disagreement about the value of Human Figure Drawings (HFDs) in both clinical practice and clinical research. Adler (1970, p. 52) concluded that

> of all available psychological testing instruments, HFDs . . . are second only to the Rorschach in frequency of use in hospitals and clinics in the U.S. [Sundberg, 1961]. At the same time, reviews of the HFD literature (Harris, 1963; Roback, 1968; Swensen, 1968) are almost universally pessimistic about the validity of this instrument as commonly used in clinical practice.

Part of the difficulty with HFDs in prior clinical research is that the drawings have frequently been used as they are in clinical practice, that is, "evaluated by the holistic intuitive judgment of the clinician" (Swensen, 1968). Our analyses of HFDs, in contrast, use two well-articulated, objective, quantitative scales to assess changes in HFDs over the course of long-term treatment: the Goodenough–Harris (GH) and the Robins Balance-Tilt (RBT) scales.

Research on HFDs is consistent with broader considerations about the role of projective techniques in research (particularly the Rorschach and the Thematic Apperception Test [TAT]) and the need to develop systematic methods for the assessment of object relations and object representation for studying the effects of the therapeutic process (Blatt, 1975; Blatt & Wild, 1976). Therapeutic progress should be accompanied by increasing articulation, differentiation, and integration of self and object representations (Blatt, Wild, & Ritzler, 1975). Mayman and Krohn (1975, p. 159) noted that an object relations approach to projective measures "holds real promise as a measure of personality change effected by psychotherapy," and they encouraged "adaptation of tests other than the Rorschach to object-relations theory."

Analysis of HFDs has the potential to contribute to the growing body of research on the use of projective tests to assess self and object representation. Schafer (1954, 1967) with the Rorschach, Phillipson (1955) with the Object Relation Test, and Krohn (1972) with dreams all noted significant relationships among important dimensions of the clinical process and the quality of object representation in dreams, early memories, and psychological tests. HFDs may provide yet another way to assess clinically relevant aspects of this representational world. Research on HFDs as a method for assessing the quality of object relations and representations, however, has yielded inconclusive results. Swensen (1968) cited mostly negative results in his review of the literature on HFDs, whereas Machover (1949, 1953, 1960), Wille (1954), Hammer (1958), Witkin, Dyk, Faterson, Goodenough, and Karp (1962), and Koppitz (1968) reported more positive findings. Witkin et al. (1962) found a highly significant positive correlation between the degree of differentiation in cognitive style (i.e., the "perceptual index" that includes "field dependence–independence") and the degree of differentiation in HFDs. Lord (1971), based on the study of the body concept in HFDs (Witkin et al., 1962), found significant correlations between early memories and an active–passive stance in the HFDs of adolescent boys. Modell (1951, p. 595) found that more regressed psychiatric patients had a "loss of sexual identification of body image" on HFDs. Haworth and Normington (1961, p. 447), studying the sexual differentiation of children, found that girls, in contrast to boys, "consistently show greater emphasis on own sex figures." Robins (1980) also found evidence that female patients consistently drew more differentiated female HFDs than male HFDs; but when an individual has a disturbed same-sex parent, the individual's drawing of a human figure of that sex was disrupted.

Despite a rather extensive literature on HFDs, it is noteworthy that they have never been used in the assessment of psychotherapy change. The purpose of the present analysis is to examine whether systematic assessment of HFDs early and later in the treatment process can provide some understanding of changes that occur in the long-term intensive treatment of seriously disturbed young adults.

Of the 90 seriously disturbed adolescents and young adults in our total sample, 32 patients had complete HFDs at admission (Time 1) and again on average about 15 months later (Time 2) in the treatment process. Of these 32 patients (14 females and 18 males), 15 were independently judged to be primarily anaclitic and 17 to be primarily introjective. As with the total sample of 90 subjects, approximately two-thirds of the anaclitic patients were female (9 of 15, or 60%) and two-thirds of the introjective patients were male (12 of 17, or 70%).

CHANGES IN DEGREE OF DIFFERENTIATION AND ORGANIZATION

The HFDs were assessed with two objective scoring systems. The degree of differentiation was assessed by procedures developed originally by Goodenough (1926) and later revised by Harris (1963), and the degree of organization was assessed by procedures developed by Robins (1980) based on concepts of the balance and tilt of figure drawings. (See pages 63–65 for a detailed presentation of these scoring procedures.)

The GH scores for male and female figures drawn at Time 1 and at Time 2 are highly intercorrelated in both anaclitic and introjective subjects ($r > .78$). The RBT scores for male and female figures at Time 1 and Time 2 are also highly intercorrelated for introjective subjects ($r = .76$ and .73, respectively) but not for anaclitic subjects at Time 1 or at Time 2 ($r = .04$ and .37, respectively). Correlations between GH and RBT at Time 1 and Time 2 for the entire sample ranged from .40 to .61, indicating that these two scores are somewhat independent.

Table 6.1 presents two-way analyses of variance (ANOVA) for a repeated measures design of the GH and the RBT measures for male and female figures drawn by anaclitic and introjective patients at admission and later in the treatment process.[?] The data indicate significant change; HFDs in the second testing, as compared with the initial testing, were

TABLE 6.1

Two-Way Analysis of Variance of Differentiation and Organization in Human Figure Drawings of Anaclitic and Introjective Patients at Time 1 and Time 2

| | Means | | | | ANOVA ($df = 1.30$) F values (repeated measures) | | |
| | Anaclitic | | Introjective | | | | |
	T1	T2	T1	T2	A/I	T1/T2	A × B
Goodenough–Harris							
Total score	−.068	.215	−.573	.444	.05	7.90**	2.51
Male drawing	−.022	.095	−.316	.251	.04	5.85*	2.53
Female drawing	−.046	.120	−.257	.192	.04	7.73**	1.64
Robins Balance-Tilt							
Total score	.322	.193	−1.243	.789	.35	2.86†	3.68†
Male drawing	.400	−.263	−.530	.410	.06	.14	4.60*
Female drawing	−.078	.457	−.713	.379	.73	6.15**	.72

†$p<.10$ *$p<.05$ **$p<.01$

TABLE 6.2
Matched *t* Tests and Effect Size for Differences in Human Figure
Drawings of Anaclitic and Introjective Patients at Time 1 and Time 2

	Matched *t* tests		Effect size		
	Anaclitic patients (*n* = 15)	Introjective patients (*n* = 17)	Total sample (*n* = 32)	Anaclitic patients (*n* = 15)	Introjective patients (*n* = 17)
Goodenough–Harris					
Total score	−.14	−3.11*	.36	.16	.51
Male drawing	−.97	−2.58*	.36	.13	.53
Female drawing	−1.04	−2.61*	.32	.17	.44
Robins Balance-Tilt					
Total score	1.06	−2.97**	.36	.05	.74
Male drawing	.73	−2.52*	.10	.03	.71
Female drawing	−1.25	−2.62*	.56	.40	.68

*p<.05   **p<.01

significantly more fully articulated and differentiated (as indicated by
the GH scores) and significantly more centered and organized in space
(as indicated by the RBT scores). In addition to these significant main
effects over time, there was a significant (*p*<.05) interaction on the
balance-tilt measure for the drawing of a male figure, indicating that the
drawing of a male figure by introjective subjects became significantly
more centered and organized at Time 2 (*p*<.01), whereas the drawing of
a male figure by anaclitic patients changed to a nonsignificant degree in
the opposite direction. As indicated in Table 6.2, matched *t* tests for both
the GH and RBT scores within the anaclitic and introjective groups
indicate that the significant improvement in the GH and RBT scores of
the HFDs at Time 2 occurred primarily in introjective and not in anaclitic
patients. The effect size of these changes in introjective patients is substantial for both the GH and RBT measures of the HFD. The finding of
significant improvement over time, especially for introjective patients, is
consistent with the findings based on variables derived from the analyses of clinical case records, the Rorschach, the intelligence test, and the
TAT protocols reported in prior chapters. Significant positive change
over long-term treatment occurs primarily in introjective patients.

As indicated in Tables 6.3 and 6.4, these changes noted in GH and
RBT over treatment are relatively independent of any confounding variables such as the level of therapist experience, the use of medication, the
level of premorbid social adjustment, the severity of psychopathology,

TABLE 6.3

Two-Way Analyses of Covariance Assessing Effects of Potentially Confounding Variables on Change in Level of Differentiation (Goodenough–Harris) of Human Figure Drawings from Time 1 to Time 2

	Covariate means		F ratio (df = 1.27)		
	Anaclitic (n = 15)	Introjective (n = 17)	A/I	Variable	Interaction
Therapist experience	*> 6 yr* −1.07 / *< 6 yr* .34	*> 5 yr* .99 / *< 6 yr* .20	4.07**	.40	5.02**
Medication	*Meds* −.52 / *No meds* .37	*Meds* .79 / *No meds* .36	1.68	.20	.19
Premorbid level					
Goldstein	*Good* .05 / *Poor* −.05	*Good* .88 / *Poor* .31	1.51	.48	.24
Phillips	*Good* −.05 / *Poor* .00	*Good* 1.54 / *Poor* .03	3.23*	2.66	3.05*
Sex	*Male* .16 / *Female* −.11	*Male* .42 / *Female* 1.17	2.44	.20	1.06
Severity of pathology	*Psychotic* −.21 / *Borderline* .14 / *Neurotic* —	*Psychotic* .21 / *Borderline* .84 / *Neurotic* 2.08	1.38	1.12	.09

*p < .05   **p < .01

TABLE 6.4

Two-Way Analyses of Covariance Assessing Effects of Potentially Confounding Variables on Change in Level of Organization (Balance-Tilt) of Human Figure Drawings from Time 1 to Time 2

| | Covariate means | | F ratio (df = 1.27) | | |
	Anaclitic (n = 15)	Introjective (n = 17)	A/I	Variable	Interaction
Therapist experience	> 6 yr −1.88 < 6 yr .51	> 6 yr 1.29 < 6 yr .76	2.35	.70	1.82
Medication	Meds −5.40 No meds .66	Meds −1.68 No meds 1.68	3.79*	16.85***	1.35
Premorbid level					
Goldstein	Good 1.44 Poor .63	Good 1.24 Poor .99	.18	.41	.27
Phillips	.68 −.49	1.97 .40	1.00	1.61	.03
Sex	Male −1.56 Female .87	Male .85 Female 1.53	2.04	1.99	.68
Severity of pathology	Psychotic −1.09 Borderline .63 Neurotic —	Psychotic .48 Borderline 1.30 Neurotic 3.34	1.08	1.22	.19

*p<.05   ***p<.001

and the sex of the patient. The level of therapist experience had a significant interaction with the anaclitic–introjective distinction on the GH score such that anaclitic patients with less experienced therapists appeared to have more substantial improvement in GH scores ($p<.06$) at Time 2 (controlling for the score at Time 1) than did anaclitic patients with more experienced therapists. The reverse pattern, although not statistically significant, occurred with introjective patients. Also, introjective patients with better premorbid social adjustment tended ($p<.10$) to have more improved GH scores than introjective patients with poorer premorbid adjustment. In terms of the RBT score, there was a significant ($p<.001$) main effect in the use of medication such that both anaclitic and introjective patients not receiving medication had substantially improved RBT scores at Time 2 in comparison with anaclitic and introjective patients who received medication. This finding was especially significant for anaclitic patients ($p<.001$), but for introjective patients ($p<.03$) as well.

Interestingly, these assessments of the degree of articulation (GH) and organization (RBT) in HFDs do not have consistent significant correlations with the various other measures derived from the clinical case records and from the Rorschach, the intelligence test, or the TAT at Time 1 or at Time 2. Thus, it appears that HFDs provide a unique and independent dimension for assessing therapeutic change. Although aspects of HFDs are inconsistently related to other assessment methods at both Time 1 and Time 2, analyses of change in HFDs come to essentially the same conclusions about the nature of therapeutic change in seriously disturbed young adults as found with other measures (i.e., assessment of clinical case reports, aspects of Rorschach and TAT protocols, and intelligence test scores). The analyses of the HFDs and other assessments of change indicate that statistically significant, constructive change occurs primarily with introjective rather than anaclitic patients. Why change seems more manifest in the introjective patients is an interesting and important question. The multidimensionality of the findings that change is consistently more substantial for introjective than for anaclitic patients on a wide variety of assessment procedures, however, suggests that this finding is not a consequence of modes of assessment that may be biased toward the more ideational introjective patients. Rather, the significantly greater change over treatment in introjective patients may be an important consideration when evaluating the therapeutic process with seriously disturbed patients, especially because these findings run counter to the oft-noted expectation that hysteric patients have a better prognosis for treatment.

In summary, the analyses of HFDs indicate that the degree of articulation and differentiation of body details and clothing in HFDs (as measured by the GH) and the stabilization of the "slant" and "footing" of the figure (as measured by the RBT) can be measured reliably. Both these variables provide valuable independent measures of therapeutic change in seriously disturbed patients. The organization of the drawing of the male figure (RBT) appears problematic, however, for anaclitic patients, yielding results that run counter to the overall pattern of greater differentiation and organization of HFDs from Time 1 to Time 2.

ILLUSTRATIVE CLINICAL EXAMPLES

The following clinical examples elaborate some of the changes noted in the HFDs of patients over the course of the treatment process.

Patient 91: Improved Introjective Male

The male HFDs

	Time 1	Time 2
Goodenough–Harris	23	39
Robins Balance-Tilt	18	15

The GH scores for the male drawings (Figure 6.1) show a marked improvement of 16 points. At Time 2 the patient adds outline and proportion to the head and face, with a projection of a chin; ears in proper position; fingers, hands, wrists, ankles, and feet in proportion; and knee joints. The RBT also shows slight improvement.

The male drawing at Time 1 looks like an infantile blob doll, with poor boundaries and proportions, helpless arms ("flippers"), no hands, and a posture suggestive of passivity and dependence. At Time 2, the male figure is erect, with a very clear, definite shape, a young man in proper form and proportion, with a protruding chin and accented knees, suggesting movement, activity, and assertion. The dim, unassertive line quality at Time 1 changes to a more forceful, defined execution at Time 2. The patient commented to the examiner that the Time 1 figure "looks a little screwy," which could be due to the asymmetrical facial features. At Time 2, the face is definitely symmetrical, modeled to show pronounced facial features. The patient also commented at Time 1 that the figure was "missing genitals"; the Time 2 figure continues to be without genitals, possibly suggesting the need for further sexual integration in subsequent therapy.

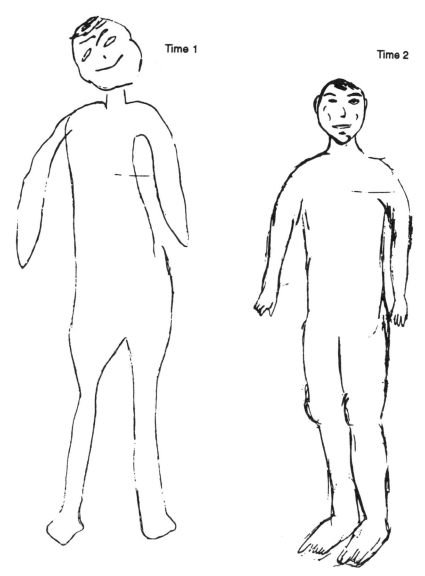

FIG. 6.1. Patient 91: Male Human Figure Drawings.

The female HFDs

	Time 1	Time 2
Goodenough–Harris	21	34
Robins Balance-Tilt	15	12

Time 1   Time 2

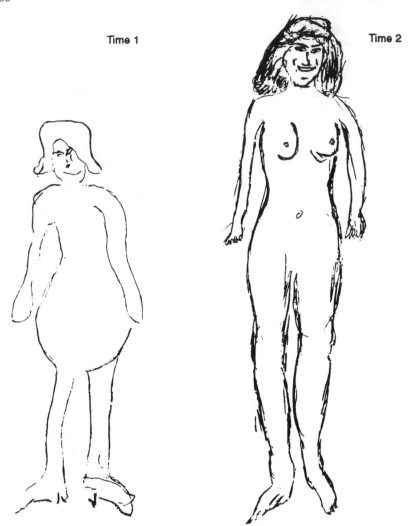

FIG. 6.2. Patient 91: Female Human Figure Drawings.

The female figure also has a substantial 13-point improvement on the GH from Time 1 to Time 2 (see Figure 6.2). At Time 2, the patient had increasingly elaborated the head and neck (eyes, cheeks, both chin and forehead, line of jaw, and definite hairstyle), and the hands and fingers; the figure also has a definite waist, and the waist, breasts, and hip contour are proportionate. The improvement in balance and tilt (from 15 to 12), although slight, implies less pathology in the female figure at Time 2 than at Time 1.

The female figure at Time 1 is vague, grossly distorted, devoid of details, and has poorly defined boundaries; the figure at Time 2 has striking detail and well-defined boundaries. The figure at Time 1 lacks important body parts that deal with self-definition as well as a capacity for communication with others (e.g., the face, eyes, and mouth, as well as the hands and fingers). The figure at Time 1 is totally lacking sexual differentiation (e.g., her legs do not meet in the crotch area), but at Time 2 the figure has an appropriate juncture of the crotch, a waist, a convex curve of the hips, breasts, nipples, and a feminine hairstyle. At Time 1 the figure is bent to one side; at Time 2 the figure is erect. At Time 1 her face is obscure, without definition; at Time 2 her face is intentionally shaped with a protruding chin, cheeks, a definite nose, eyes, and a smiling mouth. The figure has become much more human. The quality of the lines at Time 1 is very weak; at Time 2 the figure is drawn much more forcefully, with pencil pressure intentionally being applied to accentuate various body parts.

The patient commented to the examiner at Time 1 that the "woman" was "not very pleasant," and that she was "missing various parts, like breasts." This contrasts strikingly with the figure at Time 2, who appears rather pleasant (smiling) and with prominent breasts.

In sum, the patient appears to have a less vague and a more mature and benevolent representation of a woman at Time 2.

Patient 14: Improved Anaclitic Male

The male HFDs

	Time 1	Time 2
Goodenough–Harris	45	64
Robins Balance-Tilt	13	5

Patient 14 had a substantial increase over the course of treatment in the articulation and differentiation (GH) with which he drew human figures and in the degree to which they were presented in a balanced and integrated way (RBT). For the male figures (see Figure 6.3), the GH scores increased from 45 to 64, and the Robins Balance-Tilt score decreased from 13 to 5, reflecting better balance and integration of the human figure.

The 19-point increase on the GH in the drawings of the male figure from Time 1 to Time 2 signals a remarkable improvement. Individual items added at Time 2 include the projection of a chin and of a line for the jaw, stylized hair, correct number of fingers, opposition of the thumb, proportion of head to body, enhanced motor coordination in execution of the lines, and an anatomically correct head, body, and

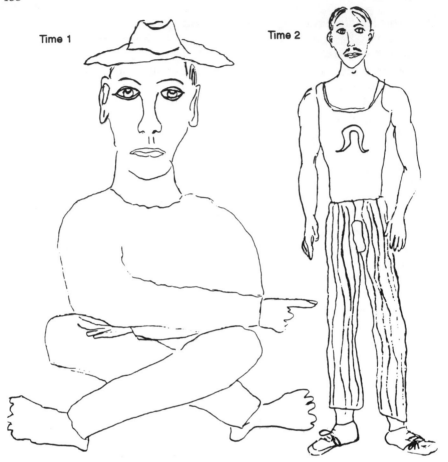

FIG. 6.3. Patient 14: Male Human Figure Drawings.

limbs. The RBT change from 13 to 5 indicated that the figure at Time 2 is more well balanced, without the vertical slant found at Time 1.

The male figure at Time 1 is seated, with nondescript clothing, an exaggerated large head, an inappropriately small hat, and a poorly formed chin, hands, and feet. The male figure at Time 2 is standing erect, showing his entire body; he has definite athletic clothing complete with an identifying logo on his shirt, an appropriately sized head, and remarkably accurate structural anatomical proportions (e.g., well-formed musculature of shoulders and forearms, as well as hands and feet drawn in perspective).

It is noteworthy that at Time 1 the eyes are highlighted with very dark surrounding lines, an elaboration commonly attributed to patients with paranoid issues (Levy & Machover, cited in Hammer, 1958), a hypothesis corroborated by this patient's diagnosis. In this context, it may be all the more significant that at Time 2 the eyes are accurately portrayed, which could signal the diminution of paranoid issues. The figure at Time 1 is sedentary and slumped and appears passive compared with the active erect stance of the athlete at Time 2. The patient commented that the figure at Time 1 is "not a real person, just a drawing," whereas at Time 2 the figure now appears as a real person and even had some kind of "name" (the symbol of identity on the shirt that appears to be an "omega").

The Time 2 figure exhibits an important change in sexual differentiation: the protruding chin, muscle tonus, moustache, Adam's apple, and fly on the pants all suggest the patient's taking his stand as a male. Finally, the darker quality of lines shown at Time 2 also suggests a more active, engaged, and aggressive person than at Time 1.

In sum, the marked increase in the GH and the moderate improvement in the RBT of the drawings of the male figure suggest that this patient has made major constructive changes in the treatment process.

The female HFDs

	Time 1	Time 2
Goodenough–Harris	46	54
Robins Balance-Tilt	10	5

The differentiation of the female figure at Time 2, as compared with Time 1, increased by 8 points (46 to 54), a clear indicator of positive change (see Figure 6.4). The Time 2 figure now possesses two definite hands, feet drawn correctly and in proportion, a neckline on her clothing, indications of a feminine waist and hip contour, and a definite type of garb. The figure also is drawn with better motor coordination of junctures and lines than the figure at Time 1. The RBT score improves from 10 to 5, indicating a clear improvement in the female figure's posture.

What is immediately striking about the female figures is that they are the same person. Note also that the female figure at Time 1 has marked elaboration of the eyes and that at Time 2 this elaboration has been omitted. The Time 1 figure draws attention to her eyes and face (in her unusually large head), whereas the focus of the Time 2 figure seems to be the entire head–body gestalt.

The sedentary, passive postural figure with deformed feet at Time 1 also suggests that she may be nude from the waist up, a detail that

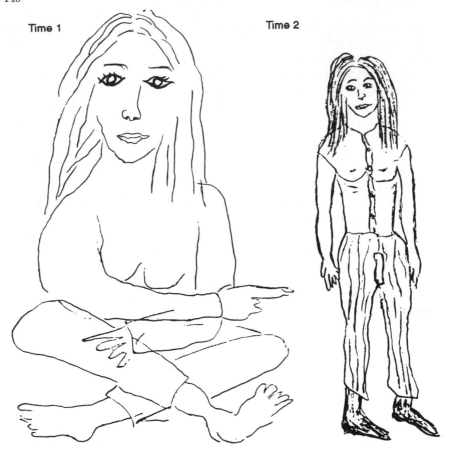

Time 1   Time 2

FIG. 6.4. Patient 14: Female Human Figure Drawings.

probably has dynamic meaning. The active, standing figure at Time 2, clearly clothed over her breasts, may suggest some super-ego internalization. Although the female figure at Time 2 is much more differentiated sexually than at Time 1 (with better-formed breasts, nipples, convex hips, hairstyle, specific type of blouse, and more feminine musculature of arms), there is still some sexual ambiguity because of the presence of the fly on the pants.

Patient 19: Improved Introjective Male

The male HFDs

	Time 1	Time 2
Goodenough–Harris	41	49
Robins Balance-Tilt	8	12

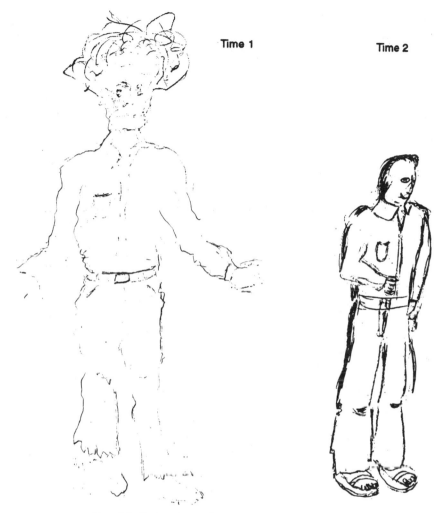

FIG. 6.5. Patient 19: Male Human Figure Drawings.

The GH shows clear improvement at Time 2 (8 points), including greater detail in the eyes, a nose drawn in two dimensions, a mouth, the bridge of the nose, fingers, feet (sandals, toes), and complete clothing, as well as more coordinated lines and junctures (see Figure 6.5). The RBT change from 8 to 12 indicates a slight regression and a minor loss of vertical uprightness. This could also be due to the "quarter-side" stance of the figure at Time 2 as compared with the "full-face" stance at Time 1.

The Time 1 male is extremely vague and incomplete; the lines are so light that they conceal as well as suggest the presence of this figure. At

Time 1, the figure has no discernible feet and hands. The Time 2 male is a different person, with much clearer defining lines, especially detailed feet that are capable of supporting the entire person.

The face at Time 1 is an undifferentiated enigma, with barely the suggestion of a mouth. The entire figure at Time 1 is wispy, spread out in a passive, defenseless way as compared with the tighter, more substantial, on-his-feet and smiling figure at Time 2 with knee joints suggesting he is ready for action. At Time 1, the wrinkled, ragged clothes with wild hair give the impression of a homeless "bag man"; conversely, the impression at Time 2 is of an appropriately dressed young man with stylish bell-bottoms and sandals.

At Time 1, the crotch area is vacant, whereas at Time 2 the crotch area is quite elaborated, with closure of the upper thighs as well as a fly on the pants. At Time 1, the patient commented to the examiner that this drawing was a "self-portrait." Time 2 shows considerable change in how he perceives his own solidity and standing as a male.

In sum, the improvement in articulation and differentiation of the male figure signals a positive change in the patient's perception of the male figure, which implies that this patient has been working on his identity as a male. The loss of vertical uprightness at Time 2, however, suggests the possibility that much work remains to be done to establish his identity so that it provides him with some sense of stability.

The female HFDs

	Time 1	Time 2
Goodenough–Harris	40	47
Robins Balance-Tilt	14	0

The female figure at Time 2 also clearly improves on the GH (7 points); it possesses a neck, eye detail, more styled hair, proper attachment of arms and legs, neckline, collar, head outline, and some hip contour (see Figure 6.6). The change in RBT from 14 to 0 signals the achievement of perfect balance-tilt, a major improvement in the Time 2 female figure.

The figure at Time 1 is extremely vague, an almost eerie figure with floating arms, perhaps due to its ill-defined boundaries. The figure at Time 2 is much more well defined; although she is still the same person with the contorted "Cupid's bow" lips, she now has discernible arms, hands, and feet. The distorted Cupid's bow may represent a key dynamic issue for this patient: Alluring, seductive lips that are associated with speaking and affection are experienced as exaggerated and distorted. The fact that the figure at Time 1 may also be nude from the waist up

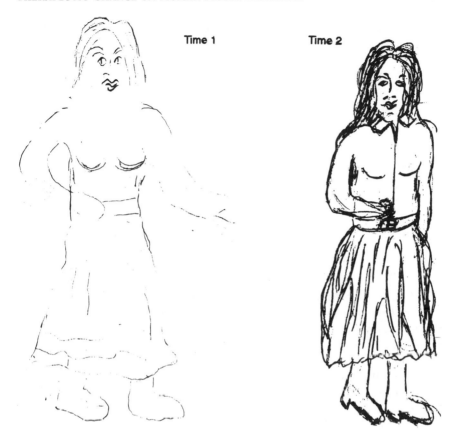

FIG. 6.6. Patient 19: Female Human Figure Drawings.

strengthens the impression of seductiveness. Also, at Time 1, the breasts are outlined two or three times, but at Time 2, the breasts are appropriately covered with a blouse, which could indicate some growth in super-ego integration. After drawing the female figure at Time 1, the patient commented to the examiner: "This is my mother when she was younger. Guess I have an oedipal thing still." The poignancy of his comment is borne out by the fact, alluded to in his case summary, that there is some indication that at 14 years of age he had sexual intercourse with his mother. It is also interesting to note the similar positions of the Time 2 male and female upper bodies (right arm bent, left arm at the side). Because the patient names the female figure "Mom" (who was also hospitalized for psychiatric difficulties), could their similar stances denote the patient's identification with his mother as a psychiatric patient (especially because the patient identified the male figure as his "self-portrait")?

In sum, both the male and female figures have generally improved, but the female figure is much improved on the RBT, whereas the male is slightly regressed. Also, both the male and female figures become much more distinct and differentiated at Time 2, indicating significant therapeutic gain.

Patient 56: Improved Introjective Female

The male HFDs

	Time 1	Time 2
Goodenough–Harris	23	53
Robins Balance-Tilt	18	0

Similar changes are noted in this female patient's drawing of the male figures (see Figure 6.7). Striking positive change on the GH for the male figure includes increased articulation of the eyebrow, lips and nose in two dimensions, projection of a chin, elaborate hairstyle, correct finger detail, a knee joint (suggesting movement), outline and proportion of the head and face, and an elaboration of clothing. This 30-point increase in differentiation is indicative of considerable change. The change in RBT from 18 to perfect 0 also indicates constructive change in the male figure at Time 2.

The male figure at Time 1 is an off-balance figure with a primitive circle for the head; a distorted eye pupil; a bland childish smile; short, helpless arms (also poised so as to be "picked up," as in the female figure); unarticulated fingers; and an unrealistic stance with the feet pointed out. All this contrasts strikingly with the perfectly balanced, moving figure at Time 2. The conventional hairstyle and articulated facial features at Time 2 are consistent with the image of a substantial person—a person with shaped buttocks, thighs, and lower legs, who is in motion with foot extension and flexion, suggesting tendon and muscular connections. This is a far cry from the precarious, side-leaning figure at Time 1. The outstretched hand at Time 2 may also suggest a more benevolent social attitude, a friendlier figure than the infantile, wispy character at Time 1.

In sum, this patient's depiction of "the male" has changed substantially, from an undifferentiated, infantile, helpless, vapidly grinning figure to an active, sexual, muscular, stylish man on the move.

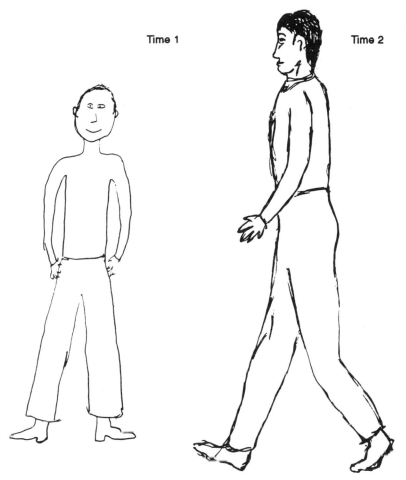

Time 1

Time 2

Fig. 6.7. Patient 56: Male Human Figure Drawings.

The female HFDs

	Time 1	Time 2
Goodenough–Harris	21	43
Robins Balance-Tilt	15	4

The female figure shows a substantial 22-point improvement on the GH (see Figure 6.8). At Time 2, the head is no longer a primitive circle but an ovoid structure denoting facial contour and more humanlike

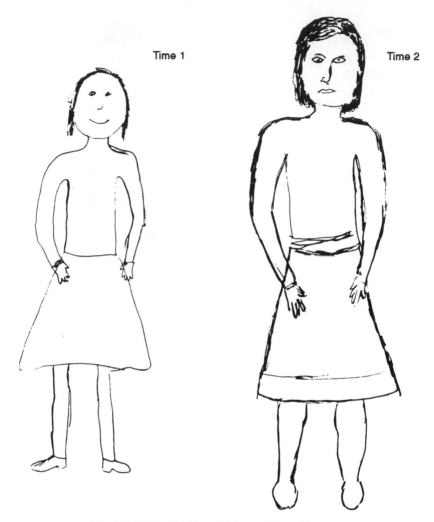

Time 1   Time 2

FIG. 6.8. Patient 56: Female Human Figure Drawings.

features. This female patient has added greater eye detail (pupil, eyebrow) and proper eye proportion, lips in two dimensions, the bridge of the nose, and a definite hairstyle to her drawings of the female figure. A belt is also added at Time 2; opposition of the thumb is more clearly shown; the stance of the feet is more realistic, facing frontward; and the inside angle of the legs suggests the presence of a crotch. The change from 15 to 4 in balance and tilt is also substantial and is further evidence of less pathology in the female figure at Time 2.

The female figure at Time 1 seems generally more primitive and immature than the figure at Time 2. The face at Time 1 communicates only a vapid, primitive smile with little or no differentiated communication, whereas the face at Time 2 is more human but more disturbed. An infantile quality at Time 1 is conveyed by the helpless arms (shorter than at Time 2), as well as the crude depiction of the position of the feet and the parallel lines describing the inner thighs, suggesting that there is no crotch under her skirt. At Time 1, the figure appears more as a passive, happy face doll wanting to be picked up. This positioning of the arms (making an angle of more than 10 degrees with the vertical axis of the trunk) is most common in drawings of very young children (Harris, 1963). The passive helplessness and the "pick me up" angles of the arms and trunk at Time 1 are replaced at Time 2 by a sense of active power in the forward stance of the feet; "shaped" legs, suggesting active calf muscles; and an elaboration of the thumb–forefinger opposition, expressing a capacity for grasping.

After completing the drawing of the figure at Time 2, the patient commented to the examiner: "There's still a residue of the old [patient's name]." "The old" here ironically refers back to "the young," the infantile, innocent, passive, nonsexual self.

The change in the drawings of the two female figures suggests that this patient appears to be less passive and less helpless and has become a more active, articulated, and sexual person. The change also suggests, however, that the patient is a more troubled or perplexed (judging from the facial expression and asymmetry of the pupils), more mature woman.

Summary

In summary, the empirical data clearly indicate that HFDs show reliable and consistent change with treatment. The clinical examples illustrate the changes that occurred in the articulation and organization in the HFDs of many patients over the course of treatment, as well as how these changes seem to express some of the dynamic issues central to the treatment process. The HFDs are another useful assessment procedure for evaluating therapeutic gain, especially when comparing change from initial drawings. The clinical and research utility of the HFD appears to be augmented considerably by consideration of changes within patients over time.

NOTES

1. This chapter derives from a paper by Robins, Blatt, and Ford (1991) in the *Journal of Personality Assessment*.
2. Scores on the GH and RBT scales for the drawings of the male and female figures were transformed to standard (*z*) scores and then combined for each subject to give a Total GH and a Total RBT score for each subject at Time 1 and Time 2. Scores for the RBT score were reversed so that negative scores indicate greater deviation from vertical.

Configurations of Therapeutic Change

Analyses of variance and covariance as well as matched t tests were used to evaluate overall group changes in clinical case records and psychological test protocols. Within these overall group comparisons at Time 1 and Time 2, however, different individuals may change to varying degrees and in different directions on separate variables. While analyses of variance and t tests assess group effects over time, they evaluate only the relationship of change in different variables across individuals that are consistent within the total group. To the extent that different individuals may change to varying degrees and in different directions on separate variables, these different effects may cancel each other out and not be evident in various analyses of group effects. To examine possible patterns of change in different spheres of functioning within individuals, we correlated change on psychological test variables with change on the ratings of the clinical case records. In evaluating these correlations (or covariations) between change scores in different sets of variables, we sought to identify patterns of change as individuals progress or regress during the treatment process. Independent of the changes noted for total groups on separate variables, the correlation of change scores among different variables from independent sources permits us to examine whether there are particular configurations of variables that indicate both progressive and regressive change for different types of patients. These configurations of change can be identified by studying the relationships among the various measures of change from independent sources of data—the ratings made on the clinical case records (the Menninger Scales of Interpersonal Relations, the Strauss–Harder Clinical Symptom Scales, and the Fairweather Scale of Interpersonal Communication) and the independent scoring of the psychological test protocols (thought disorder, concept of the object and Mutuality of Autonomy on the Rorschach, and intelligence test scores). In this chapter, we will present the correlations among change scores (Time 1 minus Time 2) of variables obtained from these two data sources—the objective behavioral observations reported in the clinical case records and the subjective cognitive, affective, and interpersonal dimensions assessed in psychological test protocols—and consider the implications of these findings for understanding therapeutic process and change.[1]

Table 7.1 presents the correlations between changes in the composite thought disorder score derived from the Rorschach and the various ratings made from the clinical case records. Changes in thought disorder covaried to a highly significant degree with changes in the assessment of clinical symptoms on the Strauss–Harder. Decrease in total thought disorder correlated significantly ($p<.05$) with decreases in all four Strauss–Harder symptom scales. This relationship between thought disorder on the Rorschach and independent rating of different types of clinical symptoms in the case records was significant for both anaclitic and introjective patients, but this relationship was predominant for introjec-

TABLE 7.1

Correlation of Changes in Case Record Ratings with Changes in Total Composite Thought Disorder on the Rorschach

	Total sample ($n = 90$)	Anaclitic patients ($n = 42$)	Introjective patients ($n = 48$)
Menninger Scales			
Factor I (Interpersonal relatedness)	−.18†	−.15	−.24†
Motivation for treatment	−.19†	−.24	−.17
Sublimatory capacity	−.003	.04	−.15
Superego integration	−.17†	−.08	−.23
Object relations	−.19†	−.19	−.18
Factor II (Impulsivity)	−.11	−.10	−.11
Fairweather	.11	.04	.23
Interpersonal communication			
Strauss–Harder symptoms			
Neurotic	.33**	.28†	.34**
Psychotic	.31**	.16	.45***
Labile Affect	.36***	.39**	.34**
Flattened Affect	.29*	.33*	.19

†$p<.10$ *$p<.05$ **$p<.01$ ***$p<.001$

TABLE 7.2
Correlation of Changes in Case Record Ratings
with Changes in Intelligence (Full Scale IQ)

	Total sample (n = 90)	Anaclitic patients (n = 42)	Introjective patients (n = 48)
Menninger Scales			
Factor I (Interpersonal relatedness)	.12	−.03	.22
Motivation for treatment	.04	.10	−.01
Sublimatory capacity	.02	.12	.11
Superego integration	.17	.02	.27†
Object relations	.13	−.11	.30*
Factor II (Impulsivity)	−.05	.28†	−.26†
Fairweather			
Interpersonal communication	−.20	−.21	−.20
Strauss–Harder symptoms			
Neurotic	−.27**	−.16	−.36**
Psychotic	.01	.24	−.09
Labile Affect	−.14	−.04	−.23
Flattened Affect	−.27**	−.02	−.47***

†$p<.10$ *$p<.05$ **$p<.01$ ***$p<.001$

tive patients. Changes in thought disorder in introjective patients correlated significantly primarily with changes in Labile Affect and neurotic and psychotic symptoms. In anaclitic patients, the significant correlations between changes in thought disorder and clinical symptoms occurred primarily with those symptom scales measuring affect disturbances (Flattened and Labile Affect). Despite these highly significant relationships between changes in thought disorder on the Rorschach and changes in a variety of different types of clinical symptoms, there were no significant correlations between changes in thought disorder and changes in manifest social behavior as assessed by the Menninger and Fairweather scales for either anaclitic or introjective patients.

Table 7.2 presents the correlation between changes in IQ scores and changes in clinical symptoms and interpersonal and social behavior rated from case records. Highly significant correlations were found between changes in IQ and changes in clinical symptoms. Increases in Full Scale IQ significantly correlated with decreases in several types of clinical symptoms, especially for introjective patients. There were no consistent and significant relationships, however, between changes in IQ and social behavior for anaclitic patients, and only marginal ones for introjective patients.

Tables 7.3 and 7.4 present the correlations between the developmental index (weighted sum) and the developmental mean, respectively, of the concept of the object on the Rorschach for accurately (OR+) as well as for inaccurately perceived (OR−) human responses and ratings made from clinical case records. Consistent with earlier findings (Blatt et al., 1976b), changes in both the developmental index and the developmental mean of accurately perceived human responses (OR+) do not correlate significantly with changes in the clinical case records of these seriously disturbed inpatients. In this study, consistent with our earlier research (Blatt et al., 1976b) with seriously disturbed inpatients, only one significant relationship was found between the concept of the

TABLE 7.3

Correlation of Changes in Ratings of Case Records with Changes in the Quality of Object Representation (Developmental Index) on the Rorschach

	OR Factor Plus (OR+)			OR Factor Minus (OR−)		
	Total ($n = 90$)	Anaclitic ($n = 42$)	Introjective ($n = 48$)	Total ($n = 90$)	Anaclitic ($n = 42$)	Introjective ($n = 48$)
Menninger Scales						
Factor I (Interpersonal relatedness)	.02	.13	−.09	−.21*	−.45**	−.17
Motivation for treatment	−.01	−.001	−.04	−.17†	−.29†	−.17
Sublimatory capacity	−.01	.16	−.16	−.14	−.43**	−.06
Superego integration	.02	−.03	.04	−.22*	−.40**	−.20
Object relations	.07	.27†	−.14	−.14	−.35**	−.10
Factor II (Impulsivity)	−.13	−.16	−.10	.14	.16	.14
Fairweather						
Interpersonal communication	−.13	−.09	−.16	.14	.13	.17
Strauss–Harder symptoms						
Neurotic	−.07	−.08	−.05	.27**	.19	.36**
Psychotic	−.13	−.16	−.10	.22*	.22	.25†
Labile Affect	−.15	.07	−.41**	−.03	−.01	−.04
Flattened Affect	−.12	−.20	−.03	.09	.30*	.03

†$p<.10$ *$p<.05$ **$p<.01$

TABLE 7.4
Correlation of Changes in Ratings of Case Records with Changes in the Quality
of Object Representation (Developmental Mean) on the Rorschach

	OR Factor Plus (OR+)			OR Factor Minus (OR−)		
	Total (n = 90)	Anaclitic (n = 42)	Introjective (n = 48)	Total (n = 90)	Anaclitic (n = 42)	Introjective (n = 48)
Menninger Scales						
Factor I (Interpersonal relatedness)	−.06	−.05	−.09	−.24*	−.28†	−.27†
Motivation for treatment	−.13	−.11	−.17	−.16	−.18	−.18
Sublimatory capacity	−.04	.07	−.09	−.35***	−.28*	−.41**
Superego integration	.03	−.11	−.04	−.15	−.19	−.16
Object relations	.06	.13	.02	−.14	−.26†	−.09
Factor II (Impulsivity)	−.21†	−.13	−.27†	.26**	.31*	.24†
Fairweather						
Interpersonal communication	.01	.00	.01	−.03	.12	−.15
Strauss–Harder symptoms						
Neurotic	−.03	.09	−.11	.01	−.05	.11
Psychotic	−.07	.02	.09	.03	.19	−.03
Labile Affect	−.07	−.13	−.02	−.05	−.09	.04
Flattened Affect	−.11	−.01	−.23	.12	.25	.01

†p<.10   *p<.05   **p<.01   ***p<.001

object on accurately perceived human responses on the Rorschach
(OR+) and ratings made from the clinical case records, and this was
with introjective patients. In these patients, an increase in the developmental index for accurately perceived responses correlated significantly
($p<.01$) with a reduction in labile affect. An increase in the developmental mean also correlated significantly ($p<.05$) with a decrease in impulsivity. Given the large number of comparisons made with the OR+
measures, however, these two significant findings are probably due to
chance.

In our prior research with another sample of seriously disturbed
inpatients (Blatt et al., 1976b), we found that the differentiation, articulation, and integration of inaccurately perceived human responses (OR−)
were significantly related to the severity of psychotic symptoms among
seriously disturbed inpatients. Here, too, in this sample of seriously
disturbed inpatients, highly significant correlations were found between
the developmental index and developmental mean of inaccurately perceived human responses (OR−) and ratings of various aspects of the
clinical case records. As indicated in Table 7.3, increased investment
(higher developmental index) in inaccurately perceived human representations on the Rorschach (OR−) correlated significantly with increases in neurotic and psychotic symptoms primarily for introjective
patients, and with flattened affect in anaclitic patients.

Most noteworthy, however, are the highly significant relationships
between the degree of investment in inaccurately perceived human representations (OR−) (as measured by both the developmental index and
the developmental mean) and the quality of interpersonal relationships
as rated on the Menninger scales. For anaclitic patients, decreased investment in inaccurately perceived human representations (lower OR−
scores) correlated significantly ($p<.05$) with increases in Menninger Factor I and several of the individual Menninger scales.[2] Thus, for anaclitic
patients, decreases in the investment of inaccurately perceived human
responses appear to be a particularly valuable measure of progressive
change during the treatment of seriously disturbed patients, especially
as expressed in changes in their interpersonal behavior. As disturbed
anaclitic patients improve, they begin to relinquish investment in inappropriate or autistic fantasies about interpersonal relationships. Because
therapeutic progress was generally less apparent in the group of anaclitic patients, it is not surprising that the object representation scores did
not show an overall significant improvement from Time 1 to Time 2 for
the total group of patients, or even for anaclitic patients considered
separately. But object representation scores, especially those for inaccurately perceived human responses (OR−), appear to be a sensitive

measure of progressive and regressive changes in the seriously disturbed anaclitic patients who participated in this investigation of therapeutic change.

As discussed earlier, the Mutuality of Autonomy (MOA) is a complex measure that derives from the degree of malevolence portrayed in interactions on the Rorschach. The mean MOA score is a complex measure that is significantly related to independent measures of both the degree of thought disorder and the quality of interpersonal relations (Blatt, Tuber, & Auerbach, 1990). Thus, as indicated in Table 7.5, change in the mean MOA score for the total sample correlates significantly with change in some of the Menninger scales of interpersonal relations (Motivation for Treatment, Superego Integration, and Object Relations) and with all four Strauss–Harder symptom scales. These significant relationships occur primarily with introjective patients, but significant correlations were also obtained in anaclitic patients between changes in the mean MOA score and the two affect regulation scales on the Strauss–Harder (Labile and Flattened Affect). As the mean MOA score changed toward the representation of more benevolent and reciprocal interactions, the quality of interpersonal relations improved and a range of clinical symptoms decreased, primarily for introjective patients.

TABLE 7.5
Correlation of Changes in Case Record Ratings
with Change of the Mean MOA Score on the Rorschach

	Total ($n = 90$)	Anaclitic ($n = 42$)	Introjective ($n = 48$)
Menninger Scales			
Factor I (Interpersonal relatedness)	−.32***	−.24	−.39**
Motivation for treatment	−.32***	−.18	−.47***
Sublimatory capacity	−.18	−.19	−.18
Superego integration	−.26**	−.14	−.37**
Object relations	−.24*	−.27	−.18
Factor II (Impulsivity)	−.02	−.03	−.02
Fairweather			
Interpersonal communication	.10	.03	.17
Strauss–Harder symptoms			
Neurotic	.28**	.20	.37**
Psychotic	.32***	.24	.40**
Labile Affect	.30**	.36*	.16
Flattened Affect	.29**	.38**	.13

*$p<.05$ **$p<.01$ ***$p<.001$

In summary, there appear to be significant clusters of variables derived from case records and psychological test protocols that covary differentially with changes in anaclitic and introjective patients during treatment. Change (improvement and regression) in the more ideational introjective patients is reflected primarily in changes in clinical symptoms noted in the case records and changes in cognitive processes such as thought disorder on the Rorschach and intelligence test scores. Change (improvement and regression) in the more interpersonally oriented anaclitic patients, in contrast, is reflected more consistently in changes in case record ratings of interpersonal relationships (the Menninger scales) and the developmental level of the concept of the object for inaccurately perceived human responses on the Rorschach. For the seriously disturbed anaclitic patient, decreased investment in inaccurately perceived human forms on the Rorschach (that is, decreased investment in previously gratifying autistic fantasies about relatedness) correlated significantly with increases in the quality of the interpersonal relations independently noted in the case records. Change in the more multidimensional MOA scale on the Rorschach, however, correlates significantly with change in both interpersonal behavior and clinical symptoms, primarily in introjective patients.

The design of this study and the nature and quality of the data in it provided a unique opportunity to study the process of change. Data analyses thus far have explored two aspects of this process: (1) Analyses of variance (and covariance) as well as matched t tests enabled us to identify variables on which the entire group or subgroups of patients changed over time, and (2) correlations of change scores broadened this search and enabled us to identify patterns of covariation between changes in psychological test variables and dimensions of independent assessments by the clinical staff for the entire group and for subgroups of patients.

Both the analyses of variance and the correlation of change scores are descriptive analytic approaches. They describe what kinds of changes have occurred in the case records and psychological test protocols during treatment. Without a control group of randomly equivalent people receiving some other kind of intervention (or no treatment at all), however, it is not possible to specify precisely what contributed to these changes. But given the consistent findings obtained in the analyses of variance and correlations of change scores, substantial changes appear to have occurred in this sample of patients in multiple independent measures of both their psychological functioning (as measured by test protocols) and their overt behavior (as assessed in the evaluation of their clinical case records).

To exemplify the quality of these clinical changes noted in the statistical analyses of our data, Chapter 8 presents clinical vignettes of four patients who were judged by the clinical staff to have improved markedly. We present two females and two males (one each judged to have had an anaclitic or an introjective form of psychopathology), and we contrast segments of their Rorschach protocol at Time 1 and Time 2 to illustrate aspects of their therapeutic change as it appears in the psychological test protocols.

NOTES

1. The correlation of change scores is a simple and helpful screening device for the preliminary exploration of relationships among variables in a longitudinal data set. Caution needs to be exercised, however, in the interpretation of correlated change scores because they can be misleading in a number of ways. It is possible for the relationship between change scores of two variables to be spurious. If, for example, patients were selected for inclusion in the study (i.e., hospitalized) because of their impaired psychological functioning and behavior, then all measures, because they are likely to be exaggerated at first testing, are subject to regression toward the mean (i.e., to move toward more modulated scores). This statistical artifact could generate spurious correlations among change scores. Similarly, two measures that are both influenced by an unidentified and unmeasured third factor could result in a spurious correlation of change scores. Also, the synchronous correlation between two variables at either Time 1 or Time 2 can generate significance in the correlations of change scores. Despite these cautions, correlation of change scores provides an opportunity to assess patterns of change within individuals as they progress and regress during treatment.
2. This relationship between change in OR− scores and change in social behavior in anaclitic patients occurs with both the developmental index and the developmental mean of inaccurately perceived human representations, even though these two variables are only marginally interrelated. The developmental mean and the developmental index of OR+ correlate .38 and .22, and these two measures of OR− correlate .68 and .29, for anaclitic and introjective patients, respectively.

Chapter 8

Illustrative Clinical Cases

In the research presented in this book, we have taken a binocular view. We have looked at the same patients through two separate lenses: (1) through the systematic evaluation of clinical observations presented in narrative case reports and (2) through the precise delineation of psychological test variables, especially from the Rorschach, whose reliability and validity have been documented in a number of prior cross-sectional research investigations. We rated data from each of these points of view without knowledge of the other, in order to demonstrate the validity of both approaches to clinical assessment.

In relation to careful and systematic clinical observation, we have been able to validate two specific Rorschach dimensions as effective measures of change: (1) types of formal thought disorder first articulated by Rapaport, Gill, and Schafer (1945) and later placed within an integrative theoretical model by Blatt and his colleagues (Blatt & Ritzler, 1974; Blatt & Wild, 1976; Blatt, Wild, & Ritzler, 1975); and (2) the concept of the human form, for which a complex and comprehensive methodology has been developed (Blatt et al., 1976a). The present research has added significantly to knowledge about the specific effectiveness of these two dimensions; namely, we have learned to pay close attention to change over time in the extent of disordered thinking and in the *fantastic* elaboration of the human figure on the Rorschach, that is, to changes in how seriously disturbed patients elaborate the human figure *without* support from consensually perceived properties of the inkblot (OR−).

The general understanding of such investment in thought disorder and in unrealistic human form on the Rorschach is that they represent privately held, personalized fantasies designed to ward off painful reality (Blatt, Schimek, & Brenneis, 1980). The purpose of this chapter is to place selected Rorschach responses side by side with clinical descriptions in order to suggest why, for some patients, giving up thought disorder and private elaborations of the human form on the Rorschach might be related to independent evidence of concomitant positive change.

Thus, we turn to detailed descriptions of four inpatients in an effort to identify some of the more prominent relationships that exist between the psychological test measures and the independent clinical evaluation of therapeutic change. Here we reverse the research process that has occupied much of this book so far. Instead of abstracting and reducing the complexity of the individual case in order to develop constructs applicable across many patients, we now take our identified and validated psychological test constructs, especially those derived from the Rorschach, and demonstrate their rich resonances within the single case.

Two of these inpatients, a man and a woman, presented primarily introjective configurations of psychopathology. The other two, also a man and a woman, had primarily anaclitic disorders. These broad, contrasting diagnostic categories of anaclitic and introjective disorders represent a basic dichotomy used throughout this research. Patients manifesting mainly introjective psychopathology reveal primarily over-ideational symptoms; their preoccupations are with issues of anger, aggression, and self-definition. By contrast, patients with mainly anaclitic psychopathology focus on issues of affection, intimacy, and attempts to establish and maintain satisfying interpersonal relations (Blatt, 1974, 1990b; Blatt & Shichman, 1983). For the anaclitic patients, in accordance with our theoretical formulations and research findings, we will look at changes in both the elaboration of the representation of the human figure on the Rorschach and its relation to consensual reality; for the introjective patients, correspondingly, we will concentrate on shifts in thought disorder.

Each of these four patients was considered to be markedly improved. The estimates of improvement were made from case reports prepared by the clinical staff at two points in the treatment process, soon after admission and then after approximately 15 months of treatment. Using selected Rorschach responses obtained at these same two points, juxtaposed with selected excerpts or summaries of relevant case descriptions, we attempt to suggest why, for the two anaclitic patients, progress is marked by evidence of diminished investment in the unrealistic representation of the human figure and why, for the two introjective patients, progress is marked by evidence of lessened thought disorder.

CASE I: IMPROVED ANACLITIC MALE

Mr. F, a man in his early twenties, was diagnosed at admission as having a "schizophrenic character disorder" (what would now be termed a Schizotypal Personality Disorder in DSM III-R) with "depressive and paranoid features." He had always been a marginal performer, feeling himself different from other people, lonely, directionless, and an object of ridicule. His earliest memories center around his beating up smaller children or being attacked himself by bullies.

His father, a self-made executive from an impoverished background, largely withdrew from his family for fear that any open opposition to his wife would precipitate psychotic episodes in her. During the patient's adolescence, the father experienced a severe identity crisis centering on ambivalence toward his own overachievement. The patient's mother, described as a "cold, tight, probably chronically paranoid, schizophrenic woman," had strong protective feelings toward the patient whom she saw as a damaged child because of his long-standing timidity.

At admission, Mr. F revealed a range of moods from angry, violent, bitter hatefulness to a sensitive softness and vulnerability. Despite the easy exercise of stereotypic, overlearned verbal skills that enabled him to simulate clear thinking, his capacity for attention or conceptual precision was frequently marred by a substrate of vagueness. In unstructured or emotionally stimulating situations, his thinking became more openly disorganized. Although tending in the patient community to be either isolated or involved in hostile collusion around illicit drugs, he came regularly to his initial therapy sessions, did not want to leave, and told his therapist that he had ideas he was too anxious to reveal. It was thought at the initial case conference that any intensified transference experience with his female therapist would arouse in him fear that he would drive her mad; he might therefore cover up and withdraw from involvement.

Rorschach Protocol of Mr. F: Initial Testing

RORSCHACH CARD I AT TIME 1

(Mr. F is using the entire blot in all five associations.)

1. Looks like somebody, reminds me of someone riding a horse or motorcycle, colliding with two people walking down the street. They are jumping out of the way.

(Someone?) Two figures look like people and I sense a type of motion in symbolism of people and another figure behind them.

2. Looks like a bug maybe after I stepped on it.

(Bug?) It just looked like a mess. All of it. (Stepped?) Just something that came to my mind.

3. Maybe a smudge of oil or grime.

(Smudge?) It looks smudge just like somebody had grease on a cloth and wiped it out. (Oil?) The darkness is like black motor oil.

4. An explosion within one's mind.

(Explosion?) Looking from the center to the sides separating out. The hands in the center are trying to escape from the two negatives on the side.

5. Two winged people trying to carry a woman off into the sky.

(People?) Looked like wings and heads, like the shape of a woman's body in the center.

On Card I of the Rorschach at Time 1, we have clear evidence of aggressive, damaging impulsivity (Response 1: "someone riding a . . . motorcycle, colliding with two people") followed later by depressive content (Response 3: "a smudge of oil or grime") followed by defensive, hypomanic content attempting to restore what is destroyed (Response 5: "two winged people trying to carry a woman off . . ."). Of particular importance is Response 4 ("an explosion within one's mind"), for it is here that our scoring technology captures the nuances of this young man's object representation. The key phrase is "the hands in the center are trying to escape from the two negatives on the side." Although the "hands" in question are readily identified in the upper center of the blot, this response, because of the merger of the "hands" with the "two negatives on the side" (previously identified as a "smudge" or a "mess"), is scored as a "spoiled form" response and therefore as a poor or inaccurate form. Clinically, it is evident that in Response 1, the patient has projected the same destructive impulse that in Response 2 ("a bug after I stepped on it") is introjected. It is from this introjected conflict—namely, the presumed search for closeness, leading to murderous feelings following deprivation, leading to introjected dysphoric feelings, leading to a flight into a manic defense—that he seeks to flee in Response 4. An "explosion in one's mind" aptly characterizes his isolated, subjective experience, where he is left alone with weakened resources to escape from largely unmodulated overstimulation. Response 4 condenses into a single response both his high level of impulsive, destructive affect and his cutoff, limited, and isolated resources for control. Contact with others is so dangerous that he must escape into fantastical thought. He is left simply with "hands . . . trying to escape. . . ."

The following is summarized from the therapist's reporting of the course in treatment for Mr. F: For several months, the therapy was marked by a heavy, oppressed mood that both patient and therapist shared. When he did talk, Mr. F gave long recitals of his violent feelings and his sense of being oppressed. He was often condescending and refused to talk to his therapist about what was on his mind. Seven months into the treatment, he began to bring in some everyday problems, particularly his alienation among the other patients. Patient and therapist began to deal with his transference to the institution, particularly Mr. F's ambivalence about its craziness and the fact that for him it was home. Nine months into the treatment he raised the question of a change of therapist, which focused on the therapist's disinclination to urge activity. "He seemed," wrote his therapist, "to be saying that he wanted to hear that I could tolerate his depression, craziness, and lack of accomplishment." This sequence led to increased initiatives by Mr. F in the patient community and in activities. Finally, at 14 months, he began an intense, and in some ways helpful, relationship with a female patient, which he discussed openly. In the case conference at Time 2, the therapist made the following comment about the transference: "I think until the last month I hadn't thought there was any transference with me at all. I'm not sure what it was or where I was; it was like I was being kept someplace. But in the last month he comes in, he notices, he's observing what's in my office, a new picture, talking about it, asking me how I am . . . and its' suddenly like I'm *there*, which I haven't really been before."

Rorschach Protocol of Mr. F: Second Testing

RORSCHACH CARD I AT TIME 2

I see all kinds of things.

1. This could be somebody waving.

(Waving?) Like a hand, a person's head, a cape. Nothing there that really represents an arm.

2. This sort of reminds me of an elephant with big ears.

(Elephant?) These look sort of like ears. A nose on the bottom with a trunk.

3. Like a human sitting on a throne or chair. (Card is being held upside down.)

(Human?) This is a person with arms. This is a crown or large hat.

The contrast between the responses at Time 1 and Time 2 is clear on Rorschach Card I: There is marked reduction in the urgency to cope with intense, destructive impulses. Rather than a triad involved in violent moves toward separation, he now perceives a single person. His association of "somebody waving" suggests a marked reduction in both the scope and intensity of the previous internal press to push people apart. The responses convey a sense of a slowing, a toning down of urgent needs and fears, and much less of an anxious scanning for the already decided on clues concerning separateness. Rather, his style is more controlled and sequential. In Response I, for example, he allows himself a pause in order to make critical assessments concerning perceptual support in the blot ("nothing there that really represents . . ."). He reveals a less pressured associational content that does not elaborate beyond available perceptual support. Thus, in terms of our research measure, he is relinquishing an intense investment in unrealistic, autistic fantasy (OR−) and is beginning to establish a more accurate conception of interpersonal reality. He can allow more neutral, even vague content (Response 2: "an elephant with big ears"). Dysphoric affect is absent, and although there are still hypomanic strivings (Response 3: "a human . . . on a throne . . . a crown . . ."), there is also evidence of modulation and control of these strivings ("a human, sitting . . . " as opposed to the "colliding" of Time 1).

The most pertinent response for our purposes involves the same "hands" in Response 4 of Time 1. These hands, which were seen as disconnected and fleeing from overstimulating and unmanageable experience at Time 1, are now seen as connected (albeit with no "arm" in evidence) and "waving." Having been subordinated to the fourth response at Time 1, the association to hands becomes the first response at Time 2. This first response at Time 2 suggests both greater internal control and evidence of a willingness to initiate contact with an as yet undefined other ("somebody waving . . . like a hand . . .").

This sequence from Response 4 at Time 1 of disembodied "hands . . . trying to escape" to Response 1 at Time 2 of "somebody waving . . . a hand" constitutes an example of an anaclitic patient's relinquishment of an autistically elaborated and poorly perceived human form for a more reality-based but less elaborated human representation. Such a relinquishment is identified by our empirical results as evidence of positive therapeutic change.

In the case conference at Time 2, several discussants commented on "the simple, matter-of-fact, clear-cut, rather unemotional . . . yet warm . . . presentation" of the therapist. One noted "the structure which is being provided while also letting the patient go his own rather isolated way." Another spoke of the therapist as "standing by and being available, as a person to whom Mr. F can come regularly and just be with." But perhaps the most apposite comment for our purposes was from a senior member of the clinical staff who said, "I think it is . . . evidence of Mr. F's strength that the therapist hasn't felt that there was a transference of any kind. For this patient to succeed in keeping out of expression, and probably out of awareness, any of the feelings that he's placing onto his therapist from his very disturbed and destructive mother who would be a principal source of the transference, *is* transference, with a reverse twist that reflects Mr. F's strength."

Although one might not have inferred such information about the transference from the Rorschach data in isolation, the summary construct that the patient imposes on the blot of "somebody waving" aptly and rather entirely captures the essence of the necessarily distant but nonetheless positive transference that Mr. F had thus far been able to develop with his therapist.

CASE II: IMPROVED ANACLITIC FEMALE

Ms. I is a woman in her late teens for whom the severity of the diagnosis at admission was uncertain. She showed hysterical, obsessional, and paranoid qualities, and the degree of her interpersonal withdrawal at least suggested a schizophrenic reaction. The general working diagnosis at admission was of a long-standing depression in a hysterical character with serious borderline features. At the Time 2 case conference, it was thought that Ms. I possessed the inner conflicts of a hysteric—specifically the longing to be intruded on sexually together with the fear that anyone who does so will overwhelm her—but that weaknesses in her family structure did not allow her to manifest the symptoms of a hysteric. When Ms. I was 8 years old, her mother threw her 17-year old sister out of the house because of the sister's promiscuity. Her parents subsequently divorced. At age 16, a year before her mother remarried, Ms. I gave birth to a child, placed it for adoption, and probably suffered a postpartum psychotic reaction.

At admission, Ms. I's depression was expressed as a pervasive sense of emptiness, emotional deadness, and defectiveness rather than as acute grief or pain. She felt passive and helpless. She was better able to function in situations that required passive repetition and was much less able to integrate actively. She was constricted and unsure about her own emotional experience and appeared as a wistful, conventional little girl who externalized responsibility and was in search of responses, particularly enacted emotional responses. In therapy, she sat with her legs open and often screamed that she was nothing. She tended to be isolated in the patient community but was more clinging and seeking of time with her therapist than persons described as schizophrenic. She manifested a depressive's typical attempts to control the therapist through a pathetic, grasping helplessness. At the same time, others experienced her as profoundly passive, amorphous, and difficult to understand.

Rorschach Protocol of Ms. I: Initial Testing

RORSCHACH CARD IV AT TIME 1

1. Some kind of woolly creature. It's got really big feet. (Ms. I is using the entire blot.)

2. And this part in here (small, white area in the center) sort of looks like a fetus. It's got an umbilical cord, sort of misplaced a little, I think. A fetus with wings. (She laughs.) Like it's an angel fetus.

(Angel fetus?) The head and the little ass, and its feet were sort of coming down; they weren't curled up. I guess it couldn't be inside the womb in that position. It was a little high up but it was attached to something in the center.

In her first response to Card IV of the Rorschach at Time 1, Ms. I manages only a minimal differentiation and integration of the entire blot. She begins with the edge of the card ("woolly") and the most evident detail ("big feet") and stops her delineation there. By contrast, in Response 2, she gives considerable elaboration to a small, white space embedded in the center of the blot. These elaborate associations to a humanoidlike figure are imposed on a small inner area of the blot that does not support them; it is a response involving poor form. At the same time, the response is extensively differentiated and integrated, including a serious fabulized combination (much like a contamination tendency) ("angel fetus," "fetus with wings").

This second response is clearly important and highly overdetermined. It is an idealized, fantasy-based image of the child she lost to adoption. For our purposes, however, the emphasis here is on her own self-image in relation to her therapist. In locating this image within the inner confines of the "woolly creature," she tries to defend against her incipient anxiety about being intruded on and instead becomes the one doing the intruding. However, she must retreat as far as possible from any hint of aggressive impulse; thus she urgently seeks a most extreme description of benign impotence ("an angel fetus"). At the same time in this complex response, she is equally able to capture the tenacious and potent clinging inherent in her passive-dependent, depressive position. This is indeed a patient who gets under the therapist's skin! First she discovers herself securely embedded in some larger, undefined, but protective surround. From that position, one can sense in her a certain glee as she makes fine differentiations hinting at aggressive potential (the "feet" that "were curled up" but "were sort of coming down" and "the little ass"). In retrospect, one might even perceive a positive prognostic sign in her willingness to use the protective surrounding as a base for initiative. But the hinting at such initiative is weak.

Her therapist reported Ms. I's extensive attacks on his privacy, complemented by his own constant inability to create any lasting meaning between them, as well as a steady impotence in his efforts to fill her up and satisfy her by his presence. A major turning point occurred 8 months into the therapy when the therapist set down an emphatic refusal to tolerate further coercive regression; at this point, Ms. I, outside the therapy, began to shift away from interpersonal isolation. Her subsequent sexual promiscuity and her taking of trips away from the hospital seemed indicative of an ambivalently expressed initiative. On one hand, her therapist felt isolated and abandoned as Ms. I engaged in an extensive liaison with a young man outside the hospital, a liaison resulting in pregnancy and an abortion. On the other hand, the therapist directly experienced her as somewhat less defensive and repetitive and a little warmer.

At the case conference at Time 2, one discussant commented on this patient's preoccupation with the making of ornamented boxes. He noticed that in her semideliberate regression in the therapy, as well as in her history of giving away her baby at age 16 and in her more recent abortion, Ms. I enacts the identity of someone who once contained something worthwhile only to have that valuable thing taken away and herself left empty.

Rorschach Protocol of Ms. I: Second Testing

RORSCHACH CARD IV AT TIME 2

1. There's his feet. He's like a big animal; big feet. I don't know what you call him; just a monster. His feet, his head, his arms, his hands.

(Big feet?) Furry, like a gorilla, I guess. (Furry?) Here (Ms. I points to edge of blot). Because it's not smooth; it's shaggy. The edge and the inside, too. Mostly the edge, I think.

5. I see a person.
(Person?) Some man. Who, I don't know. He's not pretty.

The first part of her Rorschach at Time 2 suggests a modulation in her experiences of abandonment. The initial Time 1 response of "woolly creature" (that creature that surrounds and contains a tiny "angel fetus") now at Time 2 receives two new definitions: The "creature" becomes more accessible ("furry") and more humanoid ("gorilla"). Thus, at Time 2, the environment that surrounds the tiny creature in the inner white space becomes integrated into a slightly more available context, although that environment is still ambivalently welcoming and not yet clearly human. These new definitions may represent both nascent positive experiences of the therapist and some shifting in her own self-evaluation.

But the major change is in Response 5, where the heavily described and securely ensconced "angel fetus" at Time 1 now, at Time 2, becomes an unenclosed, largely undefined "person."

At the conference at Time 2, a discussant described two identity fragments available to this patient. Historically important here, once again, is the fact that when Ms. I was 8 years old, the mother threw the patient's 17-year old sister out of the house because of her promiscuity. In the long beginning phase of the therapy, Ms. I behaved as if she were a small child, requiring the therapist to enact the role of protective parent. However, when the therapist refused to tolerate her coercive regression, Ms. I swung abruptly from being a clinging child to becoming a promiscuous woman, albeit without much feeling and without clear definition.

Returning again to the Rorschach, the "angel fetus" of Time 1, which is a percept of poor form heavily invested with autistic definition, is perceived as wholly inside and contained by the surrounding "creature." At Time 2, by contrast, this same percept emerges as a full person in the outer world, albeit someone who lacks clear definition and is "not pretty." This Rorschach human form response may thus be seen as presenting in summary fashion both some possible transformations in the patient's experience of her therapist and a second stage (that of ill-defined promiscuity) in Ms. I's effort to develop a feminine identity.

This example constitutes a second illustration of how, in an anaclitic patient, a decrease in the elaboration of the representation of an inaccurately perceived human form (from the highly defined but ineptly located "angel fetus" to the far less defined and still ineptly located "person") might be related to clinical observation of partial improvement.

CASE III: IMPROVED INTROJECTIVE MALE

Mr. B, a man in his early twenties, described himself as fearing he was "going to fall apart" or "go over the edge." The general picture on admission was of a severely anxious young adult with uncoalesced identity fragments who was struggling against a regressive pull from a destructive and very disturbed mother. In the past, Mr. B had feared punishment or indifference from his father; recently, he had sought closeness with him but then perceived him as ridiculed and "spineless." Mr. B's diagnosis was of a narcissistic character with borderline and obsessive features.

Mr. B revealed large gaps when trying to recall some of the previous year's events. He could be articulate and coherent, but often the sessions became a tumble of themes, with the urgency of an emerging new thought interrupting the prior theme that he had just begun to discuss. He possessed a degree of self-observation but was steadily concerned he might inadvertently "let out" material that would lead to strong shame or guilt. When he stumbled into inappropriately revealing responses, he mobilized ineffective, obsessional-like defenses during which he offered everything he could think of in a desperate manner. To minimize the pressured intensity of his inner experience, he spent much of his energy censoring, doubting, and denying his feelings and impulses.

Rorschach Protocol of Mr. B: Initial Testing

RORSCHACH CARDS I AND IX AT TIME 1

Card I

2. Two hands reaching out. Like you're looking down on something flying, with two hands reaching out.

(Hands?) Looks like it's flying. Because of the line down the body. It looks like a bird. The line looks like a spine.

I don't know why I saw it looking down, because it could be looking up, too. (fabulized combination-serious)

3. A woman with a shirt, with hands, but her head is screwed up. Her skirt is bell-shaped.

(Woman?) The head is messed up. There shouldn't be two mounds. It's not my idea of a woman's head. Hands reaching up, like a peasant woman dancing, from behind. I wonder why I see it from behind? It could just as well be from the front. I see something else: a woman from behind. A woman's ass. Because her feet are going off at any angle. It's sort of a round shape of her rear. This is interesting! Wow!

Card IX

1. This is like a psychic spirit; very hazy and it's blue. This figure here. This tall, thin thing. There's a blue aura around it. Oh, wow! Down here it's red and here it's green. Green is like a learning stage you go through. There is blue: the head. It shows psychic growth.

The whole development of the spirit. It's like moving. The orange is broken away. It's rising and will break away and be completely free. It will vanish, with a oneness, realizing a part of everything and not exist as a self. It will go into everything. It won't need to exist as a separate thing. As soon as a person says a word, he must realize it becomes part of everything—realizes his own oneness. (confabulation; contamination tendency)

Consistent with the obsessive features of his primarily introjective personality organization, Mr. B emphasized on Card I the instability of his own point of view: Is he below or above, behind or in front? He was likewise unable to control the integration of percept and association: He perceived "hands" (and, by inference, "wings"), which he introduced in order to justify the serious fabulized combination of "flying," which fits his subjective sense of instability. Then, as if to emphasize this instability, he retreated to the *terra firma* of the center "line" and produced the ill-fitting association of "spine." (We recall his reaching out to his "spineless" father.)

Continuing on Card I, Mr. B latched onto the relatively conventional and popular percepts "woman with a shirt" and (again) "hands." But then, as his associations outran his percepts, he could not integrate the "messed up" head. He gave voice to his renewed disorientation by locating the confusion in himself as viewer. (Is he "in front" or "behind"?) Finally, he revealed further loss of control by indicating his subjective experience of the blot unfolding, as it were, before his eyes ("I see something else. . . . Wow!).

Mr. B's display of a rapid associative movement from "flying" to "bird" to "spine," and his barely modulated sense of being unstably located within his entire associative world, reveal his desperate dilemma: how to resist the powerful, seductive pull of his "messed up" mother when he has no other position or place in which to anchor himself.

Under the pressure of Card IX's combined stimuli of color and dedifferentiation, Mr. B revealed his most extreme loss of control over subjective experience. He behaved as if the blot possessed an initiative of its own; no longer could he maintain a sense of himself as author or agent: "It's like moving. The orange is broken away. It's rising and will break away. . . . It will vanish." Initially, he tried to ground himself by focusing on boundaries defined by the colors. But he rapidly became incoherent, using language that evoked an experience of merger.

One way to understand this thought-disordered material is to consider it as representing Mr. B's great difficulty, when subjected to simultaneous overstimulation and dedifferentiation, in holding onto an internalized other of sufficient clarity and stability to enable his own self-definition. Thus, his subjective sense of self as organizer, as delineator and unifier, simply fragments and "vanishes."

Early in treatment, Mr. B developed a positive, idealizing transference with his male therapist: "I want to stay with you; here is important, outside is not." "I like how straight and calm you are." But then, in what turned out to be a repeated pattern, he anticipated being controlled. In response, he attempted to control all the ways in which he might engage the therapist. He noted, "I'm covering over more and more. I was ready to let things go when I first came."

Mr. B then proceeded to explore a range of experiences with his therapist: wishing to compete with him, arouse his envy, place him in the role of uniting his parents or excluding them. He began to worry about becoming competitive and mean. At the same time, he started to discover others as both critical of him and too dangerously powerful to be confronted directly. Throughout this period, he consciously feared more serious disorganization.

Although oedipal issues seemed to be prominent, it became clear that the primary pathway of change was in Mr. B's revision of the internalization of his father: He moved from experiencing his father/therapist both as omnipotent and coercive, on the one hand, and as someone he could defeat, on the other, to realizing his father as someone who might hurt him and whom he might hurt. This latter alternative he would achieve both through heavy criticism and by being disappointing. These processes led to some fearful, extremely tentative explorations of his longings for merger with his mother. But such concerns were summarily curtailed in favor of more introjective issues around vocational identity and discharge. Mr. B actively began to consolidate a part identity of someone able to work; here he consciously modeled himself on an aspect of his father's early vocation. Mr. B's emphasis on establishing and maintaining a viable self-concept—in contrast to the focus of anaclitic patients on interpersonal relations and feelings—illustrates a major concern of introjective patients. This consolidation led to marked oscillations between seeing himself as still helpless to control and modulate his impulses and experiencing himself as having developed a sufficiently stable and functional identity that would enable him to move on.

Rorschach Protocol of Mr. B: Second Testing

RORSCHACH CARDS I AND IX AT TIME 2

Card I

2. In the middle there's a dancer with a translucent, see-through dress, with her hands reaching forward, and we're looking at it from behind. It's really distorted and out of proportion.

(Dancer?) We're looking at the back. Hips, legs, they're together. Her tunic is way too long. I saw these bumps and thought of two heads, but now I see one head: this dark part here, with the shoulders and hands going out. (Translucent?) You can see her hips, the outline. Like it's translucent. It's big, billowy dress, way too big. It's out of proportion, with trunk too long and the dress too big. (Dancer?) More the hands made me think of a dancer and the silhouette of the legs and hips.

Card IX

1. I see first—have the feeling—my vocabulary isn't good—something dreamlike or ethereal. What does ethereal mean? In the middle, there's a tall silhouette of a spirit that's very hazy.

(Silhouette?) This section here that's light blue and green—sort of hazy—with the spirit kind of thing. It's very hazy.

(Light blue or green?) There are no sharp lines. It looks like the spirit forms out of the pink and green into the top part. Sort of the spirit rising. This pale blue–green here could be an aura around the spirit.

On Card I at Time 2, Mr. B is much firmer about his own point of view. The established association of "something flying with two hands reaching out" is now no longer in evidence. He is more certain, in comparison with Time 1, about his anchored viewpoint as observer ("We're looking at it from behind"). The use of the collaborative "we" suggests a sense of sharing, participation and identification with a stabilizing other. Moreover, he is able to integrate, without the earlier evidences of disequilibrium, his two originally separated percepts of "skirt" and "woman's ass" into one: "a dancer with a translucent, see-through dress." Although the associative material remains sexually provocative, his characterization at Time 2 of the single human percept as a "dancer" places the figure, despite its open sexuality, in a more modulated and better-defined context.

Further evidence of his growing sense of stability is found in his more critical evaluation at Time 2 of the fit between association and percept ("It is really distorted and out of proportion"). His assumption that the blot is at fault may represent an intermediate step between his earlier state of great uncertainty about the stability of what he sees and an as yet unrealized capacity for relaxed self-criticism.

Similarly, on Card IX, although the basic content is not much different from the earlier testing, his language suggests a considerably increased sense of himself as the originator of his percepts. He no longer appears so strenuously tasked by Card IX's combination of exciting color and confusing dedifferentiation. Rather, he is now consciously imposing his own definitions and is aware that he is the author of what he sees. Although he remains unable to define and integrate whatever is "dreamlike or ethereal," "very hazy," and with "no sharp lines," he does not now have to flee the field of inquiry into incoherence. The severe thought disorder noted in this response at Time 1 has significantly diminished.

In sum, the evidence offered in this example suggests a degree of recovery in Mr. B's subjective sense of stability and control. As a consequence, he is somewhat better able to demarcate his own inner experience; he can thus relinquish the protection of a thought-disordered retreat.

At the Time 2 case conference, it was evident that Mr. B was planning to be discharged and wanted to continue with his therapist on a private basis. Some discussants at the case conference wondered whether his choice of work identity was premature and would limit further exploration. Others thought that at this point, having come through a deeply disturbed emotional state and still concerned with psychological survival, he could not possibly now be prepared to solidify a more inclusive identity.

CASE IV: IMPROVED INTROJECTIVE FEMALE

Ms. K, a woman in her mid-twenties, had experienced a growing sense of futility, depression, and detachment. Becoming seriously confused, she was no longer able to function in the daily tasks of work and living. Her diagnosis at admission was of decompensation in a longstanding, severe obsessive character disorder with depressive and masochistic features.

Sad and angry looking, she hid her femininity. Clearly, she was depressed, but the manner in which she withdrew, with her face appearing tense and flushed, made her look as if she were in a rage. Rarely spontaneous, and with a restrained and careful manner consistent with her primary introjective personality organization, she described herself as having two parts: her controlled, ordinary self, and "something else." She feared she could become violent.

At her most depressed, Ms. K described herself as being completely detached and without feelings. Yet she became upset, even furious, when she could not keep a tight control over her wants and longings. She revealed great sexual confusion and was very much frightened by the prospect of intimacy.

When she allowed the expression of some hope, she said that she wanted to establish a more effective identity—to be in contact with herself, to be a woman and not an overgrown child, that is, not always having to become whatever person she happened to like at a particular time.

Rorschach Protocol of Ms. K: Initial Testing

RORSCHACH CARDS I AND VIII AT TIME 1

Card I

1. It looks like two devils or demons. They're pulling, fighting over a woman. They're trying to take her away, and she's fighting them.

(Devils?) They're wearing big, black cloaks, and they have on pointed hats. They might be magicians. In any case, they're evil. (Evil?) Just because they look like devils, magicians. (Anything else?) No. Just—they're trying to take the woman away, standing above her, pulling on her. (fabulized to confabulation) (Woman?) It just looked like a woman because a dress on and two heads. I can't explain the two heads, but she looks like a woman. (Taking her away?) They were taking her away to become a prostitute. (Prostitute?) Yes. (Anything else?) No. (fabulized combination-serious)

Card VIII

2. This thing up here is a genie.

(Genie?) Partly because it's a peculiar-looking thing coming up behind two curtains, as if it might come out of a bottle. An ethereal sort of thing. That much is behind the curtain. (confabulation tendency)

3. The rest of it is some kind of curtain—except for his head and arms—that he's hiding behind. I don't know what he's doing.

(Curtain?) It doesn't particularly, but it's just something that the genie is coming out of. (Out of?) No, I mean he's coming over the top of it. Kind of like the wizard in *The Wizard of Oz*. The wizard comes out from behind the curtain. (fabulized combination-regular)

Ms. K clearly presents themes of masochistic helplessness, the projection of sadistic intent, and the coalescing of destructive violence with sexual desire. On the one hand, she is hapless victim; on the other, she projects powerful, uncontrolled, fused sexual and aggressive impulses. It is as if she can discover no sufficient locus of modulating control, either inside herself or from another, to bind and master unacceptable impulses that threaten to "come up out of a bottle" or "[come] over the top." Her thought-disordered, overelaborated responses, in which the spatial contiguity of two percepts is taken as creating a coalesced relationship between the percepts ("a woman because a dress on and two heads . . . They were taking her away to become a prostitute"), become an appropriate means to describe the marked absence of sufficient boundaries lodged within her experience.

Her course in treatment, as evaluated in summary terms at her second case conference, was characterized as having proceeded well. Crucial elements in the therapy were seen to be her male therapist's flexibility, playfulness, and willingness to accept, in a nonpressuring manner, Ms. K's growing capacity for childlike behavior. The therapist appeared to have been for Ms. K highly visible, available for gradual attachment, and steadily usable for an increasing number of partial identifications.

Rorschach Protocols of Ms. K: Second Testing
KORSCHACH CARDS I AND VIII AT TIME 2

Card I

1. You want me to look at it top-side up? (Ms. K rotates card.) It's what I saw before if I hold it [top-side up]. I remember what I saw before seemed like a woman in the middle, perhaps with two heads, and on either side of her were satanic, winged creatures pulling at her. (fabulized combination-serious; confabulation)

2. But it also looks like some kind of bird flying (the entire card), either way (Ms. K holds the card top-side up and then upside-down). That's all on that one. (Ms. K turns card over.)

(Very big?) It looks as though it has a massive body and wings up like this and I'm looking at it. (First part of "wing" is seen; rest of "wing" is obscured.) (Bird?) I hadn't thought of what kind of bird, except it might be an eagle or albatross, except that the albatross is all white.

Card VIII

2. Upside-down it looks like a torso, opened, so it's flat and these two things that were bears (i.e., in the previous response) are lungs, and

some ribs in the middle, and that's (at bottom) a pelvis, and this, the spine (Ms. K runs her finger up the middle of the card), and that's (blue) muscles in the back, and this part (orange) muscles in front, and these two (center pink) are breasts, and it hasn't got a heart. That's unfortunate.

(See something like this?) Perhaps in my science lab when I was in ninth grade. I can't think of any place since then. I have in my mind a fancy anatomy textbook with plastic layers in it (Ms. K describes the kind of book) and all done in bright colors.

Among the most available evidence of change is Ms. K's greater control over the urgency of her associations. At Time 1 she experienced herself either as participating as actor (Card I: "they're pulling," and "she's fighting") or, under the greater stimulation of color, as reacting helplessly to an unfolding drama (Card VIII: "it's a peculiar-looking thing coming up . . . I don't know what he's doing"; "he's coming over the top of it . . ."). At Time 2, she experienced the stimulus less as impinging on her and more as under her control (Card I: "I remember what I saw"; "I'm looking at it"; Card VIII: "I have in my mind a fancy anatomy textbook with plastic layers in it").

On Card VIII at the first testing, Ms. K avoided altogether the evocative stimulation of color (i.e., of emotion). Now, still avoiding, she chooses the metaphor of anatomy, suggesting a curiosity about what is inside. With less fearfulness and self-doubt, she begins to turn the pages, as it were, in a beginning, weak attempt to locate names for her feelings. Her search for a more stabilized identity includes attempts to articulate affective experiences more fully. Clearly, she has a way to go before she can transform her emerging feminine identity and her still inchoate emotions into initiatives toward intimacy. But she seems aware of the work ahead—and at the same time makes a playful bow to *The Wizard of Oz* (". . . it hasn't got a heart. That's unfortunate"). Although she remains unable yet to probe her emotional experience, as evidenced on Card VIII by her continuing inability to integrate color, she also is much less threatened by her previous capacity to dissociate this same experience, as evidenced by her subjective sense at Time 1 of being out of control. Thus far, the pressure of unintegrated (projected) impulses is lessened, and with it, a relinquishing of some disordered thinking. How she will proceed to reorganize her experience is as yet unclear.

The general attitude of the clinical staff at Ms. K's Time 2 case conference was that she was just beginning to enter into a wider appreciation of her feeling states. Some of the more negative aspects of these feelings still needed to be clarified; she possessed reservoirs of hostility that she did not yet understand. She had much work to do experimenting with feminine and maternal identifications and had yet to become attached to a man other than her therapist. Given her difficulties, it was thought that Ms. K's psychological development was proceeding appropriately and that nothing should be rushed.

SUMMARY

These four case illustrations, typical of the range of material in this rich body of clinical data, provide detailed examples of two of the major findings of this research: (1) how, for anaclitic patients, observed improvement correlates with decreased investment in inappropriate or autistic fantasies about human relationships, and (2) how, for introjective patients, observed improvement correlates with decreased reliance on disordered thinking.

Thus, for the anaclitic Mr. F, his Time 1 Rorschach presentation of a fantastically elaborated human relationship revealed him as inchoately embedded in—and then barely escaping—chaos. By Time 2, he used this same area of the blot to represent a human figure distantly engaged in vague contact with an as yet undefined other. These responses fit well with Mr. F's extremely tentative efforts to come closer to a benign female therapist who represented the dangerous and engulfing madness of his mother.

The anaclitic Ms. I, at Time 1, autistically elaborated a tiny human figure discovered first as symbiotically ensconced within a largely undefined other and then revealed as powerfully passive, grandiose, and helpless. By Time 2, Ms. I used this same area of the blot to reveal an impoverished representation of an undesirable adult figure in ambiguous relationship to a somewhat more benign, humanoid surround. This shift in human representation corresponds well with Ms. I's movement from a primitive merger transference to a relatively more distant, more separated involvement with her therapist, a movement partially disguised by her reawakened adolescent promiscuity.

The resonances for introjective patients between a reduction in thought disorder on the Rorschach and improved clinical behavior are more subtle and less dramatic even though these findings are well documented in the empirical data presented in earlier chapters. Relinquishment of thought disorder for a particular area of a Rorschach blot does not usually result in easily identifiable residues. The patient's referents instead often become vague or unrevealingly conventional as the patient attempts to reestablish contact with reality.

The introjective Mr. B, urgently seeking psychic structuring to facilitate his separation from a dangerously seductive mother, revealed a style of thinking at Time 1 characterized by instability, permeable boundaries, and an unintegrated, vulnerable definition of self and others. At Time 2, following the tentative rearousal and reworking of identity fragments deriving from his father, Mr. B was able to represent a more stable, delimited, but still often vague array of self and other definitions to the same areas of the Rorschach.

Similarly, the introjective Ms. K, initially struggling to maintain a tight control over her internal emotional states, expressed on her Time 1 Rorschach the arousal of projected destructive violence and inchoate sexual urges. By Time 2, following her growing ability to use her therapist for an increasing number of partial identifications, Ms. K used the same areas of the Rorschach to indicate that the pressure of the unintegrated, projected impulses had lessened, and with it the need to resort so intensively to her original levels of disordered thinking.

It seems altogether appropriate that these subtle shifts in the imaginative worlds of these patients, as assessed on the Rorschach, should be related to constructive behavioral change. These parallel changes in imagination and in behavior reveal the efforts of these seriously disturbed patients to relinquish deeply established, maladaptive efforts to find a sense of safety by avoiding and distorting and, instead, to become more realistically and appropriately involved, even if tentatively, with people who are now the central figures in their lives.

CHAPTER 9

The Prediction of Therapeutic Change

One of the more fascinating and important questions in psychotherapy research is the prediction of who is likely to gain from the treatment experience. Still applicable today is Frank's (1979) comment:

> After decades of research, the amount of well-established, clinically relevant knowledge about psychotherapeutic outcome still remains disappointingly meager. Although some relationships between determinants and outcome have attained statistical significance, few are powerful enough to be clinically relevant, and most of [these] . . . are intuitively obvious. An example is the finding that patients who begin therapy at a high level of functioning terminate at higher levels than those who begin at lower levels. In other words, the healthier one is to start with, the healthier one is at the end (Garfield, 1978). . . . [R]esearch . . . to date suggest that the major determinants of therapeutic success appear to lie in aspects of patients' personality and style of life (pp. 310, 312).

Although sociodemographic variables such as age, sex, race, social class, education, intelligence, and marital status may influence to some extent who gets selected for therapy, these factors generally have little direct effect on therapeutic outcome (Lambert & Asay, 1984). The psychological qualities a patient brings to the therapy situation are probably the most important factors determining the outcome of therapy (Garfield, 1978; Lambert, 1979; Lambert & Asay, 1984; Luborsky, 1975b; Luborsky et al., 1980; Meltzoff & Kornreich, 1970; Strupp, 1980a), especially the patient's capacity to become involved in a therapeutic relationship (Gomes–Schwartz, 1978).

The establishment of a therapeutic relationship was initially viewed in psychotherapy research as primarily a function of the therapist's interpersonal skills like empathy, positive regard, and authenticity (e.g., Rogers, 1957, 1959; Truax, Tunnell, Fine, & Wargo, 1966; Truax et al., 1967). Later research (e.g., Strupp, 1980a, b, c, d) indicated, however, that differences in outcome are more often a result of the patient's capacity to enter into a therapeutic alliance (Hartley & Strupp, 1983). Strupp (1980b, p. 716) commented:

> If the patient is a person who by virtue of his past life experience is capable of human relatedness and therefore is amenable to learning mediated within that context, the outcome, even though the individual may have suffered traumas, reverses, and other vicissitudes, is likely to be positive. . . . If, on the other hand, his early life experiences have been so destructive that human relatedness has failed to acquire a markedly positive valence, and elaborate neurotic and characterological malfunctions have created massive barriers to intimacy . . . chances are that psychotherapy either results in failure or at best in very modest gains.

Various studies indicate that the severity of a patient's psychological disturbances at the outset of treatment is another major factor influencing therapeutic outcome. A large number of studies report that more-integrated and less-disturbed patients are more likely to have a positive therapeutic outcome (e.g., Barron, 1953; Garfield, 1978; Katz & Solomon, 1958; McNair, Lorr, Young, Roth, & Boyd, 1964; Rogers, Gendlin, Kiesler, & Truax, 1967; Luborsky, Chandler, Auerbach, Cohen, & Bachrach, 1971; Luborsky, Mintz, & Christoph, 1979). Luborsky et al. (1971), in an early review of this literature, found 31 studies that reported a positive relationship between adequacy of prior adjustment and therapeutic outcome, 1 study that reported a negative relationship, and 23 studies that were inconclusive or reported nonsignificant findings. Luborsky et al. (1971, p. 146) concluded that "initially sicker patients do not improve as much with psychotherapy as the initially healthier." Lambert and Asay (1984, p. 335), however, noted that a significant body of knowledge also supports the opposite view that more seriously disturbed patients show the greatest amount of therapeutic gain (e.g., Ewing, 1964; Frank, 1974; Kernberg et al., 1972; LaBarbera & Cornsweet, 1985; Nichols & Beck, 1960; Smith, Sjoholm, & Nielsen, 1975; Stone, Frank, Nash, & Imber, 1961; Truax et al., 1966). Other studies indicate that there is no relationship between degree of maladjustment and therapeutic gain (e.g., Cappon, 1964; Cartwright & Roth, 1957; Frank, Gliedman, Imber, Nash, & Stone, 1957; Klein, 1960; Seeman, 1954). It seems that when initial disturbances are assessed by self-report (e.g., Ewing, 1964; Nichols & Beck, 1960; Stone et al., 1961) or by psychological tests (e.g., LaBarbera & Cornsweet, 1985; Truax et al., 1966), the results generally suggest that patients who indicate greater psychological disturbance and distress, but who also have the least amount of overt behavioral disruption, are likely to show greatest therapeutic improvement. An inverse relationship between level of initial disturbance and therapeutic outcome, however, seems to occur in studies that use more general clinical evaluations (e.g., diagnosis, type of onset, degree of social impairment) (e.g., Patrick, 1984) rather than psychological assessment procedures for evaluating initial level of disturbance. Lambert and Asay (1984) concluded that although the bulk of the research indicates that better therapeutic outcome is obtained with less-disturbed patients, there are frequent contradictory findings. "Although better adjusted patients bring more personal resources to the therapeutic situation, they do not necessarily show more therapeutic gain" (Lambert & Asay, 1984, p. 340).

Luborsky, Crits–Christoph, Mintz, and Auerbach (1988), in an update of an earlier extensive review (Luborsky, Chandler, Auerbach, Cohen, & Bachrach, 1971) of the literature and of their own research, concluded that the "final outcomes of psychotherapy are predicted significantly but only modestly from some types of initial information about the patient, while information about the therapist apart from the treatment adds relatively little to predictability" (p. 133). Luborsky et al. (1988) found the best pretreatment predictors were psychological health (clinicians' ratings of patients on the Health–Sickness Rating Scale) and the patient's degree of emotional freedom and overcontrol (both rated on the Prognostic Index Interview). But "these pretreatment indicators represent only a few of the many potential predictors that were tried . . . and they explained only 5–10% of the outcome variance" (p. 269). Luborsky et al. (1988) concluded that most studies find that "greater psychological health [as measured by global measures such as the . . . severity of diagnosis, etc.] at the start of treatment is associated with greater benefits" (p. 281). Similar, but somewhat more equivocal, findings are obtained when psychological health is measured by psychological tests (e.g., Minnesota Multiphasic Personality Inventory [MMPI], Thematic Apperception Test [TAT], Barron Ego Strength Scale, and Rorschach Prognostic Scale). Some of these differences in results may be a function of the fact that interview evaluations of severity of psychological disturbance may be influenced by the patient's capacity to establish an appropriate working relationship with the interviewer, whereas test data may provide assessments of pathology that are less influenced by the patient's interpersonal capacities. It is also noteworthy in this regard that high levels of initial negative affect (anxiety and depression) as well as subjective distress are also predictive of better outcome. Thus, it is possible that the relationship between severity of disturbance and therapeutic outcome may be a consequence of how the severity of disturbance is assessed. Severity of disturbance may have a positive or negative relationship to outcome, depending on which dimensions are assessed and the method through which the assessment is conducted.

Lambert and Asay (1984), in their extensive review of this literature, stressed the need for greater methodological rigor in evaluating the relationship of severity of disturbance to treatment outcome. Important methodological considerations complicate the investigation of predictors of therapeutic outcome such as the effect of initial levels on subsequent measurement and the tendency for centripetal drift in which test scores, on repeated measures, tend to regress toward the mean. These methodological considerations result in the possibility that more seriously disturbed patients, those with extreme pretreatment test scores, have greater potential to display improvement than do less disturbed individuals because pretherapy scores may correlate with change scores (Beutler & Hamblin, 1986). Fiske et al. (1970) proposed the use of residual gain rather than raw gain scores to control for these effects of initial levels by statistically partialling out pretherapy levels from posttherapy test scores. Cronbach and Furby (1970, p. 74), however, argued that this procedure may discard a portion of what may be "genuine and important change in the person." Barrett–Lennard (1962) developed an alternative procedure for controlling for these statistical problems by dichotomizing his sample into mildly and severely disturbed groups on the basis of pretherapy test scores and then considering change within the more restricted range of each of the two groups. Although this procedure may diminish these statistical issues to some degree it does not eliminate them, because the pretherapy scores still remain an issue within each subgroup (Eckert, Abeles, & Graham, 1988). The statistical technique of path analysis, however, allows for more effective and systematic control of the effects of initial levels by treating them as continuous variables and by accounting for the partial correlations among the measures.

In addition to these statistical issues, measures of level of initial disturbance and of therapeutic change and outcome need to be carefully defined and precisely assessed in order to predict therapeutic outcome (Frank, 1979; Garfield, 1978; Mintz, 1972; Mintz, Luborsky, & Christoph, 1979). The results of the Menninger Psychotherapy Research Project (e.g., Kernberg et al., 1972), for example, indicate that patients need "some degree of ego strength" in order to establish and maintain a therapeutic alliance and to tolerate the frustrations and anxiety involved in dynamic psychotherapy. But it may not be ego strength per se that is important in determining therapeutic outcome, but the capacity to enter into, and to maintain, a therapeutic alliance. In their extensive literature of factors predicting therapeutic outcome, Lambert and Asay (1984) concluded that the most important variables to consider in evaluating a patient's capacity to gain from psychotherapy are those variables that directly assess the patient's capacity to participate in the therapeutic relationship.

In the analyses presented in this chapter, we use Rorschach protocols obtained early and later in the treatment process to assess systematically the patient's capacity and potential for establishing meaningful interpersonal relationships as well as the severity of the patient's psychopathology. We use these assessments to test empirically if psychological test variables obtained from the Rorschach at the beginning of treatment can provide effective predictors of therapeutic change as assessed by clinicians' evaluations of patient's behavior after a substantial period of long-term, inpatient treatment of seriously disturbed adolescents and young adults.

Thus, a fundamental question that can be answered from this investigation of therapeutic change is the value of data about the patient's cognitive, affective, and interpersonal experiences as assessed by psychological test evaluations obtained at the beginning of treatment, as prognostic indicators of the eventual level of clinical symptoms and social functioning after a substantial period of intensive treatment. The answer to this question lies in the database of this study but requires going beyond our initial analyses of the data that used repeated measures analyses of variance and the correlations of change scores. This question requires a more comprehensive statistical analysis that isolates the predictive relationships among pretreatment variables and posttreatment outcomes from the autocorrelations and synchronous correlations among the various assessment measures.[1]

Path analysis is a statistical procedure that partials out synchronous and autocorrelated relationships and expresses the residual relationships between psychological test predictors at Time 1 (T_1) and clinical behavior at Time 2 (C_2). Unlike a simple cross-logged correlation model which tests the strength of the T_1C_2 correlation against the C_1T_2 correlation, the path analysis approach statistically removes the effects of confounding relationships (such as C_1C_2, T_1T_2, T_1C_1, and C_2T_2 correlations) to provide a path coefficient which reflects the part of the T_1C_2 relationship which is not accounted for by any of the other relationships in the model. Through a series of partial correlations, path analysis isolates the causal effect of one variable or set of variables on another by statistically controlling for specified intervening or concomitant variables such as autocorrelations and synchronous correlations (Blalock, 1964, 1967;

Duncan, 1969; Tukey, 1954; Wright 1934, 1960). Although this is a well-founded statistical procedure used widely in biometrics and sociological research, its application is relatively new to clinical psychology.

Like all statistical techniques, path analysis is subject to limitations. The following assumptions underlie path analysis:

1. It cannot control for the effects of additional variables that have not been measured and that are not included in the model. Although extraneous variables do not invalidate the observed relationship among measured variables, they could alter the casual inference.

2. The particular causal factors and causal order specified in any path analysis model are arbitrary; the specific path model tested is one among many that could fit the data. The choice is not the result of optimization nor is it mathematically determined; it is instead an operationalization of the investigator's hypotheses. The decisions about which paths or linkages to include or exclude from the model, and whether those linkages are nonrecursive (unidirectional) or recursive (bidirectional), are based on the researcher's conceptualization of the probable relationships among the variables. In this study, we can draw causal inferences about the relation of variables at Time 1 on variables at Time 2 based on the assumptions that time is a unidirectional, linear process and that psychological processes are enduring traits that influence manifest behavior. Because we hypothesized that psychological traits at admission are predictive of later clinical outcome, we assumed that all paths between Time 1 and Time 2 are unidirectional and that psychological traits, as assessed by test variables at Time 1 and Time 2 (T_1, T_2), can affect manifest behavior as assessed by case record variables at Time 1 and Time 2 (C_1, C_2). These assumptions produce the path model illustrated in Figure 9.1.

3. Like other multivariate techniques, path analysis is subject to spuriousness; as the number of variables tested approaches the number of cases, there is an increased risk that among the many possible combinations of variables, some of the variables predict well by chance alone.

In path analysis, the residualized regression coefficient is not only a relative indicator of the strength of the relationship, but its absolute meaning is the proportion of variance in one variable that is uniquely explained by the other(s) within the assumptions of the arbitrarily chosen model. The model is judged to be complete to the extent that the

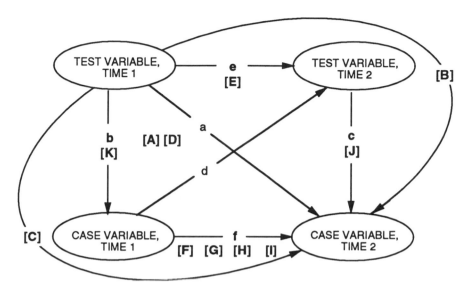

FIG. 9.1. Prototype for path analysis.

Definition of Correlations: **a.** test-case cross-lagged correlation; **b.** test-case synchronous correlation, Time 1; **c.** test-case synchronous correlation, Time 2; **d.** case-test cross-lagged correlation; **e.** test autocorrelation; **f.** case autocorrelation.

Definition of Path Coefficients. [A] direct effect of test 1 on case 2; [B] indirect effect of test 1 through test 2 on case 2; [C] indirect effect of test 1 through case 1 on case 2; [D] sum of paths A, B, & C. The closer this value is to the test-case cross-lagged correlation, the more confidence in the adequacy of the path model; [E] direct effect of test 1 on test 2 (equals test autocorrelation); [F] direct effect of case 1 on case 2; [G] spurious effect of test 1 on relationship between case 1 and case 2; [H] spurious effect of test 1 and test 2 on relationship between case 1 and case 2; [I] sum of paths F, G, and H. Compare to case autocorrelation; [J] direct effect of test 2 on case 2; [K] direct effect of test 1 on case 1.

path coefficients account for the observed correlations. (If path coefficients in a given model fail to account for the correlation, either the model is not optimal or external unmeasured variables are generating spurious relationships among the measured variables.)[2]

A path model, using conventional multiple regression techniques, yields separate estimates of direct, indirect, and spurious effects. A *direct effect* is the variance in one variable directly attributable to another. An *indirect effect* of one variable on another is mediated by one or more intervening variables, while a *spurious effect* between two variables is the result of a common relationship with another variable (or variables). The direct effect, therefore, is that portion of the relationship between two variables after adjustment for the contributions of indirect and spurious effects. As illustrated in Figure 9.1, the model yields estimates of five direct paths, two spurious paths, and two indirect paths. The spurious and indirect paths can be computed as compound paths (products of direct paths):

Spurious paths

1. $P_{t_1c_1}P_{t_1c_2}$ That portion of the relationship between C_1 and C_2 that results from T_1 as a common source of variance [Path G].

2. $P_{t_1c_1}P_{t_1t_2}P_{t_2c_2}$ That portion of the relationship between C_1 and C_2 that results from the stability of test variables over time and the static relationship of test variables with case record variables at each measurement point [Path H].

Indirect paths

1. $P_{t_1c_1}P_{c_1c_2}$ That part of the relationship between T_1 and C_2 due to T_1's effect on C_1 and C_1's effect on C_2 [Path C].

2. $P_{t_1t_2}P_{t_2c_2}$ That part of the relationship between T_1 and C_2 due to T_1's effect on T_2 and T_2's effect on C_2 [Path B].

The correlation between C_1 and C_2 can be decomposed into three paths

$$r_{c_1c_2} = P_{c_1c_2} + P_{t_1c_1}P_{t_1c_2} + P_{t_1c_1}P_{t_1t_2}P_{t_2c_2}$$

one direct and two spurious, while the correlation between T_1 and C_2 can be decomposed into one direct and two indirect paths

$$r_{t_1c_2} = P_{t_1c_2} + P_{t_1c_1}P_{c_1c_2} + P_{t_1t_2}P_{t_2c_2}.$$

These three paths are substantively interpretable, although the direct path is of primary interest, since it represents the causal relationship between test records at Time 1 (T_1) and case records at Time 2 (C_2). The partial correlation, that is the coefficient of the path $T_1 \rightarrow C_2$, expresses the variance accounted for in the relationship between these two variables. We set a path coefficient of $|.100|$ as our cutoff score; that is, we considered as statistically significant a path coefficient that accounted for greater than 10% of the variance (what would be equivalent to a zero order correlation of approximately .32, with a sample size of 90, $p<.005$).

RESULTS

Based on a priori theoretical expectations, a limited number of pairs of test and case variables were analyzed according to the path model illustrated in Figure 9.1. In all, 35 pairs of test and case variables were examined, comprised of five test variables and seven case variables.[3] The five Rorschach test variables studied were the extent of thought disorder (TD), the degree of reality testing (F+%), the mean developmental score of accurately and inaccurately perceived human responses (mean OR+, mean OR−),[4] and the average Mutuality of Autonomy (MOA) score, which assesses the quality of the interactions attributed to people, animals, and objects on the Rorschach. The seven case variables were the extent of clinical symptoms of psychosis, neurosis, and labile and flattened affect (as assessed on the Strauss–Harder Case-Record Rating Scales), the quality of interpersonal relations (Menninger Factor I), the degree of impulsivity (Menninger Factor II), and the extent of interpersonal communication (Fairweather). The strength of the 35 $T_1 \rightarrow C_2$ paths ranged from near 0 to .342, and, as indicated in Table 9.1, there were 16 pairs in which the absolute value of the $T_1 \rightarrow C_2$ path coefficient was $|.1|$ or greater. In addition, the sum of paths accounting for the relationship between T_1 and C_2 (the direct path plus both indirect paths) was compared with the simple zero order correlation $r_{t_1 c_2}$ and the differences were almost always minimal. This indicates that the variables included in the model are exhaustive and that the specified path is adequate to account for the relationships among the variables over time.

As indicated in Table 9.1, sixteen of the 35 paths explored had substantial predictive value, with path coefficients $\geq |.100|$, accounting for more than 10% of the variance. Of the five test variables explored, the only Rorschach test variable that failed to have substantial predictive value was the degree of reality testing (F+%). The other four Rorschach test variables had substantial value for predicting clinical status at Time 2 as measured by several of the seven criterion variables derived from the clinical case record.[5]

The most effective psychological test predictor at Time 1 appears to be the mean MOA score. As indicated in Table 9.2, the mean MOA score at Time 1 was predictive of all seven clinical case record variables at Time 2 (both the level of clinical symptoms and the quality of interpersonal relations). The mean developmental levels of accurately and inaccurately perceived human figures (mean OR+, mean OR−) on the Rorschach were also predictive, but primarily of the quality of interpersonal relationships (Menninger Factor I and Fairweather) at Time 2. These two psychological test variables that assess the developmental level of the differentiation, articulation, and integration of human figures on the Rorschach (mean OR+ and mean OR−), however, did not predict the level of clinical symptoms at Time 2. The extent of thought disorder on the Rorschach, in contrast, predicted three of the four clinical symptoms scales at Time 2 (Neurotic and Labile and Flattened Affect) as well

TABLE 9.1

Path Analyses of Rorschach Variables at Time 1 Predicting Ratings of Clinical Case Records at Time 2

(Ranking by Absolute Value of Path $t_1 \longrightarrow c_2$)

Rank	$t_1 \longrightarrow c_2$ Path coefficient	Test variable	Case variable	(A) r t_1 c_2	(B) Sum of paths	A–B differences
1	.342	MOA mean*	Menninger Factor I	.230	.230	.00
2	-.299	MOA mean	Strauss-Harder Psychotic	-.157	-.156	-.001
3	-.260	MOA mean	Strauss-Harder Neurotic	-.199	-.199	.00
4	.251	Developmental mean OR-	Menninger Factor I	.099	.098	.001
5	-.244	MOA mean	Strauss-Harder Flattened Affect	-.138	-.138	.000
6	-.222	Developmental mean OR+	Fairweather Communication	-.247	-.261	.014
7	-.175	MOA mean	Menninger Factor II	-.156	-.158	.002
8	-.172	Thought disorder	Strauss-Harder Labile Affect	.023	.027	-.004
9	-.167	MOA mean	Strauss-Harder Labile Affect	-.065	-.066	.001
10	-.157	Thought disorder	Fairweather Communication	-.121	-.117	-.004
11	-.144	Thought disorder	Strauss-Harder Neurotic	-.088	-.105	.017
12	-.138	MOA mean	Fairweather Communication	-.097	-.046	-.051
13	.120	Developmental mean OR+	Menninger Factor I	.112	.112	.00
14	-.108	Thought disorder	Strauss-Harder Flattened Affect	.046	.046	.00
15	-.105	Developmental mean OR-	Menninger Factor II	.002	-.007	.009
16	-.100	Reality testing (F+%)	Fairweather Communication	-.109	-.109	.00

19 other pairs of variables had $t_1 \longrightarrow c_2$ path coefficients <|.100|

*Mean MOA score at Time 1 also has substantial path coefficients (ranging from .344 to .229) with each of the four Menninger scales at Time 2 (Motivation for treatment, I Sublimatory capacity, Superego integration, and Object relations) that comprise the Menninger Factor I score.

TABLE 9.2
Path Coefficients $(T_1 \rightarrow C_2) > |.100|$ for Five Test Variables
by Seven Clinical Case Variables

Case variables (Criteria)	Test variables (Predictors)				
	MOA mean	OR+ mean	OR− mean	Thought disorder	F+%
Strauss–Harder symptoms					
Psychotic	−.299				
Neurotic	−.260			−.144	
Labile Affect	−.167			−.172	
Flattened Affect	−.244			−.108	
Menninger Scales					
Factor I (Interpersonal relations)	.342	.120	.251		
Factor II (Impulsivity)	−.175		−.105		
Fairweather					
Interpersonal communication	−.138	−.222		−.157	−.100

as the Fairweather Scale of interpersonal communication. Thus, the mean MOA score seems more comprehensive in that it predicted both interpersonal behavior and clinical symptoms, whereas the extent of thought disorder on the Rorschach predicted primarily clinical symptoms, and the concept of the object predicted primarily the quality of interpersonal relationships. Thought disorder and the concept of the object on the Rorschach appear to be more focused measures than the mean MOA scale, predicting primarily clinical symptoms and the quality of interpersonal relationships, respectively (see Blatt, Tuber, & Auerbach, 1990, for an elaboration of this point about the multidimensionality of the mean MOA score).

The strongest relationships were found between the mean MOA score at Time 1 (degree of malevolence attributed to the interactions of people, animals, and objects on the Rorschach) and the quality of interpersonal relations (Menninger Factor I) (a path of .342), the degree of interpersonal communication (Fairweather) (a path of −.138), the extent of psychotic and neurotic symptoms at Time 2 (paths of −.299 and −.260, respectively), and the quality of affect and impulse control (Flattened and Labile Affect and Menninger Factor II [Impulsivity] scores) (paths of −.244, −.167, and −.175, respectively). Substantively, this means that the more an individual reports perceiving malevolent, destructive, unilateral interactions between people, animals, and/or objects on the Rorschach at Time 1, the better the interpersonal relations and interpersonal communication, the less severe and frequent the clinical symptoms, the better the affect tone, and the lower the impulsivity at Time 2, controlling for the level of these variables at Time 1. Quantitatively, it means that, in terms of standardized variables, a difference of 1 unit in the mean MOA score at Time 1 produces a difference of .342 units in the Menninger Factor I score, −.138 units of the Fairweather score, −.299 and −.260 units in the Psychotic and Neurotic symptoms scales, and −.244, −.167, and −.175 in the Flattened and Labile Affect scores and the Menninger Impulsivity score, respectively, at Time 2.[6]

The indirect paths for predicting the Menninger Factor I scale at Time 2 are of little consequence for these variables (−.035 for the effects of mean MOA at Time 1 on Menninger Factor I at Time 2 through Menninger Factor I at Time 1, and −.076 for the indirect path mediated by mean MOA at Time 2). It is also noteworthy that the magnitude of the path between Menninger Factor I at Time 1 and at Time 2 (.353) suggests that there is not a strong unified pattern of change across the patient population on this measure. Menninger Factor I at Time 2 is predicted almost as well by the mean MOA score at Time 1 as by the Menninger Factor I score at Time 1. Furthermore, the synchronous correlations (at both Time 1 and Time 2) between the mean MOA score and the Menninger Factor I score are quite low. Altogether this makes the strength of the predictive relationship between mean MOA score at Time 1 and Menninger Factor I at Time 2 quite remarkable.[7] The same is true for the mean MOA at Time 1 predicting psychotic and neurotic symptoms at Time 2. The two indirect paths in predicting psychotic and neurotic symptoms are quite low (.088, .055 and .001, .060, respectively); the path of the autocorrelations between psychotic and neurotic symptoms at Time 1 and Time 2 are each moderate or low (.249 and .003, respectively); and the synchronous correlations of each of these two clinical variables with the MOA score at Time 1 and at Time 2 are also low. Thus, the mean MOA at Time 1 is remarkably effective in predicting the extent of major clinical symptoms at Time 2.

In summary, the mean MOA score on the Rorschach at Time 1 appears to have considerable prognostic value for predicting clinical behavior at Time 2. Seriously disturbed inpatients who portrayed interactions on the Rorschach as disrupted, malevolent, destructive, and unrelated or unilateral early in the treatment process appear clinically more intact later in the treatment process. After a considerable period of treatment, they have fewer and/or less severe manifest clinical symptoms and appear to be more constructively engaged with others, including clinical staff and other patients.

TABLE 9.3

Path Coefficients ($T_1 \rightarrow C_2$) of Most Malevolent
and Most Benevolent MOA Response at Time 1 with Criterion Measures
of Interpersonal Behavior and Clinical Symptoms at Time 2

	Most malevolent	Most benevolent
Interpersonal behavior		
Menninger Factor I* (Interpersonal relations)	.336	−.013
Menninger Factor II (Impulsivity)	−.305	.130
Fairweather	−.239	−.104
Clinical symptoms		
Strauss–Harder		
Neurotic	−.308	.090
Psychotic	−.373	−.002
Labile Affect	−.078	−.038
Flattened Affect	−.198	.014

*Path analyses of the four scales that comprise this first factor of the Menninger Scales (Motivation for Treatment, Sublimatory Capacity, Superego Integration and Object Relations) all have substantial path coefficients with the level of the most malevolent MOA response, ranging from |.224| to |.386|, but insubstantial path coefficients (<|.100|) with the level of the most benevolent MOA response.

To explore further the mean MOA score as a predictor of therapeutic progress, we examined whether the prognostic value of the MOA score was due to a lack of giving at least one response that is more benevolent or the tendency to give at least one response that has highly malevolent content. Thus, we used as predictor variables at Time 1 the value of the single most benevolent and the single most malevolent response given by each subject. As indicated in Table 9.3, the value of the single most benevolent response had a substantial path (>|.100|) in only two of the seven path analyses calculated for predicting the ratings of clinical behavior at Time 2. In contrast, the value of the single most malevolent interaction portrayed on the Rorschach had a substantial path (>.|100|) for six of the seven criterion measures evaluating clinical behavior at Time 2. The more severe the single most malevolent response at Time 1, the better the interpersonal relationships and the less intense and/or frequent the clinical symptoms much later in the treatment process.

The mean and the single most malevolent MOA scores were the most effective predictors of clinical status and functioning much later in the treatment process. Another test variable that was an effective predictor was the mean developmental level of inaccurately perceived human forms on the Rorschach (OR−). As discussed earlier, and as indicated in

Tables 9.1 and 9.2, this test variable at Time 1 was predictive of interpersonal relationships and social interactions at Time 2, but not of clinical symptoms. The path between the mean developmental level of inaccurately perceived human forms (OR−) at Time 1 and the Menninger Factor I score at Time 2 is .251. (The higher the developmental level of inaccurately perceived responses at Time 1, the better the interpersonal relations at Time 2.) This path coefficient does not seem to be attenuated by indirect paths, although there are moderate autocorrelations between C_1 and C_2 and T_1 and T_2. The mean developmental level of inaccurately perceived responses (OR−) also tended to predict impulsivity as measured by the Menninger Factor II score ($T_1 \rightarrow C_2 = -.105$). The mean developmental level of accurately perceived human responses (OR+) was also predictive of interpersonal behavior later in the treatment process. The higher the developmental mean on the Rorschach at Time 1, the better the interpersonal relationships at Time 2 as measured by the Fairweather Scale ($T_1 \rightarrow C_2 = -.222$) and the Menninger Factor I ($T_1 \rightarrow C_2 = .120$), and neither of these $T_1 \rightarrow C_2$ paths seems to be substantially attenuated by indirect paths, although the autocorrelations are moderate. In sum, a higher mean developmental level of human responses on the Rorschach, whether accurately or inaccurately perceived, was predictive of more appropriate interpersonal behavior at Time 2. The mean developmental level of accurately or inaccurately perceived human responses at Time 1, however, did not predict clinical symptoms at Time 2.

Thought disorder on the Rorschach at Time 1, on the other hand, predicted primarily the severity of clinical symptoms at Time 2. Thought disorder had substantial path coefficients ($T_1 \rightarrow C_2$) with the Labile Affect, Neurotic, and Flattened Affect scales of the Strauss–Harder (path coefficients were −.172, −.144, and −.108, respectively). The higher the thought disorder on the Rorschach at Time 1, the less frequent and/or severe the clinical symptoms reported in the clinical case records at Time 2. The indirect paths in these relationships were minimal, as was the autocorrelation C_1–C_2, although the T_1–T_2 autocorrelation was substantial. Thought disorder also had a substantial path coefficient (−.157) with the Fairweather Scale of Interpersonal Communication. The greater the thought disorder at Time 1, the better the interpersonal communication at Time 2. The level of thought disorder at Time 1, however, did not have a substantial path with the psychotic scale of the Strauss–Harder.

The application of the path analytic method to the ratings derived from clinical case records and psychological test protocols yielded impressive test predictions of therapeutic change. In this statistical procedure that removes the effects of auto, synchronous, indirect, and spurious relationships, there remained remarkably strong residual effects of psychological test variables derived from the Rorschach at Time 1 predicting aspects of clinical behavior at Time 2. Most noteworthy was the consistent finding that patients who had a better clinical picture at Time 2 were those who communicated disruptive, malevolent, unilateral interactions (MOA) on the Rorschach at Time 1. These patients had fewer and/or less severe clinical symptoms of neurosis, psychosis, and flattened affect as well as more appropriate and intact interpersonal behavior at Time 2, controlling for the initial level of each of these variables at Time 1. The path analyses also indicate that the greater the thought disorder on the Rorschach at Time 1, the less the clinical symptoms of labile and flattened affect and of neurosis at Time 2. It is impressive that both the content of Rorschach responses as assessed by the MOA and the formal or structural disturbances in thinking as assessed by the degree of thought disorder on the Rorschach indicated that those seriously disturbed patients who are willing and/or able to communicate disturbed and disrupted thinking are those who seem to profit more fully from the therapeutic experience. Positive therapeutic change, however, was also related to the degree to which patients were able at the first testing to represent human figures on the Rorschach (accurately and inaccurately perceived) that were more fully human, that were more elaborated and well-articulated with physical and functional attributes, and that were portrayed in congruent and appropriate action and interaction. Generally, the capacity to represent accurately perceived human figures on the Rorschach as well elaborated and engaged in appropriate and constructive activity is viewed as an indication of the capacity for constructive interpersonal relationships (Blatt et al., 1990).

In summary, severely disturbed patients who appear to benefit most over the course of 15 months of comprehensive inpatient treatment, including intensive individual psychotherapy four times a week, are those who at admission are able and/or willing to express disrupted thinking and portray interactions as malevolent and destructive, but who at the same time are able to maintain the structure of human representations at a high developmental level. In contrast, the capacity for reality testing, at least as assessed in the traditional way on the Rorschach by the accuracy of the perceived forms, appears to be unrelated to the degree of therapeutic change and outcome.

In terms of the value of the various ways of assessing Rorschach responses used in the present study, the MOA scale appears to predict therapeutic gain in the capacity to establish meaningful interpersonal relations and to change symptomatically. These results are consistent with earlier findings (Blatt, Tuber, & Auerbach, 1990) that indicated that the MOA is a broad-gauge measure that assesses disruptions both in cognitive processes and in the quality of interpersonal relatedness. The assessments of thought disorder on the Rorschach (Blatt & Berman, 1984; Blatt & Ritzler, 1974) and of the concept of the human object (Blatt et al., 1976b), in contrast, appear to be more specific and focused assessment procedures. Thought disorder on the Rorschach predicted primarily change of clinical symptoms as assessed by the Strauss–Harder rating scales. The concept of the human object on the Rorschach predicted change primarily in the quality of interpersonal behavior as assessed on the Menninger and the Fairweather rating scales. Thus, while the MOA scale is more effective as a general predictor of outcome, the findings with thought disorder and the quality of object representation have important theoretical implications in articulating the factors that contribute to change in particular dimensions or domains.

In general, the results indicate that psychological processes assessed on the Rorschach are predictive of the capacity of seriously disturbed adolescents and young adults to be responsive to an extensive and intensive, long-term, inpatient therapeutic experience conducted in an open inpatient treatment facility. Subsequent research needs to be directed toward examining whether these dimensions are predictive of the responses of other types of patients in other clinical settings, and whether other psychological parameters can also be effective in predicting therapeutic response. But consistent with some prior reports, the ability of seriously disturbed adolescents and young adults to share with others their disordered thinking and representations of disruptive and destructive interpersonal interactions, as well as indications of a capacity to form constructive interpersonal relations, is an important prognostic indicator of a patient's capacity to respond constructively to therapeutic intervention. It seems that what initially would be considered both positive and negative factors each contributed to prognosis, suggesting that the apparent inconsistencies in the literature about prognostic indications of potential therapeutic change may be a function of the methods of measurement, the nature of the patient sample, the type of treatment, and the oversimplification of multiply determined outcomes. But these data suggest that there are lawful relationships in the responses of seriously disturbed patients to long-term, intensive inpatient treatment. The results of these data analyses could potentially contribute to the decision-making process in selecting those seriously disturbed patients who might benefit more fully from intensive therapeutic interventions.

NOTES

1. Autocorrelations are the correlations between two measurements of the same variables at different points in time (e.g., the correlation between Rorschach scores obtained 15 months apart, as well as the correlations between variables derived from clinical evaluations also conducted 15 months apart). Synchronous correlations are the conventional correlations between measurements of different variables at the same point in time (e.g., the correlation between test variables and clinical case record ratings at admission, as well as the test-case record correlations 15 months later).

2. The adequacy of a model can be tested by comparing the path coefficients with the simple correlations, but failing that test, there is no mechanical procedure that guides the construction of a better model. Trial and error may yield a better model, or one may be forced to conclude that relationships among measured variables contain large components of spuriousness from unmeasured variables.

3. The variables from the TAT were not included in these data analyses because they are sex linked. Including TAT variables would require considering males and females separately, thereby reducing the sample size below an acceptable level. Variables from the analyses of the HFDs were also not included in these analyses because this material was available on only a limited number of patients.

4. An alternate measure of object representation is the developmental index— the weighted sum of accurately and inaccurately perceived human responses. Results with these two summary measures of object representation essentially replicate the findings with the mean developmental level of accurately perceived and inaccurately perceived human responses on the Rorschach. The developmental mean, rather than the developmental index, was used in these analyses because the developmental index of inaccurately perceived responses (OR−) correlated significantly with the measure of thought disorder ($r = .67$), whereas the developmental mean of inaccurately perceived responses (OR−) was relatively statistically independent of the level of thought disorder ($r = .21$). Generally the developmental mean scores seem to provide a more accurate estimate of the quality of object representations and to be somewhat more effective predictors of outcome than the developmental index scores.

5. The seven criteria of clinical change were relatively independent at the first evaluation. The intercorrelation of the four Strauss–Harder symptom scales ranged from .25 to .42. The Menninger Factor I score was minimally correlated with the Menninger Factor II score but highly correlated with the Fairweather Scale ($r = −.64$). The Menninger Factor I score and the Fairweather were only moderately correlated with the four Strauss–Harder symptom scales ($r = .17$ to .45). The Menninger Factor II score was independent of the four Strauss–Harder scales ($r = .03$ to .18).

The five test predictor variables were also relatively independent at initial assessment. The developmental mean for the concept of the object for OR+ and for OR− were minimally intercorrelated with each other ($r = .28$) and with the three other test variables (correlations ranged from .06 to .33). Thought disorder correlated significantly with degree of reality testing (F+%) ($r = -.47$) and the MOA mean ($r = .49$). Degree of reality testing also correlated significantly with MOA mean ($r = -.41$).

At the second evaluation, the Strauss–Harder symptom scales were moderately intercorrelated ($r = .19$ to .47). Menninger Factor I (Interpersonal Relations) correlated significantly ($r = -.62$) with Menninger Factor II (Impulsivity), with the Fairweather Scale of Interpersonal Communication ($r = -.50$), and with the Strauss–Harder Neurotic and Psychotic scales ($r = -.42$ and −.47, respectively), but only moderately with Labile and Flattened Affect (−.23 and −.29, respectively). The Fairweather Scale correlated significantly with the Strauss–Harder Psychotic Scale ($r = .61$) but only moderately with the other three Strauss–Harder scales ($r = .26$ to .37). Menninger Factor II had only moderate correlations with the four Strauss–Harder symptom scales ($r = .20$ to .37).

At the second evaluation, the five test variables were minimally intercorrelated. The two concept of the object developmental means for OR+ and OR− were minimally intercorrelated with each other ($r = .10$) and with the three other test variables ($r = .02$ to .18). Thought disorder had moderate correlations with degree of reality testing ($r = -.28$) and MOA mean ($r = .48$), and the degree of reality testing had minimal correlation ($r = -.16$) with the MOA mean.

6. The MOA is a 7-point scale, and the scores ranged from 1.00 to 5.67 at Time 1 and from 1.00 to 6.00 at Time 2. The change of mean MOA scores from Time 1 to Time 2 ranged from −4.00 to +2.50. The MOA is a reverse scale; thus, negative scores indicate positive change.

7. To specify more precisely the source of the relationship between the mean MOA score and interpersonal relations (the Menninger Factor I score), analyses were conducted between the mean MOA score at Time 1 and the four component scales that make up Menninger Factor I. The results indicate that the relationship between the mean MOA score at Time 1 and the Menninger Factor I score at Time 2 is determined equally by all four Menninger scales: Motivation for Treatment, Sublimatory Capacity, Superego Integration, and Object Relations (the primary $T_1 \rightarrow C_2$ path coefficients were .344, .229, .263, and .287, respectively). These data indicate that the more an individual reports malevolent, unilateral interactions on the Rorschach at Time 1, the greater his or her constructive involvement with the treatment staff, including the therapist; the better regulated his or her behavior; and the more appropriate his or her interpersonal relationships at Time 2.

CHAPTER 10

Conclusion

In this study we have found consistent evidence of highly significant behavioral and psychological change in 90 seriously disturbed young adults who had been hospitalized in a long-term, open clinical facility dedicated to psychodynamically informed treatment, including psychotherapy at least four times per week. The evidence for significant progress in these patients was observed in systematic and reliable ratings made on clinical case records prepared at admission to the hospital and again some 15 months later (on average 10 months before discharge from the hospital) and on variables independently derived from several different types of psychological assessment procedures (i.e., Rorschach, Thematic Apperception Test [TAT], human figure drawings, and Wechsler intelligence tests) also obtained at these same two times. Evidence of significant therapeutic progress appeared in these multiple independent sources of data, indicating that overall, after 15 months of treatment, the entire group of seriously disturbed young adults manifested significantly less frequent and/or severe clinical symptoms; better interpersonal relations; increased intelligence; a reduction in thought disorder; a decrease in fantasies about unrealistic, possibly autistic, interpersonal relations on the Rorschach; decreased defensiveness on the TAT; and more differentiated and organized representations in drawings of the human figure. Derived from clinical case records and independently administered and scored psychological tests, these data not only point to the effectiveness of the treatment program but also indicate that psychological tests can be reliable and valid sources of data for assessing aspects of the therapeutic process and of therapeutic outcome. These methods for evaluating psychological tests (Rorschach, TAT, and human figure drawings) derived in large part from an object relations perspective. The significant findings indicate that this new approach to the analysis of psychological tests, one based on theories of representation rather than theories of perception (Blatt, 1990a), can make important contributions to clinical research.

These consistent and significant indications of clinical improvement during the treatment process in this total group of patients are congruent with the findings of Plakun (1989), who conducted a follow-up study of patients hospitalized at the Austen Riggs Center from 1950 to 1976. From an original sample of 878 patients, questionnaires were mailed to the 89 male and 148 female former patients who could be located and who were willing to participate (252 former patients could not be located, 262 failed to respond to requests for participation, 33 refused participation, and 94 had died). The average age at admission to the Riggs Center of the 237 patients who participated in the follow-up study was 24.5 years (SD ± 7.7), and they were hospitalized for an average of 16.6 months (SD ± 10.6). The average length of time following discharge from the hospital to participation in the follow-up study was 13.6 years (SD ± 6.6). Comparing this sample with those patients who did not participate in the follow-up study on a large number of baseline variables, Plakun and his colleagues (Plakun, Burkhardt, & Muller, 1985) were assured of the representativeness of their sample. Applying DSM III-R criteria to evaluate retrospectively the clinical case records of these patients, Plankun et al. identified 19 patients (20%) as psychotic, 50 patients (53%) with a diagnosis of severe personality disorder (borderline or narcissistic), and 26 patients (27%) with a major affective disorder. Plakun (1989) and his colleagues (Plakun et al., 1985) reported detailed analyses of the responses of these 95 patients to a follow-up questionnaire.

Plakun's sample overlaps substantially with the patients we evaluated in our study of therapeutic change. The patients in our sample had been hospitalized at the Riggs Center during the same time period as Plakun's sample. In fact, 40 of our 90 patients were included in Plakun's final sample. In addition, the composition of our total sample corresponds closely to Plakun's sample in terms of basic demographics as well as diagnoses. Our sample contained somewhat more patients diagnosed as having a severe personality disorder (70%), with fewer patients (10%) diagnosed as having a major affective disorder. But the percentage of psychotic patients (20%) in both samples is identical. Thus, the findings of Plakun's follow-up study—conducted with former patients some 13.6 years, on average, after their discharge from the Riggs Center— provide a good approximation of the level of overall adaptation of our patients many years subsequent to their discharge from the therapeutic program at the Riggs Center.

Plakun's sample had an average Global Adjustment Scale (GAS) at follow-up of 64.4 (formerly psychotic patients = 59.3; formerly severe personality disorders = 65.0; and major affective disorder = 65.0). GAS scores between 61 and 70, according to Endicott et al. (1976),[1] indicate mild symptoms (e.g., depressive mood and mild insomnia) or some functional difficulty in several areas of functioning, but generally good functioning, with some meaningful interpersonal relationships. Most untrained people would not consider the person as disturbed (Endicott et al., 1976). The majority of these former patients were living in private residences apart from their parents (76% to 92%, depending on original diagnosis). They reported having at least one close friend (72% to 88%) and satisfactory relations with the opposite sex (65% to 92%). A substantial number (59% and 73%, respectively) of the former affective and severe personality disordered groups (but only 37% of the former psychotic group) had been or were married following discharge. Approximately 75% of the sample had posthospital psychotherapy for a substantial period (3.7 to 6.6 years). The former severe personality disordered group had relatively few subsequent psychiatric hospitalizations ($x = 0.3$) and these were relatively brief (<2 months), while the former psychotic patients had an average of 2.6 subsequent hospitalizations for a total average of 6.2 months. In summary, given the severe disturbances that led to the initial long-term hospitalization at the Riggs Center (mean GAS score of 34 at admission), our patients appear to be leading relatively intact lives and functioning on a relatively effective level some 13 years, on average, following their long-term, intensive inpatient treatment. Thus, the behavioral and psychological changes noted in the patients in our sample after 15 months of treatment and hospitalization appear to have resulted in significant improvement in general adaptation that has been sustained for over 13 years, on average, since their discharge from the hospital.

In addition to evaluating behavioral and psychological changes as a consequence of long-term intensive treatment in our sample as a whole, we sought to evaluate the nature of therapeutic change in two types of patients. Based on theoretical and clinical considerations, we differentiated reliably two different types of patients: (1) anaclitic patients who have disturbances focused primarily on difficulties in forming satisfying interpersonal relationship and who use primarily avoidant defenses (e.g., denial and repression); (2) introjective patients who have disturbances focused primarily on issues of self-definition, autonomy, self-worth, and identity and who use primarily counteractive defenses (e.g., doing and undoing, projection, reaction formation, overcompensation, intellectualization). Significant change was consistently noted in the introjective patients; significant progress was also noted in anaclitic patients, but their change seemed more subtle and less manifest than the changes noted in introjective patients. Interpersonal relations improved significantly in both groups, but significant symptom reduction occurred primarily in introjective patients, that is, in patients preoccupied with issues of self-definition and self-worth.

Independent of positive changes noted in both anaclitic and introjective patients, there were particular configurations of variables that indicated unique changes in the anaclitic and introjective patients. Change in the more ideational introjective patients was noted most systematically in the correlations between changes in clinical symptoms in the case record and changes in cognitive functioning as measured by the intelligence test and by the presence of thought disorder on the Rorschach. A decrease in clinical symptoms was significantly related to a decrease in thought disorder on the Rorschach in both anaclitic and introjective patients, but this relationship was most apparent with introjective patients. These significant relationships between decreases in manifest clinical symptoms and in thought disorder on the Rorschach occurred for a wide range of symptoms. In addition, a decrease in clinical symptoms correlated highly with an increase in intelligence test scores, again primarily for introjective patients. Thus, there appears to be a significant relationship between changes in manifest clinical symptoms as assessed from the clinical case records and different aspects of cognitive functioning as assessed on psychological tests (e.g., thought disorder and intelligence), primarily with introjective patients.

Change in anaclitic patients, by contrast, was most consistently noted in the correlations between changes in the ratings of interpersonal behavior as reported in the case records (motivation for treatment, capacity for sublimatory activity, the level of super-ego integration, and the quality of object relations) and the concept of the human object on the Rorschach. Changes in the quality of interpersonal relationships in anaclitic patients as assessed from the clinical case reports correlated significantly with decreases in the elaboration of inaccurately perceived human responses on the Rorschach (OR−)—that is, in the investment in inappropriate or autistic fantasies about human relationships. The lack of significant correlations between changes in the various ratings based on the clinical records and changes in accurately perceived human forms on the Rorschach (OR+) is consistent with earlier findings (Blatt et al., 1976b) that indicate that it is primarily the extent of the elaboration of inaccurately perceived human forms (OR−) that has significant relationships to severity of psychopathology with seriously disturbed inpatients. In this study, as in earlier research, it was only decreased investment in inaccurately perceived human forms (decreased investment in inappropriate or autistic fantasies of human relationships) that was significantly correlated with increases in the quality of interpersonal behavior of seriously disturbed inpatients, especially in anaclitic patients.

Thus, patients with anaclitic and introjective psychopathology appear to change in different ways. Clinical change in anaclitic patients appears primarily in the quality of their interpersonal relationships, paralleled by changes in the quality of their representation of the human figure on the Rorschach. Introjective patients change clinically primarily in the degree to which they demonstrate manifest symptoms of psychosis, neurosis, and affect disturbances, paralleled by changes in the quality of their cognitive processes, as measured by thought disorder on the Rorschach and on the Wechsler intelligence test. Changes in manifest symptoms and aspects of cognitive functioning appear to be consistent measures of therapeutic change in introjective patients.

It seems quite consistent that anaclitic patients, with their preoccupations about the quality of their interpersonal relationships, should demonstrate therapeutic change primarily in interpersonal relationships as reported in the clinical case records and in changes in their conception of the human figure on the Rorschach. Likewise, it seems quite consistent that the overideational introjective patients, with their preoccupations about self-definition and self worth, should demonstrate change primarily in the reports of manifest symptoms in their case records and on psychological test measures of cognitive functioning and thought disorder.

Thus, the data indicate that seriously disturbed anaclitic and introjective patients change in different ways, at least in earlier phases of the treatment process. In assessing change in anaclitic patients, one must be attentive to changes in the quality of their interpersonal behavior and conception of people rather than clinical symptoms and cognitive functioning. To the contrary with introjective patients, manifest symptoms and ideational processes are the primary dimensions along which progression or regression is likely to occur. These findings indicate the importance of distinguishing between patients with anaclitic and introjective psychopathology and of expecting them to demonstrate change, at least initially, along different dimensions. Patients appear to change primarily along the dimensions that are most salient in their personality organization.

These findings not only have important implications for the study of therapeutic change but also raise important questions about the nature of the treatment process, at least with the types of seriously disturbed adolescent and young adult patients included in our study. It is important to consider whether the different changes that occurred in anaclitic and introjective patients reflect differences in the treatment process or whether the differences in the nature of therapeutic change indicate that these two different types of patients come to therapy with different problems, needs, and expectations, and therefore experience the therapeutic process differently and gain in different ways from the treatment experience. In subsequent research, it would be important to compare dimensions of the treatment process with these two types of patients to see whether patient and therapist focus on different issues and respond in different ways because of the different predominant concerns of each of the two types of patients. Recent research (Blatt, 1992) indicates that the anaclitic–introjective distinction interacts with the type of treatment in producing significant psychological change. In a reanalysis of the data of the Menninger Psychotherapy Research Project (MPRP) that compared the effects of long-term psychotherapy with psychoanalysis, anaclitic patients seen in psychotherapy had significantly greater indications of constructive change than anaclitic patients seen in psychoanalysis. The converse was found with introjective patients; those seen in psychoanalysis had indications of significantly greater constructive change than those seen in psychotherapy (Blatt, 1992). These differences in therapeutic response of anaclitic and introjective patients to two different types of outpatient therapy (psychotherapy and psychoanalysis) were observed by evaluating the quality of patients' object representation on the Rorschach at intake and again at termination. Differential changes in these two groups of patients in these two types of treatment were expressed primarily in changes in the quality of mental representations on the Rorschach—in the mean MOA score and the concept of the object on the Rorschach (OR+). It is noteworthy that the scoring of the quality of the object representation on the Rorschach provided understanding of therapeutic change both in the study of the relative efficacy of two types of long-term treatment for outpatients in the MPRP and in this study of change in the intensive inpatient treatment of seriously disturbed young adults. It is also noteworthy that it was primarily the developmental level of accurately perceived human forms (OR+) that was sensitive to change in the study of outpatients in the MPRP (Blatt, 1992), whereas it was the developmental level of inaccurately perceived human forms (OR−) that was sensitive to differences in seriously disturbed inpatients both in this study and in prior cross-sectional analyses (e.g., Blatt et al., 1976b; Ritzler, Wyatt, Harder, & Kaskey, 1980).

The findings of the present study, as well as the findings about the differential efficacy of psychotherapy and psychoanalysis (Blatt, 1992), raise important questions about the nature of therapeutic action and the relative contributions of interpretation and the therapeutic relationship to the process of change. Most discussions of the mutative forces in intensive long-term therapy emphasize the importance of interpretation. But recent developments in psychoanalytic theory that stress the importance of object relations in psychological development strongly suggest that we must also consider the potential contributions of the therapeutic relationship to therapeutic action. If, as Mahler (1960) and Loewald (1960) and others stress, the relationship with the primary love object is essential for emotional development and the formation of psychic structures in normal development, then we must ask about the role of the therapeutic relationship in the emotional development and the formation of psychic structures that take place in the treatment process. As Loewald (1960, p. 221) noted, "The resumption of ego development in analysis, like normal ego development in the child, is contingent upon a relationship with a constructive object." Progress in psychoanalysis "is contingent on the relationship with a new object, the analyst" (p. 221). The analyst "offers himself to the patient as a contemporary object" (p. 219), as a point of attachment for the patient's unconscious transference. Psychotherapy is a constructive, affective, interpersonal relationship in which an individual with impairments and distortions in the concept of self and of others, as well as the nature of interpersonal relations, can begin to reinitiate a developmental process leading to more mature representational structures and more appropriate interpersonal interactions (Blatt & Behrends, 1987).

The changes we noted in manifest symptoms and ideational processes in introjective patients suggest that the more ideational aspects of therapy, such as interpretation, may play a more central role for this type of patient than aspects of the therapeutic relationship, at least in the earlier phases of the treatment process. The results with anaclitic patients, who come to treatment with profound concerns about disruptions of their interpersonal relationships and who appear to change primarily on interpersonal dimensions both in clinical case reports and psychological testing, suggest that the therapeutic relationship, rather than interpretation, may be of greater importance to this type of patient, at least in the earlier phases of the treatment process. Interpretation may be more central in the treatment of paranoid, obsessive–compulsive, and introjectively depressed patients; but the therapeutic relationship seems to be of greater importance for infantile, anaclitically depressed, and hysterical anaclitic patients, at least in earlier phases of the treatment process.

The results of our study of change in the intensive treatment of seriously disturbed young adults clearly indicate the importance of differentiating between patients with predominantly anaclitic and introjective forms of psychopathology. These two types of patients, at least initially, change in different ways and along different dimensions that are most congruent with their personality organization and their primary preoccupations. Change in introjective patients seems to occur more rapidly and in more manifest form. Change in anaclitic patients seems to occur more slowly and subtly, and particularly involves changes in the quality of their object relationships and object representations, but not in manifest clinical symptoms. These results do not indicate, however, that one should necessarily alter basic techniques to accommodate the different emphasis of different types of patients. Although different types of patients may initially be more responsive to dimensions of the therapeutic relationship or to interpretations, both are essential components of the therapeutic process. Interpretations can be mutative only in the context of an effective relationship, and the quality of the therapeutic relationship can grow and mature only with accurate and well-timed interpretations through which the patient feels understood. Both are central factors in the process of internalization, which is the basic mechanism through which psychological growth occurs both in normal development and in the psychotherapeutic process (Blatt & Behrends, 1987).

Although our data suggest that interpretation may be the primary basis for early therapeutic work with introjective patients, in fully effective treatment the quality of their interpersonal relationships should eventually also become of central concern for these patients. Likewise, although our data suggest that aspects of the therapeutic relationship may be the primary basis for early therapeutic work with anaclitic patients, issues of self-definition should eventually also become of concern for anaclitic patients. Thus, as therapy progresses, patients' exaggerated emphasis on one developmental line (anaclitic versus introjective or relatedness versus self-definition) should diminish, and they should begin to consider and explore issues from the neglected developmental line as well. Patients with anaclitic psychopathology should eventually begin to explore issues of self-definition and begin to consider themselves as independent and autonomous individuals with personal needs and values. Conversely, patients with predominantly introjective psychopathology should eventually begin to allow themselves to consider issues of interpersonal relatedness and the importance of experiences of intimacy and mutuality. Ideally, therapy should enable patients to reinstitute an interdependent, dialectical developmental process that leads to the capacity to establish satisfying interpersonal relationships and meaningful concepts of self. The reactivation of this disrupted developmental process should allow both of these two developmental lines to progress to higher levels of organization and integration.

In effective psychotherapy, as in normal development, the anaclitic and introjective developmental lines become integrated and result in a complex transaction and synthesis in the development of self and object representations. Psychological maturity involves the capacity to attend to and integrate issues of interpersonal relatedness as well as self-definition. In addition, psychological maturity also involves a synthesis of the higher levels of anaclitic avoidant and introjective counteractive defenses (e.g., repression as well as overcompensation and identification). The synthesis of these higher-order defenses from both the anaclitic and the introjective developmental lines leads to the development of the capacity for sublimation, in which well-modulated, socially appropriate, and personally meaningful behavior derives from and, in turn, contributes to the further development of a full sense of personal identity and purpose and the capacity to develop mutually satisfying and reciprocal interpersonal relationships (Blatt & Blass, 1990; Blatt & Shichman, 1983).

Because our data were gathered from two independent sources and at two different points in time, we were also able to use path analytic methods to examine potential causal relationships from essential correlational data. We evaluated the prognostic capacity of several psychological test measures at intake to predict level of functioning 15 months later, after a substantial period of intensive, psychoanalytically oriented inpatient treatment. Using a path analytic method, we were able to control a number of extraneous factors and examine the residual relationship of test measures obtained at Time 1 with independent clinical assessments at Time 2. The data indicate remarkably strong residual relationships in a number of areas. Most notable was the indication that patients who had made substantial clinical progress and had less frequent and/or less severe clinical symptoms and more intact social behavior at Time 2 were those patients who, on the Rorschach at Time 1, were more willing and/or able to report disrupted and malevolent interpersonal interactions (MOA scores) as well as distorted thinking (thought disorder). Substantial clinical progress was also related to indications of a capacity to establish relatively realistic, mutual, and constructive interpersonal relationships (OR+). The mean Mutuality of Autonomy (MOA) score at Time 1—the degree of malevolent and destructive interactions attributed to people, animals, or objects on the Rorschach—was especially effective as a predictor of clinical status at Time 2. Interestingly, the attribution of more malevolent, destructive, unilateral interactions at Time 1 was predictive of lower clinical symptoms and better interpersonal relations at Time 2. The extent of elaboration and investment in inaccurately perceived human figures (OR−) and the extent of thought disorder on the Rorschach at Time 1 were also predictive of better clinical status much later in the treatment process. Greater thought disorder was especially predictive of change in clinical symptoms, and greater investment in inaccurately perceived human figures (OR−) at admission was especially predictive of change in the quality of interpersonal relations. In addition, an indicator of capacity to experience more realistic and constructive interpersonal relations (OR+) at the beginning of treatment was also predictive of substantial clinical progress in the quality of interpersonal behavior at Time 2. Thus, the data indicate that within a group of seriously disturbed patients hospitalized in an open, intensive, psychoanalytically oriented treatment facility, those patients who are more able to express and communicate disrupted interpersonal experiences and distorted thinking, and who also had indications of a capacity for interpersonal relatedness on psychological tests at the initial assessment, were more likely to enter actively into therapy and gain most fully from the treatment process.

In summary, this study that examined change in a group of 90 patients during their participation in long-term intensive treatment at the Austen Riggs Center demonstrated that there are reliable and consistent ways of assessing psychological organization and functioning from clinical case records and from psychological test protocols. Particularly useful in assessing therapeutic change were newly developed methods for evaluating the quality of object representation on the Rorschach. Variables derived from each of these independent sources demonstrate that significant constructive changes occured in patients over an extended period of intensive inpatient treatment that included psychodynamically oriented psychotherapy four times weekly. Several clinical examples illustrate the changes that occurred in both psychological test protocols and clinical behavior as patients changed during the course of intensive psychotherapy. Even further, we found that two different types of patients changed along different dimensions—dimensions consistent with the nature of their initial psychopathology. Therapeutic change in these two groups of patients appeared to be independent of a wide range of potentially confounding variables such as the level of premorbid adjustment, the severity of psychopathology, the use of medication, the experience level of the therapist, and the sex of the patient. Using path analytic methods, we also found that several variables derived from psychological test protocols administered early in treatment predicted the degree of improvement expressed in the functioning of these seriously disturbed inpatients, as independently assessed from their clinical behavior much later in the treatment process.

The overall results of the study speak to the efficacy of long-term ntensive treatment of seriously disturbed inpatients in producing significant improvement in interpersonal behavior and a reduction in major clinical symptoms. The importance of these behavioral changes is supported by significant changes also noted on psychological tests. The distinction between anaclitic and introjective types of psychopathology articulated in this research facilitated the identification of these therapeutic gains. Without this distinction, the results would have been much less clear and less impressive. Together, these findings indicate that long-term, intensive treatment of seriously disturbed young adults results in important behavioral and psychological change that can be observed and documented within the treatment context. These observations of consistent and substantial behavioral and psychological change during the treatment process are consistent with follow-up study of these patients some 13 years after discharge (Plakun, 1989) that indicates that these changes have been sustained and result in markedly improved functioning in these patients in multiple domains—clinically, interpersonally, and functionally.

The differentiation of anaclitic and introjective patients not only is helpful in evaluating change within the therapeutic context but also suggests some important leads about the nature of the social matrix that might facilitate social adaptation once patients leave the therapeutic program. Anaclitic patients are likely to be particularly responsive to supportive interpersonal relations; thus, special attention should be directed to establishing supportive social networks for these patients when they return to their communities. Introjective patients, in contrast, would also benefit from supportive relationships, but particular attention should be directed to assisting them to regain functional skills such as returning to work or school. Although the results of the present investigations provide further understanding of therapeutic change within the clinical context, subsequent investigation needs to address how various therapeutic and social forces in the community can facilitate the consolidation of the behavioral and psychological gains achieved in the treatment context and enable both anaclitic and introjective patients to establish more adaptive behavior in a broader social matrix once they leave the therapeutic program.

NOTES

1. The GAS is a variant of the Health–Sickness Rating Scale (HSRS) developed by Luborsky and his colleagues (e.g., Luborsky, 1975a).

References

Adler, P. T. (1970). Evaluation of the figure drawing technique: Reliability, factorial structure, and diagnostic usefulness. *Journal of Consulting and Clinical Psychology, 35,* 52–57.

Allison, J., Blatt, S. J., & Zimet, C. N. (1968/1988). *The interpretation of psychological tests.* New York: Hemisphere.

American Psychiatric Association. (1980). *Diagnostic and statistical manual for mental disorders—DSM-III* (3rd ed.). Washington, DC: Author.

Ames, L. (1966). Changes in Rorschach responses throughout the human lifespan. *Genetic Psychology Monographs, 74,* 89–125.

Angyal, A. (1951). *Neurosis and treatment: A holistic theory.* E. Hanfmann & R. M. Jones (Eds.). New York: Wiley.

Ansbacher, H. L. (1952). The Goodenough Draw-a-Man Test and primary mental abilities. *Journal of Consulting Psychology, 16,* 176–180.

APA Commission on Psychotherapies. (1982). *Psychotherapy research: Methodological and efficacy issues.* Washington, DC: American Psychiatric Association.

Appelbaum, S. (1977). *Anatomy of change.* New York: Plenum Press.

Astrachan, B. M., Brauer, L., Harrow, M., & Schwartz, C. (1974). Symptomatic outcome in schizophrenia. *Archives of General Psychiatry, 31,* 155–160.

Athey, G., Fleisher, J., & Coyne, L. (1980). Rorschach object representation as influenced by thought and affect organization. In J. Kwawer et al. (Eds.), *Borderline phenomena and the Rorschach Test.* New York: International University Press.

Bakan, D. (1966). *The duality of human existence: An essay on psychology and religion.* Chicago: Rand McNally.

Balint, M. (1959). *Thrills and regression.* London: Hogarth Press.

Bannister, D., & Salmon, P. (1966). Schizophrenic thought disorder: Specific or diffuse? *British Journal of Medical Psychology, 39,* 215–219.

Barrett–Lennard, G. T. (1962). Dimensions of therapist response as causal factors in therapeutic change. *Psychological Monographs, 76* (43, Whole No. 562).

Barron, R. (1953). Some test correlates of response to psychotherapy. *Journal of Consulting Psychotherapy, 17,* 235–241.

Barry, J. R., Blyth, D., & Albrecht, R. (1952). Relationships between Rorschach scores and adjustment level. *Journal of Consulting Psychology, 16,* 30–36.

Beck, S. J. (1945). *Rorschach's test (Vol. 2).* New York: Grune & Stratton.

Beck, S. J., Beck, A. G., Levitt, E. E., & Molish, H. B. (1961). *Rorschach's test: Basic processes* (Vol. 1, 3rd ed.). New York: Grune & Stratton.

Behrends, R. S., & Blatt, S. J. (1985). Internalization and psychological development throughout the life cycle. *Psychoanalytic Study of the Child, 40,* 11–39.

Bellak, L., Hurvich, M., & Gediman, H. (1973). *Ego functions in schizophrenics, neurotics, and normals.* New York: Wiley.

Bem, S. L. (1974). The measurement of psychological androgyny. *Journal of Consulting Clinical Psychology, 42,* 155–162.

Berzins, J. I., Welling, M. A., & Wetter, R. E. (1987). A new measure of psychological androgyny based on the Personality Research Form. *Journal of Consulting and Clinical Psychology, 46,* 126–138.

Beutler, L. E., & Hamblin, D. L. (1986). Individualized outcome measures of internal change: Methodological considerations. *Journal of Consulting and Clinical Psychology, 54,* 48–53.

Beutler, L. E., Johnson, D. T., Morris, K., & Neville, C. W., Jr. (1977). Effect of time-specific sets and patients' personality style on state and trait anxiety. *Psychological Reports, 40,* 1003–1010.

Bieri, J., Atkins, A. L., Briar, S., Leaman, R. L., Miller, H., & Tripodi, T. (1966). *Clinical and social judgment: The discrimination of behavioral information.* New York: Wiley.

Blalock, H. M., Jr. (1964). *Causal inferences in non-experimental research.* Chapel Hill, NC: University of North Carolina Press.

Blalock, H. M., Jr. (1967). Path coefficients versus regression coefficients. *American Journal of Sociology, 72,* 675–676.

Blatt, S. J. (1974). Levels of object representation in anaclitic and introjective depression. *Psychoanalytic Study of the Child, 29,* 107–157.

Blatt, S. J. (1975). The validity of projective techniques and their clinical and research contributions. *Journal of Personality Assessment, 39,* 327–343.

Blatt, S. J. (1990a). The Rorschach: A test of perception or an evaluation of representation. *Journal of Personality Assessment, 55,* 394–416.

Blatt, S. J. (1990b). Interpersonal relatedness and self-definition: Two personality configurations and their implications for psychopathology and psychotherapy. In J. L. Singer (Ed.), *Repression and dissociation: Implications for personality theory, psychopathology and health* (pp. 299–335). Chicago: University of Chicago Press.

Blatt, S. J. (1991). A cognitive morphology of psychopathology. *Journal of Nervous and Mental Disease, 179,* 449–458.

Blatt, S. J. (1992). The differential effect of psychotherapy and psychoanalysis on anaclitic and introjective patients: The Menninger Psychotherapy Research Project revisited. *Journal of the American Psychoanalytic Association, 40,* 691–724.

Blatt, S. J. (in press). Representational structures in psychopathology. In D. Cicchetti & S. Toth (Eds.), *Representation, emotion, and cognition in developmental psychopathology.* Rochester, NY: University of Rochester Press.

Blatt, S. J., Allison, J., & Feirstein, A. (1969). The capacity to cope with cognitive complexity. *Journal of Personality, 37,* 269–288.

Blatt, S. J., & Behrends, R. S. (1987). Separation–individuation, internalization and the nature of therapeutic action. *International Journal of Psycho-analysis, 68,* 279–297.

Blatt, S. J., & Berman, W. H. (1984). A methodology for the use of the Rorschach in clinical research. *Journal of Personality Assessment, 48,* 226–239.

Blatt, S. J., & Blass, R. (1990). Attachment and separateness: A dialectic model of the products and processes of psychological development. *The Psychoanalytic Study of the Child, 45,* 107–127.

Blatt, S. J., & Blass, R. (in press). Relatedness and self definition: A dialectic model of personality development. In G. G. Noam & K. W. Fischer (Eds.), *Development and vulnerability in relationships.* Hillsdale, NJ: Lawrence Erlbaum.

Blatt, S. J., Brenneis, C. B., Schimek, J., & Glick, M. (1976a). *A developmental analysis of the concept of the object on the Rorschach*. Unpublished manual.

Blatt, S. J., Brenneis, C. B., Schimek, J., & Glick, M. (1976b). Normal development and psychopathological impairment of the concept of the object on the Rorschach. *Journal of Abnormal Psychology, 86*, 364–373.

Blatt, S. J., & Feirstein, A. (1977). Cardiac response and personality organization. *Journal of Consulting and Clinical Psychology, 45*, 115–123.

Blatt, S. J., & Lerner, H. (1983). The psychological assessment of object representation. *Journal of Personality Assessment, 47*, 7–28.

Blatt, S. J., & Lerner, H. (1991). Psychoanalytic perspectives on personality theory. In M. Hersen, A. E. Kazdin, & A. S. Bellack (Eds.), *Handbook of clinical psychology* (rev. ed., pp. 147–169). New York: Pergamon Press.

Blatt, S. J., Quinlan, D. M., Chevron, E., McDonald, C., & Zuroff, D. L. (1982). Dependency and self-criticism: Psychological dimensions of depression. *Journal of Consulting and Clinical Psychology, 50*, 113–124.

Blatt, S. J., & Ritzler, B. A. (1974). Thought disorder and boundary disturbances in psychosis. *Journal of Consulting and Clinical Psychology, 42*, 370–381.

Blatt, S. J., Schimek, J. G., & Brenneis, C. B. (1980). The nature of the psychotic experience and its implications for the therapeutic process. In J. S. Strauss, M. Bowers, T. Downcy, S. Fleck, S. Jackson, & I. Levine (Eds.), *The psychotherapy of schizophrenia* (pp. 101–114). New York: Plenum Press.

Blatt, S. J., & Shichman, S. (1983). Two primary configurations of psychopathology. *Psychoanalysis and Contemporary Thought, 6*, 187–254.

Blatt, S. J., Tuber, S. B., & Auerbach, J. S. (1990). Representation of interpersonal interactions on the Rorschach and level of psychopathology. *Journal of Personality Assessment, 54,711 728*.

Blatt, S. J., & Wild, C. M. (1976). *Schizophrenia: A developmental analysis*. New York: Academic Press

Blatt, S. J., Wild, C. M., & Ritzler, B. A. (1975). Disturbances of object representation in schizophrenia. *Psychoanalysis and Contemporary Science, 4*, 235–288.

Blatt, S. J., & Zuroff, D. (1992). Interpersonal relatedness and self-definition: Two prototypes for depression. *Clinical Psychology Review, 12*, 527–562.

Bowlby, J. (1969). *Attachment and loss* (Vol. 1). New York: Basic Books.

Bowlby, J. (1973). *Attachment and loss: Vol. 2. Separation, anxiety, and anger*. New York: Basic Books.

Bridgman, G. B. (1961). *Life drawing*. New York: Sterling.

Burdock, E. I., & Hardesty, A. S. (1968). *Ward Behavior Inventory* (manual). New York: Springer.

Byrne, D., Barry, J., & Nelson, D. (1963). Relation of the revised repression–sensitization scale to measures of self-description. *Psychological Reports, 13*, 323–334.

Cappon, D. (1964). Results of psychotherapy. *British Journal of Psychiatry, 110*, 35–45.

Cartwright, D. S., & Roth, I. (1957). Success and satisfaction in psychotherapy. *Journal of Clinical Psychology, 13*, 20–26.

Chase, J. M. (1941). A study of the drawings of a male figure made by schizophrenic patients and normal subjects. *Character of Personality, 9*, 208–217.

Chevron, E. S., Quinlan, D. M., & Blatt, S. J. (1978). Sex roles and gender differences in the experience of depression. *Journal of Abnormal Psychology, 87*(6), 680–683.

Chodorow, N. (1978). *The reproduction of mothering: Psychoanalysis and the sociology of gender*. Berkeley: University of California Press.

Coates, S., & Tuber, S. (1988). Object representations in the Rorschachs of extreme feminine boys. In P. Lerner & H. Lerner (Eds.), *Primitive mental states on the Rorschach* (pp. 647–664). New York: International Universities Press.

Cohen, J. (1984). The benefits of meta-analysis. In J. B. W. Williams and R. L. Spitzer (Eds.), *Psychotherapy research*. New York: Guilford Press.

Cohen, J., & Cohen, P. (1975). *Applied multiple regression/correlation analysis for the behavioral sciences*. Hillsdale, NJ: Lawrence Erlbaum.

Cooley, W. W., & Mierzwa, J. A. (1961). *The Rorschach test and the career development of scientists (Interim Report 5)*. Boston, MA: Harvard Graduate School of Education.

Cramer, P. (1979). The development of defense mechanisms. *Journal of Personality, 55*, 597–614.

Cramer, P. (1987). The development of defense mechanisms. *Journal of Personality, 55*, 597–614.

Cramer, P. (1991). *The development of defense mechanisms: Theory, research and assessment*. New York: Springer-Verlag.

Cramer, P., & Blatt, S. J. (1990). Changes in defense mechanisms following intensive psychotherapy. *Journal of Personality Assessment, 54*, 711–728.

Cramer, P., Blatt, S. J., Ford, R. Q. (1988). Defense mechanisms in the anaclitic and introjective personality configurations. *Journal of Consulting and Clinical Psychology, 56*, 610–616.

Cramer, P., & Carter, T. (1978). The relationship between sexual identification and the use of defense mechanisms. *Journal of Personality, 42*, 63–73.

Crockett, W. H. (1965). Cognitive complexity and impression formation. In B. Maher (Ed.), *Progress in experimental personality research*. New York: Academic Press.

Cronbach, L. J., & Furby, L. (1970). How should we measure change—or should we? *Psychological Bulletin, 74*, 68–80.

Darke, R. A., & Geil, G. A. (1948). Homosexual activity: Relation of degree and role to the Goodenough test and to the Cornell Selective Index. *Journal of Nervous and Mental Disorders, 108*, 217–240.

Davis, P. J., & Schwartz, G. (1987). Repression and the inaccessibility of affective memories. *Journal of Personality and Social Psychology, 52*, 155–162.

DesLauriers, A., & Halpern, F. (1947). Psychological tests in childhood schizophrenia. *American Journal of Orthopsychiatry, 17*, 57–67.

Draguns, J. G., Haley, E. M., & Phillips, L. (1967). Studies of Rorschach content: A review of the research literature: Part I. Traditional content categories. *Journal of Projective Techniques and Personality Assessment, 31*, 3–32.

Duncan, O. D. (1969). Some linear models for two-wave, two-variable panel analysis. *Psychology Bulletin, 72*, 177–182.

Eckert, P. A., Abeles, N., & Graham, R. N. (1988). Symptom severity, psychotherapeutic process, and outcome. *Professional Psychology, 19*, 560–564.

Ellsworth, R. B. (1970). *The Motility, Affect, Cooperation, and Communication Scale* (Revised). Beverly Hills, CA: Western Psychological Services.

Endicott, J., & Spitzer, R. L. (1972). Current and past psychopathology scales (CAPPS): Rationale, reliability, and validity. *Archives of General Psychiatry, 23*, 678–687.

Endicott, J., & Spitzer, R. L. (1979, January). Use of the research diagnostic criteria and the schedule for affective disorders and schizophrenia to study affective disorders. *American Journal of Psychiatry, 136*, 52–56.

Endicott, J., Spitzer, R. L., Fleiss, J. L., & Cohen, J. (1976). The global assessment scale: A procedure for measuring overall severity of psychiatric disturbances. *Archives of General Psychiatry, 33*, 766–771.

Epstein, S., & Fenz, W. (1967). The detection of areas of emotional stress through variations in perceptual threshold and physiological arousal. *Journal of Experimental Research in Personality, 2,* 191–199.

Erikson, E. H. (1950). *Childhood and society.* New York: Norton.

Evans, R. G. (1982). Defense mechanisms in females as a function of sex-role orientation. *Journal of Clinical Psychology, 38,* 816–817.

Ewert, L. D., & Wiggins, N. (1973). Dimensions of the Rorschach. A matter of preference. *Journal of Consulting and Clinical Psychology, 40,* 394–403.

Ewing, T. N. (1964). Changes during counseling appropriate to the client's initial problem. *Journal of Counseling Psychology, 11,* 146–150.

Exner, J. (1974). *The Rorschach: A comprehensive system.* New York: Wiley.

Exner, J. (1978). *The Rorschach: A comprehensive system: Vol. 2. Current research and advanced interpretation.* New York: Wiley.

Exner, J. E., Weiner, I. B., & Schuyler, W. (1976). *A Rorschach workbook for the comprehensive system.* Bayville, NY: Rorschach Workshops.

Fairweather, G., Simon, R., Gebhard, M., Weingarten, E., Holland, J., Sanders, R., Stone, C., & Reahl, J. (1960). Relative effectiveness of psychotherapeutic programs: A multicriteria comparison of four programs for three different patient groups. *Psychology Monographs, 74,* 171–185.

Fiske, D. W., Hunt, H. F., Luborsky, L., Orne, M. T., Parloff, M. B., Reiser, M. F., & Tuma, A. H. (1970). The planning of research on effectiveness of psychotherapy (report of workshop sponsored and supported by the Clinical Projects Research Review Committee, National Institute of Mental Health). *Archives of General Psychiatry, 22,* 22–32.

Frank, J. D. (1974). Therapeutic components of psychotherapy. A 25-year progress report of research. *Journal of Nervous and Mental Disease, 159,* 325–342.

Frank, J. D. (1979). The present status of outcome studies. *Journal of Consulting and Clinical Psychology, 47,* 310–316.

Frank, J. D., Gliedman, L. H., Imber, S. D., Nash, E. H., Jr., & Stone, A. R. (1957). Why patients leave psychotherapy. *Archives of Neurology and Psychiatry, 77,* 283–299.

Frank, S. J., McLaughlin, A. M., & Crusco, A. (1984). Sex role attributes, symptom distress, and defensive style among college men and women. *Journal of Personality and Social Psychology, 47,* 182–192.

Franz, C. E., & White, K. M. (1985). Individuation and attachment in personality development: Extending Erikson's theory. *Journal of Personality, 53,* 224–256.

Freud, A. (1946). *The ego and the mechanisms of defense.* New York: International Universities Press.

Freud, A. (1963). The concept of developmental lines. *The psychoanalytic study of the child* (Vol. 18, pp. 245–265). New York: International Universities Press.

Freud, A. (1965a). The concept of developmental lines, In *Normality and pathology of childhood: Assessments of development* (pp. 62–92). New York: International Universities Press.

Freud, A. (1965b). Assessment of pathology in childhood, In *The writings of Anna Freud* (Vol. 5, pp. 26–59). New York: International Universities Press.

Freud, S. (1900/1952). The interpretation of dreams. *Standard edition* (Vol. 5). London: Hogarth Press.

Freud, S. (1911/1958). Formulations on the two principles of mutual functioning. *Standard edition* (Vol. 12, pp. 218–226). London: Hogarth Press.

Freud, S. (1914). On narcissism: An introduction. *The standard edition of the complete psychological works of Sigmund Freud* (Vol. 14, pp. 73–102). London: Hogarth Press.

Freud, S. (1926). *Inhibitions, symptoms and anxiety.* New York: W. W. Norton.

Freud, S. (1930). Civilization and its discontents. In *The standard edition of the complete psychological works of Sigmund Freud* (vol. 21, pp. 64–145). London: Hogarth Press.

Friedman, H. (1953). Perceptual regression in schizophrenia: An hypothesis suggested by use of the Rorschach test. *Journal of Projective Techniques, 17,* 171–185.

Galin, P. (1974). Implications for psychiatry of left and right cerebral specialization: A neurophysiological context for unconscious processes. *Archives of General Psychiatry, 31,* 572–583.

Gardner, H. (1985). *The mind's new science: A history of the cognitive revolution.* New York: Basic Books.

Gardner, R. W., Holzman, P. S., Klein, G. S., Lipton, H. B., & Spence, D. (1959). Cognitive control: A study of individual consistencies in cognitive behavior. *Psychological Issues* (Vol. 4). New York: International Universities Press.

Gardner, R. W., Jackson, D. N., & Messick, S. J. (1960). Personality organization in cognitive controls and intellectual abilities. *Psychological Issues* (Vol. 8). New York: International Universities Press.

Garfield, S., & Bergin, A. (1978). *Handbook of psychotherapy and behavior change* (2nd ed.). New York: Wiley.

Gilligan, C. (1982). *In a different voice.* Cambridge, MA: Harvard University Press.

Gleser, G., & Ihilevich, D. (1969). An objective instrument for measuring defense mechanisms. *Journal of Consulting and Clinical Psychology, 33,* 51–60.

Gleser, G., & Sacks, M. (1973). Ego defenses and reaction to stress: A validation study of the Defense Mechanisms Inventory. *Journal of Consulting and Clinical Psychology, 40,* 181–187.

Goldstein, M. J. (1978). Further data concerning the relation between premorbid adjustment and paranoid symptomatology. *Schizophrenia Bulletin, 4,* 236–243.

Goldstein, M. J., Held, J. M., & Cromwell, R. L. (1968). Premorbid adjustment and paranoid–non-paranoid status in schizophrenia. *Psychological Bulletin, 20,* 382–386.

Goldstein, M. J., Rodnick, E. H., Evans, J. R., & May, P. R. A. (1975). Long-acting phenothiazine and social therapy in the community treatment of acute schizophrenia. In M. Greenblatt (Ed.), *Drugs in combination with other therapies* (pp. 35–47). New York: Grune & Stratton.

Gomes–Schwartz, B. (1978). Effective ingredients in psychotherapy: Prediction of outcome from process variables. *Journal of Consulting and Clinical Psychology, 46,* 1023–1035.

Goodenough, F. L. (1926). *Measure of intelligence by drawings.* New York: Harcourt, Brace, & World.

Graziano, W. G., Brothen, T., & Berscheid, E. (1980). Attention, attraction, and individual differences in reaction to criticism. *Journal of Personality and Social Psychology, 38,* 193–202.

Gunderson, J. G., Frank, A. F., Katz, H. M., Vannicelli, M. L., Frosch, J. P., & Knapp, P. H. (1984). Effects of psychotherapy of schizophrenia: II. Comparative outcome of two forms of treatment. *Schizophrenia Bulletin, 10,* 564–598.

Gunderson, J. G., & Gomes–Schwartz, B. (1980). The quality of outcome from psychotherapy. In J. S. Strauss, M. Bowers, T. W. Downey, S. Fleck, S. Jackson, & I. Levine (Eds.), *The psychotherapy of schizophrenia.* New York: Plenum Press.

Gunderson, J. G., & Mosher, L. R. (Eds.). (1975). *The psychotherapy of schizophrenia.* New York: Jason Arsonson.

Gur, R. E., & Gur, R. C. (1975). Defense mechanisms, psychosomatic symptomatology and conjugate lateral eye movements. *Journal of Consulting and Clinical Psychology, 29,* 373–378.

Haggard, E. A. (1978). On quantitative Rorschach scales. *Educational and Psychological Measurement, 38,* 703–724.

Hamilton, V. (1983). Information-processing aspects of denial: Some tentative formulations. In S. Brentiz (Ed.), *The denial of stress.* New York: International Universities Press.

Hammer, E. F. (1958). *The clinical application of projective drawings.* Springfield, IL: Thomas.

Harder, D., Greenwald, D., Wechsler, S., & Ritzler, B. (1984). The Urist Rorschach mutuality of autonomy scale as an indicator of psychopathology. *Journal of Clinical Psychology, 40,* 1078–1082.

Harris, D. B. (1963). *Children's drawings as measures of intellectual maturity; a revision and extension of the Goodenough Draw-a-Man test.* New York: Harcourt, Brace, & World.

Harrow, M., & Quinlan, D. M. (1985). *Disordered thinking and schizophrenic pathology.* New York: Garner Press.

Hartley, D. E., & Strupp, H. H. (1983). The therapeutic alliance: Its relationship to outcome in brief psychotherapy. In J. Masling (Ed.), *Empirical investigation of psycho-analytic theories* (Vol. 1, pp. 1–27). Hillsdale, NJ: Lawrence Erlbaum.

Harty, M. (1976). A program to evaluate intensive psychiatric hospital treatment. *Journal of the National Association of Private Psychiatric Hospitals, 8,* 3.

Harty, M., Cerney, M., Colson, D., Coyne, L., Frieswyk, S., Johnson, S., & Mortimer, R. (1981). Correlates of change and long-term outcome for intensively treated hospital patients: An exploratory study. *Bulletin of the Menninger Clinic, 45,* 209–228.

Havighurst, R. J. (1946). Environment and the Draw-a-Man test: The performance of Indian children. *Journal of Abnormal and Social Psychology, 41,* 50–63.

Haworth, M. R. (1963). A schedule for the analysis of CAT responses. *Journal of Projective Techniques and Personality Assessment, 27,* 181–184.

Haworth, M. R., & Normington, C. J. (1961). A sexual differentiation for the D-A-P test. *Journal of Projective Techniques, 25,* 441–450.

Heffner, P., Strauss, M., & Grisell, J. (1975). Rehospitalization of schizophrenics as a function of intelligence. *Journal of Abnormal Psychology, 84,* 735–736.

Hemmendinger, L. (1960). Developmental theory and the Rorschach method. In M. A. Rickers Ovsiankina (Ed.), *Rorschach psychology.* New York: Wiley.

Holt, R. R. (1962). *Manual for the scoring of primary process manifestations in Rorschach responses* (8th ed.). New York: Research Center for Mental Health.

Holt, R. R. (1963). *Manual for scoring of primary progress manifestations in Rorschach responses.* Unpublished manuscript, New York University.

Holt, R. R. (1966). Measuring libidinal and aggressive motives and their controls by means of the Rorschach test. In D. Levine (Ed.), *Nebraska Symposium on Motivation.* Lincoln, NE: University of Nebraska Press.

Holt, R. R. (1967). The development of the primary process: A structural view. In R. R. Holt (Ed.), *Motives and thought: Psychoanalytic essays in honor of David Rapaport* (pp. 345–383). New York: International Universities Press.

Holt, R. R. (1977). A method of assessing primary process manifestations and their control in Rorschach responses. In M. Rickers–Ovsiankina (Ed.), *Rorschach psychology* (pp. 375–420). Huntington, NY: Robert E. Krieger.

Home, H. G. (1966). The concept of mind. *International Journal of Psychoanalysis, 47,* 42–49.

Honigfeld, G., Gillis, R. D., & Klett, J. C. (1966). Nurses' observation scale for inpatient evaluation. *Psychological Reports, 19,* 180–182.

Horner, M. S. (1972). Toward an understanding of achievement-related conflicts in women. *Journal of Social Issues, 78,* 157–176.

Jacobson, E. (1964). *The self and the object world.* New York: International Universities Press.

Johnston, H. (1975). *Thought disorder in schizophrenic patients and the relatives.* Unpublished doctoral dissertation, University of Chicago.

Johnston, H., & Holzman, P. S. (1979). *Assessing schizophrenic thinking.* San Francisco: Jossey-Bass.

Jones, A. W., & Rich, T. A. (1957). The Goodenough Draw-a-Man test as a measure of intelligence in aged adults. *Journal of Consulting Psychology, 21,* 235–238.

Josselson, R. L. (1973). Psychodynamic aspects of identity formation in college women. *Journal of Youth and Adolescence, 2,* 3–52.

Karon, B. P. (1984). The fear of reducing medication, and where have all the patients gone? *Schizophrenia Bulletin, 10,* 613–617.

Katz, J., & Solomon, R. Z. (1958). The patient and his experiences in an out-patient clinic. *Archives of Neurology and Psychiatry, 80,* 86–92.

Kavanagh, C. G. (1985). Changes in object representations in psychoanalysis and psychoanalytic psychotherapy. *Bulletin of the Menninger Clinic, 49,* 546–564.

Kavanagh, G. (1982). *Changes in object representations in psychoanalysis and psychoanalytic psychology.* Unpublished doctoral dissertation, Adelphi University, Institute of Advanced Psychological Studies, Garden City, NY.

Keith, J. K., & Matthews, S. M. (1984). Schizophrenia: A review of psychosocial treatment strategies. In J. B. W. Williams & R. L. Spitzer (Eds.), *Psychotherapy research.* New York: Guilford Press.

Kelly, E. L., & Fiske, D. W. (1951). *The prediction of performance in clinical psychology.* Ann Arbor: University of Michigan Press.

Kelly, G. A. (1955). *The psychology of personal constructs.* New York: Norton.

Kernberg, O. (1976). Some methodological and strategic issues in psychotherapy research: Research implications of the Menninger Foundation's psychotherapy research project. In R. Spitzer & D. Klein (Eds.), *Evaluations of psychological therapies.* Baltimore: Johns Hopkins University Press.

Kernberg, O. F. (1984). From the Menninger project to a research strategy for long-term psychotherapy of borderline personality disorders. In J. B. W. Williams & R. L. Spitzer (Eds.), *Psychotherapy research.* New York: Guilford Press.

Kernberg, O., Burstein, E., Coyne, L., Appelbaum, A., Horwitz, L., & Voth, H. (1972). Psychotherapy and psychoanalysis: Final report of the Menninger Foundation's psychotherapy research project. *Bulletin of the Menninger Clinic, 36,* 1–2.

Klein, G. S. (1976). *Psychoanalytic theory: An exploration of essentials.* New York: International Universities Press.

Klein, H. R. (1960). A study of changes occurring in patients during and after psychoanalytic treatment. In P. H. Hoch & J. Zubin (Eds.), *Current approaches to psychoanalysis.* New York: Grune & Stratton.

Klerman, G. L. (1984). Ideology and science in the individual psychotherapy of schizophrenia. *Schizophrenia Bulletin, 10,* 608–612.

Kobasa, S. C., Maddi, S. R., & Kahn, S. (1982). Hardiness and personal health: A prospective study. *Journal of Personality and Social Psychology, 42,* 168–177.

Koppitz, E. M. (1968). *Psychological evaluation of children's human figure drawings.* New York: Grune & Stratton.

Korchin, S. J., & Larson, D. G. (1977). Form perception and ego functioning. In M. Rickers-Ovsiankina (Ed.), *Rorschach psychology* (pp. 159–187). Huntington, NY: Krieger.

Krohn, A. (1972). *Object representation in dreams and projective tests: A construct validation study.* Doctoral dissertation, University of Michigan.

Krohn, A., & Mayman, M. (1974). Object representations in dreams and projective tests. *Bulletin of the Menninger Clinic, 38,* 445–466.

LaBarbera, J. D., & Cornsweet, C. (1985). Rorschach predictors of therapeutic outcome in a child psychiatric impatient service. *Journal of Personality Assessment, 49,* 120–124.

Lambert, M. J. (1979). *The effects of psychotherapy* (Vol. 1). Montreal: Eden Press.

Lambert, M. J., & Asay, T. P. (1984). Patient characteristics and their relationship to psychotherapy outcome. In M. Hersen, L. Michelson, & A. Bellack (Eds.), *Issues in psychotherapy research* (pp. 313–359). New York: Plenum Press.

Lambert, M. J., Christensen, E. R., & DeJulio, S. S. (Eds.). (1983). *The assessment of psychotherapy outcome.* New York: John Wiley and Sons.

Lapidus, L. B., & Schmolling, R. (1975). Anxiety, arousal, and schizophrenia: A theoretical integration. *Psychological Bulletin, 82,* 689–909.

Lerner, H. & St. Peter, S. (1984). Patterns of object relations in neurotic, borderline, and schizophrenic patients. *Psychiatry, 47,* 77–92.

Lerner, H., Sugarman, A., & Barbour, C. (1985). Patterns of ego boundary disturbance in neurotic, borderline, and schizophrenic patients. *Psychoanalytic Psychology, 2,* 47–66.

Loevinger, J. (1976). *Ego development.* San Francisco: Jossey-Bass.

Loewald, H. W. (1960). On the therapeutic action of psychoanalysis. *International Journal of Psychoanalysis, 41,* 16–33.

Loewald, H. W. (1962). Internalization, separation, mourning, and the superego. *Psychoanalytic Quarterly, 31,* 483–504.

LoPiccolo, J., & Blatt, S. J. (1972). Cognitive styles and sexual identity. *Journal of Clinical Psychology, 28,* 141–151.

Lord, M. M. (1971). Activity and affect in early memories of adolescent boys. *Journal of Assessment, 35,* 448–456.

Lorr, M. (1961). *The psychotic reaction profile.* Beverly Hills, CA: Western Psychological Services.

Lorr, M., & Klett, C. J. (1966). *Inpatient Multidimensional Psychiatric Rating Scale* (Revised). Palo Alto, CA: Consulting Psychologists Press.

Lowenfeld, V. (1957). *Creative and mental growth.* New York: Macmillan.

Luborsky, L. (1962). Clinicians' judgments of mental health. *Archives of General Psychiatry, 7,* 407–417.

Luborsky, L. (1975a). Clinicians' judgments of mental health: Specimen case descriptions and forms for the Health–Sickness Rating Scale. *Bulletin of the Menninger Clinic, 39*(5), 448–480.

Luborsky, L. (1975b). Assessment of outcome of psychotherapy by independent clinical evaluators: A review of the most highly recommended research measures. In I. F. Waskow & M. B. Parloff (Eds.), *Psychotherapy change measures.* Washington, DC: National Institute of Mental Health.

Luborsky, L., Chandler, M., Auerbach, A. H., Cohen, J., & Bachrach, H. M. (1971). Factors influencing the outcome of psychotherapy: A review of quantitative research. *Psychological Bulletin, 75,* 145–185.

Luborsky, L., Crits–Christoph, P., Mintz, J., & Auerbach, A. (1988). *Who will benefit from psychotherapy? Predicting therapeutic outcome.* New York: Basic Books.

Luborsky, L., Mintz, J., Auerbach, A., Christoph, P., Bachrach, H., Todd, T., Johnson, M., Cohen, M., & O'Brien, C. P. (1980). Predicting the outcome of psychotherapy. *Archives of General Psychiatry, 37,* 471–481.

Luborsky, L., Mintz, J., & Christoph, P. (1979). Are psychotherapeutic changes predictable? Comparison of a Chicago counseling center project with a Penn psychotherapy project. *Journal of Consulting and Clinical Psychology, 47,* 469–473.

Luthar, S. S., & Blatt, S. J. (1993). Dependent and self-critical depressive experiences among inner-city adolescence. *Journal of Personality, 61,* 365–386.

Macfarlane, J. W. (1971). The Berkeley studies: Objectives, samples and procedures. In M. C. Jones, N. Bayley, J. W. Macfarlane, & M. P. Honzig (Eds.), *The course of human development*. New York: Wiley.

Machover, K. (1949). *Personality projection in the drawings of the human figure*. Springfield, IL: Thomas.

Machover, K. (1953). Human figure drawings of children. *Journal of Projective Techniques, 17,* 85–91.

Machover, K. (1960). Sex differences in the developmental pattern of children as seen in Human Figure Drawings. In A. I. Rabin & M. R. Haworth (Eds.), *Projective techniques with children* (pp. 238–257). New York: Grune & Stratton.

Maddi, S. (1980). *Personality theories: A comparative analysis* (4th ed.). Homewood, IL: Dorsey.

Mahler, M. S. (1960). Symposium on psychotic object relationships: III. Perceptual de-differentiation and psychotic "object relationships." *International Journal of Psychoanalysis, 41,* 548–553.

Mahler, M. S. (1968). *On human symbiosis and the vicissitudes of individuation*. New York: International Universities Press.

May, P. R. A. (1984). A step forward in research on psychotherapy of schizophrenia. *Schizophrenia Bulletin, 10,* 604–607.

Mayman, M. (1967). Object-representations and object-relationships in Rorschach responses. *Journal of Projective Techniques and Personality Assessment, 31,* 17–24.

Mayman, M., & Krohn, A. (1975). Developments in the use of projective tests in psychotherapy outcome research. In I. Waskow & M. Parloff (Eds.), *Psychotherapy change measures* (pp. 151–169). Washington, DC: National Institute of Mental Health.

McAdams, D. P. (1980). A thematic coding system for the intimacy motive. *Journal of Research in Personality, 14,* 413–432.

McAdams, D. P. (1985). *Power, intimacy, and the life story: Personological inquiries into identity*. Homewood, IL: Densey.

McCarthy, D. (1944). A study of the reliability of the Goodenough test of intelligence. *Journal of Psychology, 18,* 285–307.

McClelland, D. (1961). *The achieving society*. New York: Free Press.

McClelland, D. C. (1980). Motive dispositions: The merits of operant and respondent measures. In L. Wheeler (Ed.), *Review of personality and social psychology*. Beverly Hills, CA: Sage.

McClelland, D. C. (1986). Some reflections on the two psychologies of love. *Journal of Personality, 54,* 334–353.

McClelland, D. C., Atkinson, J. W., Clark, R. A., & Lowell, E. L. (1953). *The achievement motive*. New York: Appleton-Century-Crofts.

McFate, M., & Orr, F. (1949). Through adolescence with the Rorschach. *Rorschach Research Exchange, 13,* 302–319.

McGlashan, T. H. (1984a). The Chestnut Lodge Follow-up Study: I. Follow-up methodology and study sample. *Archives of General Psychiatry, 41,* 573–585.

McGlashan, T. H. (1984b). The Chestnut Lodge Follow-up Study: II. Long-term outcome of schizophrenia and the affective disorders. *Archives of General Psychiatry, 41,* 586–601.

McKinnon, J. (1979). Two sematic forms: Neurophysiological and psychoanalytic descriptions. *Psychoanalysis and Contemporary Thought, 2,* 25–76.

McNair, D. (1976). Discussion: Comments on the Menninger Project. In R. Spitzer & D. Klein (Eds.), *Evaluations of psychological therapies*. Baltimore: Johns Hopkins University Press.

McNair, D. M., Lorr, M., Young, H. H., Roth, I., & Boyd, R. W. (1964). A three-year follow-up of psychotherapy patients. *Journal of Clinical Psychology, 20,* 258–264.

Meissner, W. W. (1981). Internalization and object relations. *Journal of the American Psychoanalytic Association, 27,* 345–360.

Meltzoff, J., & Kornreich, M. (1970). *Research in psychotherapy.* New York: Atherton Press.

Miller, D. R., & Swanson, G. E. (1960). *Inner conflict and defense.* New York: Holt, Rinehart & Winston.

Mintz, J. (1972). What is success in psychotherapy? *Journal of Abnormal Psychology, 80,* 11–19.

Mintz, J. (1981, May). Measuring outcome in psychodynamic psychotherapy. *Archives of General Psychiatry, 38,* 503–506.

Mintz, J., Luborsky, L., & Christoph, P. (1979). Measuring the outcome of psychotherapy: Findings of the Penn Psychotherapy Project. *Journal of Consulting and Clinical Psychology, 47,* 319–334.

Modell, A. H. (1951). The holding environment and the therapeutic action of psychoanalysis. *Journal of the American Psychoanalytic Association, 24,* 285–307.

Murstein, B. I. (1960). Factor analyses of the Rorschach. *Journal of Consulting Psychology, 24,* 262–275.

Murphy, M. M. (1956). A Goodenough scale of evaluation of human figure drawing of three non-psychotic groups of adults. *Journal of Clinical Psychology, 12,* 397–399.

Nichols, R. C., & Beck, K. W. (1960). Factors in psychotherapy change. *Journal of Consulting Psychology, 24,* 388–399.

Osgood, C., Suci, G., & Tannenbaum, P. (1957). *The measurement of meaning.* Urbana: University of Illinois Press.

Parker, R., & Piotrowski, Z. A. (1968). The significance of varieties of factors of Rorschach human movement responses. *Journal of Projective Techniques and Personality Assessment, 32,* 33–44.

Parloff, M. B. (1984). Psychotherapy research and its incredible credibility crisis. *Clinical Psychology Review, 4,* 95–109.

Patrick, J. (1984). Predicting outcome of psychiatric hospitalization: A comparison of attitudinal and psychopathological measures. *Journal of Clinical Psychology, 40,* 546–549.

Phillipson, H. (1955). *The object relations technique.* London: Tavistock Institute.

Piaget, J. (1937/1954). *The construction of reality in the child.* New York: Basic Books.

Plakun, E. M. (1989). Narcissistic personality disorder: A validity study and comparison to borderline personality disorder. *Psychiatric Clinics of North America, 12,* 603–620.

Plakun, E. M., Burkhardt, P. E., & Muller, J. P. (1985). 14-year follow-up of borderline and schizotypical personality disorders. *Comprehensive Psychiatry, 26,* 448–455.

Powers, W. F., & Hamlin, R. M. (1955). Relationship between diagnostic categories and deviant verbalizations on the Rorschach. *Journal of Consulting Psychology, 19,* 120–125.

Quinlan, D. M., Harrow, M., Tucker, G., & Carlson, K. (1972). Varieties of "disordered" thinking on the Rorschach: Findings in schizophrenic and non-schizophrenic patients. *Journal of Abnormal Psychology, 79,* 47–53.

Rapaport, D., Gill, M. M., & Schafer, R. (1945–1946). *Diagnostic psychological testing* (Vols. 1 & 2). Chicago: Year Book Publishers.

Reker, G. T. (1974). Interpersonal conceptual structures of emotionally disturbed and normal boys. *Journal of Abnormal Psychology, 83,* 380–386.

Ritzler, B. A., Wyatt, D., Harder, D., & Kaskey, M. (1980). Psychotic patterns of the concept of the object on the Rorschach. *Journal of Abnormal Psychology, 89,* 46–55.

Roback, H. B. (1968). Human figure drawings: Their utility in the clinical psychologist's armamentarium for personality assessment. *Psychological Bulletin, 70,* 1–19.

Robins, C. E. (1980). *The relation between clinical descriptions of patients and their human figure drawing performance.* Unpublished doctoral dissertation, Columbia University, New York.

Robins, C. E., Blatt, S. J., Ford, R. Q. (1991). Changes in human figure drawings during intensive treatment. *Journal of Personality Assessment, 57,* 477–497.

Rofe, Y., Lewin, I., & Padeh, B. (1977). Affiliation before and after child delivery as a function of repression–sensitization. *British Journal of Social and Clinical Psychology, 16,* 311–315.

Rogers, C. R. (1957). The necessary and sufficient conditions of therapeutic personality change. *Journal of Consulting Psychology, 21,* 95–103.

Rogers, C. R. (1959). A theory of therapy, personality, and interpersonal relationships as developed in the client-centered framework in psychology: A study of science. In S. Koch (Ed.), *Formulations of the person and the social context.* New York: McGraw-Hill.

Rogers, C. R., Gendlin, E. T., Kiesler, D. J., & Truax, C. B. (Eds.). (1967). *The therapeutic relationship and its impact.* Madison, WI: University of Wisconsin Press.

Ryan, E. R. (1973). *The capacity of the patient to enter an elementary therapeutic relationship in the initial psychotherapy interview.* Unpublished doctoral dissertation, University of Michigan, Ann Arbor, Michigan.

Ryan, R., Avery, R., & Grolnick, W. (1985). A Rorschach assessment of children's mutuality of autonomy. *Journal of Personality Assessment, 49,* 6–11.

Sandler, J., & Rosenblatt, B. (1962). The concept of the representational world. *Psychoanalytic Study of the Child, 17,* 128–145.

SAS Institute, Inc. (1979). *SAS user's guide (1979 ed.).* Cary, NC: SAS Institute, Inc.

Scarlett, H. H., Press, A. N., & Crockett, W. H. (1971). Children's descriptions of peers: A Wernerian developmental analysis. *Child Development, 42,* 439–453.

Schafer, R. (1954). *Psychoanalytic interpretation in Rorschach testing.* New York: Grune & Stratton.

Schafer, R. (1967). *Projective testing and psychoanalysis.* New York: International Universities Press.

Schafer, R. (1978). *Aspects of internalization.* New York: International Universities Press.

Schaffer, J. W., Duszynski, K. R., & Thomas, C. B. (1981). Orthogonal dimensions of individual and group forms of the Rorschach. *Journal of Personality Assessment, 45,* 230–239.

Schimek, J. G. (1968). A note on the long-range stability of selected Rorschach scores. *Journal of Projective Techniques and Personality Assessment, 32,* 63–65.

Scholz, J. A. (1973). Defense styles in suicide attempts. *Journal of Consulting and Clinical Psychology, 34,* 70–73.

Schori, T. R., & Thomas, C. B. (1972). The Rorschach test: An image analysis. *Journal of Clinical Psychology, 28,* 195–199.

Schulz, C. (1975). Self and object differentiation as a measure of change in psychotherapy. In J. G. Gunderson & L. R. Mosher (Eds.), *The psychotherapy of schizophrenia.* New York: Jason Aronson.

Schwager, E., & Spear, W. E. (1981). New perspectives on psychological tests as measures of change. *Bulletin of the Menninger Clinic, 45,* 527–541.

Searles, H. (1965). *Collected papers on schizophrenia and related subjects.* New York: International Universities Press.

Seeman, J. (1954). Counselor judgments of therapeutic process and outcome. In C. R. Roger & R. F. Dymond (Eds.), *Psychotherapy and personality change.* Chicago: University of Chicago Press.

Shor, J., & Sanville, J. (1978). *Illusion in loving: A psychoanalytic approach to intimacy and autonomy.* Los Angeles: Double Helix Press.

Signell, K. A. (1966). Cognitive complexity in person perception and nation perception: A developmental approach. *Journal of Personality, 34,* 517–537.

Slough, N. R., Kleinknecht, A., & Thorndike, R. M. (1984). The relationship of the repression–sensitization scales to anxiety. *Journal of Personality Assessment, 48,* 378–379.

Smith, F. O. (1937). What the Goodenough intelligence test measures. *Psychological Bulletin, 34,* 760–761.

Smith, G. J. W., Sjoholm, L., & Nielsen, S. (1975). Individual factors affecting the improvement of anxiety during a therapeutic period of 1½ to 2 years. *Acta Psychiatrica Scandinavica, 52,* 7–22.

Smith, M. L., Glass, G. V., & Miller, T. I. (1980). *The benefits of psychotherapy.* Baltimore: Johns Hopkins University Press.

Smith, T. W., O'Keeffe, J. C., & Jenkins, M. (1988). Dependency and self-criticism: Correlates of depression or moderators of the effects of stressful events. *Journal of Personality Disorders, 2,* 160–169.

Spear, W., & Sugarman, A. (1984). Dimensions of internalized object relations in borderline schizophrenic patients. *Psychoanalytic Psychology, 1,* 113–129.

Spiegel, H., & Spiegel, D. (1978). *Trance and treatment: Clinical uses of hypnosis.* New York: Basic Books.

Spitzer, R., & Klein, D. (Eds.). (1976). *Evaluation of psychological therapies.* Baltimore, MD: Johns Hopkins University Press.

Stanton, A. H., Gunderson, J. G., Knapp, Ph.D., Frank, A. F., Vannicelli, M. L., Schnitzer, R., & Rosenthal, R. (1984). Effects of psychotherapy in schizophrenia: I. Design and implementation of a controlled study. *Schizophrenia Bulletin, 10,* 520–563.

Stewart, A. S., & Malley, J. E. (1987). Role combination in women in the early adult years: Mitigating agency and communion. In F. Crosby (Ed.), *Spouse, parent, worker: On gender and multiple roles.* New Haven, CT: Yale University Press.

Stone, A. R., Frank, J. D., Nash, E. H., & Imber, S. D. (1961). An intensive five-year follow up study of treated psychiatric outpatients. *Journal of Nervous and Mental Disease, 133,* 410–422.

Strauss, J. C., Carpenter, W. T., & Bartko, J. (1974). Part III. Speculations on the processes that underlie schizophrenic signs and symptoms. *Schizophrenic Bulletin, 2,* 61–69.

Strauss, J. S., & Harder, D. W. (1981). The Case Record Rating Scale. A method for rating symptom and social function data from case records. *Psychiatry Research, 4,* 333–345.

Strauss, J. S., Kokes, R. F., Ritzler, B. A., Harder, D. W., & Van Ord, A. (1978). Patterns of disorder in first admission psychiatric patients. *Journal of Nervous and Mental Disease, 166,* 611–625.

Strupp, H. H. (1980a). Success and failure in time-limited psychotherapy. *Archives of General Psychiatry, 37,* 595–603.

Strupp, H. H. (1980b). Success and failure in time-limited psychotherapy. *Archives of General Psychiatry, 37,* 708–716.

Strupp, H. H. (1980c). Success and failure in time-limited psychotherapy. *Archives of General Psychiatry, 37,* 831–841.

Strupp, H. H. (1980d). Success and failure in time-limited psychotherapy. *Archives of General Psychiatry, 37,* 947–954.

Sullivan, P. F., & Roberts, L. K. (1969). The relationship of manifest anxiety to repression–sensitization on the MMPI. *Journal of Consulting and Clinical Psychology, 33,* 763–764.

Sundberg, N. D. (1961). The practice of psychological testing in clinical services in the U.S. *American Psychologist, 16,* 79–83.

Swensen, C. E. (1968). Sexual differentiation on the Draw-a-Person test. *Journal of Clinical Psychology, 11,* 37–40.

Szumotalska, E. (1992). *Severity and types of depressive affect as related to perceptual style: Relationship of anaclitic and introjective depressive configuration to holistic versus analytic similarity judgments.* Unpublished dissertation, New School for Social Research, New York.

Tempone, U. J., & Lambe, W. (1967). Repression–sensitization and its relation to measures of adjustment and conflict. *Journal of Consulting Psychology, 31,* 131–136.

Todd, F. J., & Rappoport, L. (1964). A cognitive structure approach to person perception: A comparison of two models. *Journal of Abnormal and Social Psychology, 68,* 469–478.

Truax, C. B., Tunnell, B. T., Jr., Fine, H. L., & Wargo, D. G. (1966). *The prediction of client outcome during group psychotherapy from measures of initial status.* Unpublished manuscript, Arkansas Rehabilitation Research and Training Center, University of Arkansas.

Truax, C. B., Wargo, D. G., Frank, J. D., Imber, S. D., Battle, C. C., Hoehn–Saric, R., Nash, E. H., & Stone, A. R. (1967). Therapist's contribution to accurate empathy, nonpossessive warmth and genuineness in psychotherapy. *Journal of Clinical Psychology, 22,* 331–334.

Tuber, S. B. (1983). Children's Rorschach scores as predictors of later adjustment. *Journal of Consulting and Clinical Psychology, 51,* 379–385.

Tuber, S., & Coates, S. (1989). Indices of psychopathology in the Rorschachs of boys with severe gender identity disorder. *Journal of Personality Assessment, 57,* 100–112.

Tukey, J. W. (1954). Causation, regression, and path analysis. In O. Kempthorne et al. (Eds.), *Statistics and mathematics in biology.* Ames, Iowa: Iowa State University Press.

Urist, J. (1973). *The Rorschach test as a multi-dimensional measure of object relations.* Unpublished doctoral dissertation, University of Michigan.

Urist, J. (1977). The Rorschach test and the assessment of object relations. *Journal of Personality Assessment, 41,* 3–9.

Urist, J., & Shill, M. (1982). Validity of the Rorschach Mutuality of Autonomy Scale: A replication using excerpted responses. *Journal of Personality Assessment, 46,* 451–454.

Warr, P. B., & Knapper, C. (1968). *The perception of people and events.* New York: Wiley.

Waskow, I., & Parloff, M. (Eds.). (1975). *Psychotherapy change measures.* Rockville, MD: National Institute of Mental Health.

Watkins, J. G., & Stauffacher, J. C. (1952). An index of pathological thinking in the Rorschach. *Journal of Projective Techniques, 16,* 276–286.

Weinberger, D. A., Schwartz, G. E., & Davidson, J. R. (1979). Low-anxious, high-anxious, and repressive coping styles: Psychometric patterns and behavioral and physiological responses to stress. *Journal of Abnormal Psychology, 88,* 369–380.

Weiner, I. B., & Exner, J. E. (1978). Rorschach indices of disordered thinking in patient and nonpatient adolescents and adults. *Journal of Personality Assessment, 42,* 339–343.

Weiner, R. L. (1977). Approaches to Rorschach validation. In M. A. Rickers-Ovsiankina (Ed.), *Rorschach psychology* (2nd ed., pp. 575–608). Huntington, NY: Krieger.

Werner, H. (1948). *Comparative psychology of mental development.* New York: International Universities Press.

Werner, H., & Kaplan, B. (1963). *Symbol formation: An organismic–developmental approach to language and the expression of thought.* New York: Wiley.

White, M. D., & Wilkins, W. (1973). Bogus physiological feedback and response thresholds of repressors and sensitizers. *Journal of Research in Personality, 7,* 78–87.

Whiteman, M. (1954). The performance of schizophrenics on social concepts. *Journal of Abnormal and Social Psychology, 49,* 266–271.

Wiggins, J. S. (1991). Agency and communion as conceptual coordinates for the understanding and measurement of interpersonal behavior. In W. W. Grove & D. Cicchetti (Eds.), *Thinking clearly about psychology: Vol. 2. Personality and Psychotherapy* (pp. 89–113). Minneapolis: University of Minnesota Press.

Wille, W. S. (1954). Figure drawings in amputees. *Psychiatric Quarterly, 28* (Suppl.), 192–198.

Williams, J. H. (1935). Validity and reliability of the Goodenough intelligence test. *School and Society, 41,* 653–656.

Wilson, A. (1982). *A developmental approach to the assessment of levels of internal object relations in borderline as contrasted with neurotic and psychotic patients.* Unpublished doctoral dissertation, Temple University.

Wilson, A. (1985). Boundary disturbances in borderline and psychotic states. *Journal of Personality Assessment, 49,* 346–355.

Winter, D. (1973). *The power motive.* New York: Free Press.

Witkin, H. A. (1965). Psychological differentiation and forms of psychopathology. *Journal of Abnormal Psychology, 70,* 317–336.

Witkin, H. A., Dyk, R. B., Faterson, H. I., Goodenough, D. R., & Karp, S. A. (1962). *Psychological differentiation.* New York: Wiley.

Wolff, W. (1946). *The personality of the preschool child.* New York: Grune & Stratton.

Wright, S. (1934). The method of path coefficients. *Annals of Mathematics, 5,* 161–215.

Wright, S. (1960). Path coefficients and path regressions: Alternative or complementary concepts? *Biometrics, 16,* 189–202.

Zanna, M. P., & Aziza, C. (1976). On the interaction of repression–sensitization and attention in resolving cognitive dissonance. *Journal of Personality, 44,* 577–593.

Zigler, E., & Phillips, L. (1962). Social competence and the process-reactive distinction in psychopathology. *Journal of Abnormal and Social Psychology, 64,* 215–222.

The Strauss–Harder Case Record Rating Scale

1. Rater judge:
   A. Whether the patient has the experience asked about, and
   B. Whether that experience appears to be pathological.
2. If the record is contradictory, rater should use his best judgment whether the patient has had the symptoms in question.
3. If a topic (e.g., hallucinations) is not mentioned in chart, score NI (no information) for items dealing with that topic. If the topic is mentioned (e.g., affect) but a specific item (e.g., flat affect) is not, score that item 0. For example, if the record described symptoms indicating a labile affect, then flat affect (if not specifically mentioned) would be rated 0.

The following rating symbols are used: 0, 1, 2, ?, NA, NI.

   0—There is evidence that the patient does not have the experience talked about (a statement is recorded that the symptoms are absent, or a general area is mentioned but specific item is not recorded as present).
   1—Evidence that patient definitely has the experience, but no evidence that it is continuous or severe.
   2—Evidence that the patient definitely has the experience and it is clear that it is continuous or severe or both.
   ?—There is at least some evidence that symptom may be present but rater is not sure whether it is.
   NA—Question not applicable (it is not possible that patient could

SOURCE: Strauss, J. S., & Harder, D. W. (1981). The Case Record Rating Scale: A Method for Rating Symptom and Social Function Data from Case Records. *Psychiatric Research*, 4, 333–345.

have that symptom, e.g., he couldn't hear voices talking about self if he doesn't hear voices at all).
NI—No information.

SYMPTOMS AND SIGNS

0 1 2 ? NA NI

1. Depression (crying, feeling of hopelessness, depressed mood. Do not rate depressive delusions or suicide attempts here.)
   1a. Loss of appetite
   1b. Suicidal thoughts (not attempts)
   1c. Decreased energy or interests (e.g., in activities, sex, etc.)
2. Anxiety (feels anxious, trembles, heart pounds without organic cause, attacks of fear or panic)

3–4. Motor restlessness (inability to relax physically, pacing, or fidgeting. Do not rate subjective anxiety or insomnia here.)

5. Retarded speech (slow speech, long pauses before answering)
   5a. Reduced quality of speech (rate 2 only if mute for long periods)
6. Slowed movement
   6a. Reduced quality of movement
7. Hypomanic–manic behavior (overly confident, elated mood, extravagant buying. Do not rate any delusions here.)

0 1 2 ? NA NI

8–9. Belligerence, hostility, irritability (Do not rate assaultive acts here.)
10. Somatic concerns (excessively worried about physical health)
11. General suspiciousness (feels people are looking at or laughing at him, suspicious)
12. Unkempt appearance (to a pathological degree)
13. Obsessions (Rate only: repeatedly checks things, behavior rituals, some thoughts recurring and over)

14. Disorientation (Rate only: does not know age, marital status, where he is, year or month)
15. Lack of insight (patient doesn't think he has emotional problems when he really does)
16. Depersonalization–degeneralization (feeling that others, himself, or events are unreal)
17. *Delusions* of reference or persecution (sees references to himself on TV or street signs, suspiciousness of people's intentions, others are trying to harm patient—consider patient's certainty of these delusions; if patient convinced of their reality, rate 2)

0 1 2 ? NA NI

18. Grandiose *delusions* (patient feels he has special powers, special purpose in life, special religious role [like a saint]—rate according to certainty of these delusions; if patient convinced of their reality, rate 2)
19. *Delusions* of passivity (outside force influencing or controlling thoughts or actions, others know what he thinks—rate according to certainty of these delusions; if patient convinced of their reality, rate 2)
20. Depressive *delusions* (delusional feeling of guilt, worthlessness, incurable physical illness, part of body missing or rotting—rate according to certainty of these delusions; if patient convinced of their reality, rate 2)
21. Other *delusions* (fantastic experiences, sexual delusions—rate according to certainty of those delusions; if patient convinced of their reality, rate 2)

HALLUCINATIONS

For all hallucinations score:
  1—Pseudohallucinations only—recognized by subject at time of experience not to be real perceptions (through sense)

2—Hallucinations—patient convinced of their reality now or at
    time of occurrence
NA—Not applicable—e.g., if has hallucinations only under the
    influence of alcohol or drugs

                        0 1 2 ? NA NI

22. Visual hallucinations (has visions, sees
    strange shapes, shadows, etc.)
23. Auditory hallucinations (hears strange
    sounds, voices)
    23a. Patient reports hearing several voices
         talking to each other about him.
    23b. Patient reports hearing voices com-
         menting on what he was doing or
         thinking.
24. Other hallucinations (tactile, gustatory, ol-
    factory, somatic)
25. Bizarre behavior (laughs out of context,
    loss of social restraint, posturing, grimac-
    ing)
26. Withdrawal (trouble conversing, avoids
    people, distractible or apathetic during in-
    terview)

                        0 1 2 ? NA NI

27. Bizarre speech (neologisms, inappropriate
    word use or grammar perseveration)
    27a. Vagueness or concreteness of speech
28. Nonsocial speech (lips move soundlessly,
    talks to self)
29. Flat affect (expressionless face/voice)
30. Labile affect (rapid change in behavioral
    expression in response to minimal stimu-
    li)
31. Incongruous affect (emotions shown not
    congruent with subject under discussion)
32. Delusions about hallucinations (delusion-
    al notion about nature or causes of hallu-
    cination; if no hallucinations, rate NA)
33. Patient has trouble thinking clearly
34. Fears of specific situations (phobias)
35. Insomnia
36. Conversion reactions (e.g., hysterical pa-
    ralysis or anesthesia)

37. Suicidal acts
38. Assaultive acts
39. Alcohol abuse
40. Drug abuse (specify which drugs) _____

_____

                                                        0 1 2 ? NA NI

41. Other antisocial acts (e.g., truancy, theft;

    specify which _____

    _____)

42. Sexual problems (specify _____)

43. Other (specify _____

    _____)

44. Other (specify _____

    _____)

The Fairweather Ward Behavior Rating Scale

Rate "0" for "no information"
Rate "1" for the more positive rating category
(the first Fairweather option)
Rate "2" for the more negative rating category
(the second Fairweather option)

This system provides for an additive total score, with high scores indicating more disturbed behavior.

1. _____ The patient's talk is mostly sensible.
_____ The patient's talk is mostly not sensible.
2. _____ The patient makes distinctions between new and old personnel.
_____ The patient doesn't make distinctions between new and old personnel.
3. _____ The patient says more than 3 or 4 words at a time.
_____ The patient never says more than 3 or 4 words at a time.
4. _____ The patient talks about sports with personnel.
_____ The patient does not talk about sports with personnel.
5. _____ The patient answers sensibly if talked to.
_____ The patient does not answer sensibly if talked to.
6. _____ The patient often writes a letter.
_____ The patient never writes a letter.
7. _____ The patient often takes part in back and forth conversation.
_____ The patient doesn't take part in back and forth conversation.

SOURCE: Fairweather, T., Fairweather, G. W., Simon, R., Gebhard, M. E., Weingarten, E., Holland, J. L., Sanders, R., Stone, G. B., & Reahl, J. E. (1960). Relative effectiveness of psychotherapeutic programs: A multicriteria comparison of four programs for three different patient groups. *Psychological Monographs, 74*, 5 (Whole no. 492).

8. _____ The patient is seldom silent.
   _____ The patient is often silent.
9. _____ The patient starts conversations with aides.
   _____ The patient does not start conversations with aides.
10. _____ The patient often volunteers information about himself.
    _____ The patient never volunteers any information about himself.
11. _____ The patient is usually with one or more patients.
    _____ The patient is usually alone.
12. _____ The patient seldom talks to himself.
    _____ The patient often talks to himself.
13. _____ The patient usually mixes with other patients.
    _____ The patient doesn't mix with other patients.
14. _____ The patient usually talks about his family with ward person-
         nel.
    _____ The patient seldom talks about his family with ward person-
         nel.
15. _____ The patient often talks to other personnel.
    _____ The patient seldom talks to other personnel.
16. _____ The patient sometimes jokes about people or situations in the
         hospital.
    _____ The patient seldom jokes about people or situations in the
         hospital.
17. _____ The patient is frequently chatting with someone.
    _____ The patient seldom chats with anyone.
18. _____ The patient usually will reply if you speak to him.
    _____ The patient usually does not reply if you speak to him.
19. _____ The patient usually talks over happenings on the ward with
         ward personnel.
    _____ The patient seldom talks over happenings on the ward with
         ward personnel.
20. _____ The patient can take teasing.
    _____ The patient cannot take teasing.
21. _____ The patient knows the names of most of the ward personnel.
    _____ The patient does not know the names of most of the ward
         personnel.
22. _____ The patient is courteous to personnel.
    _____ The patient is not courteous to personnel.
23. _____ The patient seldom quarrels with other patients.
    _____ The patient often quarrels with other patients.
24. _____ The patient is usually playful and good-humored.
    _____ The patient is seldom playful and good-humored.

25. _____ The patient seldom complains about anything.
    _____ The patient usually complains about everything.
26. _____ The patient seldom becomes upset if something doesn't suit him.
    _____ The patient usually becomes upset if something doesn't suit him.
27. _____ The patient asks for things; he does not wait for things to be given to him.
    _____ The patient never asks for anything; he waits for things to be given to him.
28. _____ The patient makes positive suggestions when problems arise.
    _____ The patient seldom makes positive suggestions when problems arise.

The Menninger Scales for Rating Interpersonal Relations: Motivation for Treatment, Sublimatory Effectiveness, Impulsivity, Superego Integration, Quality of Object Relations

MOTIVATION FOR TREATMENT

This is a continuum that reflects several components.

1. The willingness to derive benefit from interpersonal contact.
2. A wish to win approval from others through agreeable behavior.
3. Acknowledgment of maladaptive behavior and a concern about its effect on others.
4. Conscious dissatisfaction with the present state of life and a wish to make changes.

The components are weighted differently at different levels of the scale, as the scale points indicate. For example, the lower end of the scale is

SOURCE: Harty, M., Cerney, M., Colson, D., Coyne, L., Frieswyk, S., Johnson, S., & Mortimer, R. (1981). Correlates of change and long-term outcome. *Bulletin of the Menninger Clinic, 45,* 209–228.

biased toward a capacity or willingness to accept goodness in others while the upper end has more to do with efforts at self-correction.

Definition: The degree to which the person is willing to relate to, receive benefit from, and be altered by others (particularly treatment personnel).

Scale Points

100—

95—The patient is aware of an intrapsychic problem that he wants to change. He sees his problem as affecting his experience of himself and others, his moods and temperament, and his behavior. He is fairly consistent in his efforts to master his difficulties and accepts helpful comments readily.

75—The patient is aware of some aspects of himself that go beyond overt behavior and that he wishes to change. He can often accept others' comments and confrontations to help him explore his problem areas, though his efforts at change are sporadic.

60—The patient is aware of some aspects of his behavior that interfere with his relationship to others (e.g., temper outbursts, withdrawal from others, oversleeping). He is willing to try to alter those behaviors in order to improve his relationships, but has not yet developed goals that go beyond improving the immediate situation.

45—The patient recognizes his wish for warmth, approval, and concern from treatment personnel. He is generally willing to comply with others' wishes or take their advice in order to gain approval, but does not often think of himself as undergoing beneficial change.

35—The patient sees treatment personnel as potential sources of comfort and warmth. He is somewhat aware of his wishes for their nurturance and makes efforts (perhaps awkward, demanding, and angry) to gain the closeness he wants. However, he is often unresponsive to advice, directions, and confrontations and may experience these as overly harsh criticism or unwarranted demands.

25—The patient's positive interest in treatment is expressed only in his occasionally seeking comfort through interpersonal media, such as by talking with nursing staff or remaining near other patients. These efforts are mixed with some form of retreat or withdrawal, and their meaning is usually not acknowledged.

15—The patient seems to be somewhat comforted by others' efforts to reach out to him but makes no efforts at seeking closeness or help from staff or other patients. Any wishes for comfort are stated in terms of somatic symptoms or demands for medication.

0—The patient neither asks for nor tolerates input from others. He states he is here against his will and runs away or isolates himself in his room at nearly every opportunity. Makes no demands for help or comfort in any form, even medication.

Sublimatory Effectiveness

This scale refers to the person's level of functioning at the specific time the rating is made. Capacities the person once had but has lost, or capacities the person does not now have but might develop, should not be included in the basis for this rating.

The person's interests and activities should enter into this rating to the extent that they are *not* dominated solely by the need for immediate gratification or tension release. The number and variety of interests are secondary to this consideration; thus, a person who is very "busy" with a variety of activities might still receive a low rating if the activities all seem oriented to immediate gratification, whereas a person whose interests are fewer in number might receive a higher rating if the quality of the interests shows more "neutralization" of the drive component.

The level of the person's skill or accomplishment in an activity is not crucial; what is important is the quality of the involvement.

Definition: The extent to which the person channels his psychological needs into work, recreational, and social activities that are productive and socially appropriate, and that provide him with enjoyment and satisfaction.

100—

95—The person has a range of stable interests and activities that are not oriented solely to immediate gratification; he invests himself vigorously in these pursuits, freely exercises his capacities in them, and derives lasting satisfaction from them.

75—The person has a range of interests and activities that are productive and socially appropriate, but with some restrictions on the ability to pursue and enjoy them fully. For example, interests may tend to shift frequently or to be pursued in a somewhat pressured manner. However, considerable satisfaction still is derived from these activities.

55—The person's range of interests is somewhat restricted in relation to available opportunities. He pursues some activities that involve more than immediate gratification or tension release, but effortfully and with reduced productivity and enjoyment.

40—A few interests are maintained with some consistency, but the range of such interests and the satisfaction derived from them are quite restricted. The person has difficulty investing himself in pursuits that do not provide immediate gratification, and may experience them as drudgery.

30—The person's range of interests and activities is quite restricted in relation to available opportunities, and there is much difficulty in pursuing those he does have. At times he is able to maintain some interests, although with much effort and little enjoyment; often, however, these interests are allowed to lapse.

20—Few interests that are not oriented to immediate gratification or tension release, and these are pursued erratically, unproductively, and with little enjoyment or satisfaction.

5—There is no apparent capacity for interests or activities that go beyond the satisfaction of immediate needs.

IMPULSIVITY

Note that this scale measures only one aspect of psychopathology; impulsivity should be distinguished from action taken on the basis of inaccurate or delusional beliefs, as well as from other kinds of pathology such as withdrawal, calculated exploitativeness, and confusion without impulsive behavior.

There are, however, "passive" forms of impulsive behavior, such as allowing oneself to be influenced to act rashly, or "giving in" to temptations. The crucial points are the presence or absence of anticipation and judgment, and the degree to which the behavior jeopardizes the person's overall adjustment.

Impulsivity is not the same as action–orientation; an unreflective person, more comfortable with actions than with words or thoughts, is not impulsive if he does not engage in thoughtless actions that jeopardize his adjustment.

Definition: The extent to which thoughtless action—that is, action that is taken without anticipating and judging its likely consequences—interferes with the person's ability to maintain a satisfactory life adjustment.

100—Chronic tendencies toward immediate action on any impulse, regardless of circumstances; actions so extreme that if not externally restrained they would frequently threaten the survival of the person or those around him.

85—Generalized impulsive behavior as a lifestyle, with only intermittent periods of precarious control. Occasionally the person can control the most life-threatening aspects of his behavior, but is unable to consistently maintain even ordinary social functioning.

70—General impulsivity that seriously compromises the person's social and/or sexual adjustment, even though the appearance of ordinary social functioning may be maintained in some respects (such as holding a job or maintaining a marriage). However, the person does not often engage in life-threatening impulsive behavior.

55—Impulsive behavior is frequent enough and extreme enough to have important consequences for the person's life, but does not reach life-threatening proportions and is confined to relatively circumscribed conflictual areas. In most respects ordinary social functioning is maintained (examples: impulsive sexual behavior or overindulgence in alcohol at the service of neurotic needs).

35—Occasional impulsive behavior related to circumscribed conflicts is mostly kept private and does not violate social convention. Although impulsivity may constitute a problem for the individual in terms of the inefficiency it creates or the undue effort of maintaining control, impulsive behavior does not cause irreversible change in the person's life (example: "temper tantrums" when certain neurotic needs are frustrated).

20—Impulsive behavior of any kind is rare and never constitutes a serious threat to the individual's adjustment. However, control is maintained at significant cost to the individual in terms of undue conformity, inhibition, or blandness.

0—The person consistently maintains smooth control over his urges to action, and does so without slavish conformity, undue inhibition, or emotional blandness. Under all normal circumstances, needs and tensions are acted on in ways that are socially appropriate and in harmony with the individual's total personality.

SUPEREGO INTEGRATION

Definition: The extent to which the person's behavior is regulated in accord with ethical values that are comfortably internalized, stable, and consistent, yet allow flexible response to reality circumstances.

100—The person strives consistently to behave in accord with ethical values that are fully experienced as his own and that are stable, yet flexible. Instinctual needs are gratified when appropriate, and there is tolerance for the inevitable deviations from the ideal. Normal guilt over such deviations serves as a signal for self-corrective behavior.

80—There is a stable, consistent set of values according to which the person regulates his behavior, but these are not experienced fully as a part of the self. Compliance with them may thus be somewhat effortful, ambivalent, or rigid, although normal gratifications are generally permitted. When the person in some way violates his own standards, his guilt may be somewhat exaggerated or defensively warded off.

60—There is excessively strict self-regulation to the point that satisfaction of ordinary human needs is interfered with. "Morality" may be highly prized but is conceived of mainly in terms of imposed prohibitions to which one must submit or rebel. Symptoms or character traits such as frigidity or impotence, social inhibition, or depression in the face of success may reflect such conflicts, but integrity and honesty in relationships are maintained.

50—Excessive strictness in some areas coexists with lack of normal guilt in others; moral values show some inconsistencies or "lacunae" although not to the point of permitting clearly antisocial behavior. Rebellion against overly strict moral standards, without recognizing these as internal, may be characteristic. Both shame and guilt are important in self-regulation. Inconsistent reaction formations against opposite wishes lead to puritanical and "do-gooder" character trends.

For exploitative–antisocial superego pathology: Opportunism and personal advantage, more than internalized standards, are the regulators of behavior. There is a capacity for loyalties to other individuals but not to general ethical principles; there is a prominent tendency to "go along" with whatever is convenient. The person stops short of gross antisocial behavior, but mainly to avoid shame or out of a realistic appreciation of consequences.

35—*For excessively harsh superego pathology:* The person experiences more intense personified guilt. This is accompanied by severe depressive episodes. There is also a masochistic renunciation of skills and opportunities for personal growth and development, and a pleasureless "duty-bound" cast to life. Severe compulsive trends, rituals, "undoing," tormenting self-ridicule and self-blame alternate with provocations of others who humiliate and provide external harsh controls and prohibitions over the life of the individual.

For exploitative–antisocial superego pathology: There is little evidence of internalized ethical standards: Chronic manipulativeness, lying, stealing, etc., occur without guilt, and with only momentary shame at being caught. The person's loyalties are formed and maintained on the basis of personal advantage, although dealings with others show some concessions to ordinary humaneness.

20—*For excessively harsh superego pathology:* There are delusional preoccupations with having committed unpardonable sins. Self-mutilation—burning and cutting—may occur, along with occasionally more radical self-destructive behaviors that are just short of full-blown suicide attempts. Masochistic self-renunciations and a pleasureless constriction of life are extreme. Profound depressive episodes may occur.

For exploitative–antisocial superego pathology: There is no capacity for loyalty to any individual or any value beyond personal survival and gratification. The person also demonstrates chronic antisocial behavior, aggression, and ruthless exploitation of others without any sense of guilt, shame, or concern.

For excessively harsh superego pathology: Suicide and massive depression may occur.

5—Delusions of perfection can also predominate. This results from the projection of extraordinarily harsh, punitive, and unintegrated superego nuclei as tormenting persecutors delusionally conceived of as annihilative. There is a massive renunciation of libidinal and aggressive strivings to placate superego demands.

QUALITY OF OBJECT RELATIONS

Definition: The extent to which the person can experience stable, enduring relationships, in which the expression and gratification of individual needs do not compromise the person's empathy and respect for the other.

100—The person's relationships are stable, mature, and well differentiated. He understands and empathizes with others but does not confuse their needs with his; tolerates differences without loss of regard for others; is genuinely concerned for the well-being of others; and feels gratified by his relationships without feeling guilt.

80—Relationships are stable with depth of empathy and concern. Mature elements predominate, but the ability to participate fully in relationships is hampered by neurotic inhibitions or character traits (e.g., shyness, abrasiveness, or flirtatiousness) that interfere with the ability to find intimacy.

60—Relationships are stable, with some capacity for empathy and concern, but the more significant relationships are characterized by intense ambivalence and neurotic conflicts.

40—There are significant limitations on the capacity for stable relationships, although conventional respect and regard for others are present. Either stability is maintained by the avoidance of real emotional involvement, or intensity of feeling gives rise to turbulent, unstable relationships. The person is lacking in empathy and may tend to exploit or manipulate others.

25—The capacity for relationships is seriously limited. Contacts with others may be very restricted and marked by aloofness, awkwardness, and emotional impoverishment, or else intense and chaotic, marked by serious and repeated misinterpretation of others. There are no relationships that are experienced as consistently satisfying. Manipulation and exploitativeness may be prominent features, although not flagrant violations of ordinary social conventions.

15—Relationships show little stability. The person has little or no capacity for empathy or understanding of others; he may manifest disorganization or bizarreness in his contacts with others, may be withdrawn to the point of hardly recognizing their presence, or may be chronically exploitative and manipulative with only the most superficial social adaptation. Even ordinary social conventions are usually not recognized, but there is some minimal evidence of differential response to others.

5—There is virtually no capacity for relatedness to people that recognizes their independent existence or their difference from inanimate objects; others are treated with ruthless, indiscriminate, aggressive exploitation, or are responded to in completely autistic and undifferentiated ways. There is little recognition of, or concession to, even the most basic of social conventions.

Types of Thought Disorder

Thought disorder on the Rorschach Test can be placed on a developmental continuum in terms of the severity of the disturbance of boundary articulation. This continuum ranges from responses in which there is a failure to maintain a differentiation between two independent concepts or percepts such as when they merge and fuse in an idiosyncratic or bizarre union, to responses in which there is a failure to maintain a differentiation between what is perceived and one's reactions to it (a fusion of outside and inside), to responses in which percepts or concepts are placed in some inappropriate causal relationship simply because they are contiguous in time or space. Several major types of thought disorder frequently seen on the Rorschach (Rapaport et al., 1945) can be located on this developmental continuum (Blatt & Ritzler, 1974). These types of Rorschach responses would include the following.

Self–Other Boundary Disturbance

Contamination (Score = 6). Contamination is the fusion of two independent and separate concepts or perceptions into one idiosyncratic response. Objects or concepts cannot maintain their separateness or independence and become fused in a single distorted unit (e.g., Card X, "a rabbit's hand"). The basic issue is the instability of boundaries between objects or ideas (e.g., top of Card III "is Fire Island because it is red and surrounded by water"). Contamination responses are usually pathognomic of schizophrenia, a central feature being a tendency not to differentiate oneself from others and to blur and confuse conventional boundaries (Blatt & Wild, 1976).

SOURCE: Blatt, S. J., & Ritzler, B. A. (1974). Thought disorder and boundary disturbances in psychosis. *Journal of Consulting and Clinical Psychology, 42*, 370–381.

Contamination Tendency (Score = 5).   Contamination Tendency is scored both for partial contaminations or where critical distance is maintained so that a potential contamination response is recognized as distorted and inappropriate (e.g., Card IV, "an animalistic rocket taking off—but I can't explain that very well"). A partial contamination is scored, for example, when two ideas are given to the same area of the card and there is a quality of instability to the separateness between the ideas (e.g., "they look like eggs, but they are really lions"). The instability between the ideas can be expressed by alternations or shifts in meaning. On occasion there can be confusion between inside and outside in which both views are presented simultaneously.

Fabulized Combination-Serious (Score = 5).   Two percepts that have spatial contiguity are given a coalesced relationship. A relationship is established within a single unit such that the integrity of each object is maintained in isolation but also violated by the interrelationship within the unit. Thus, two percepts are combined into one incongruous response in which there are disparate parts within a single unit (Card II, "a penguin with a man's legs" [upper red area]). The incongruous blend of partial features from two different types of objects is like a contamination tendency, but is not quite a full contamination because the integrity of each of the separate parts has not been violated.

Inner–Outer Boundary Disturbance

Confabulation (Score = 4).   The infusion of a response, sometimes accurately perceived, with extensive and arbitrary ideational or affective elaboration that has little or no justification in the percept itself. There is a loss of distance between what is perceived and one's associations to the perception, such that associations overwhelm the perception with often grandiose and highly unrealistic personal elaborations and associations (bottom of Card IX, "two fetuses, they represent good and evil, heaven and hell"). Confabulation is scored for excessive associative elaboration and not on the formal accuracy of the response.

Confabulation Tendency (including Fabulized to Confabulized) (Score = 3). Less severe confabulations in which associative elaboration is not extreme or it is accompanied by some critical appraisal or delayed recognition of the unrealistic and inappropriate nature of the associations (e.g., Card VII, "I see a door opening to Shangri-La, crazy huh?" or "two rodents climbing up a mountain that is so steep they probably won't get to the top and will want to stop").

Boundary Laxness

Fabulized Combination-Regular (Score = 2). The contiguity of two percepts is taken as indicating a relationship between the percepts. But each percept is a separate and independent image with its own definition and integrity. The disturbance in boundaries is indicated by the fact that these two independent percepts and concepts are placed in some artificial relationship or juxtaposition because of their spatial or temporal contiguity (e.g., Card X, "a rabbit with two worms coming out of its ear" or on Card VIII, "two elephants dancing on a butterfly").

Fabulized Combination-Regular Tendency (Score = 1). The relationship established between two separate objects because of their spatial contiguity is recognized as inappropriate. It is apparent that the subject is aware of the distortion and inappropriateness of the response and that he is intentionally temporarily bending reality in the formation of the response (e.g., Card III, "two women picking up a huge sea creature—they couldn't really").

A Developmental Analysis of the Concept of the Object on the Rorschach

The importance of the human response on the Rorschach has been noted often in a variety of contexts, but generally with a minimum of theoretical elaboration. Aspects of these responses may have particular relevance for the study of the development of the concept of the object and its impairment in psychopathology. This scoring system is an attempt to apply developmental principles of differentiation, articulation, and integration (Werner, 1948; Werner & Kaplan, 1963) to the study of human responses given to the Rorschach.

Differentiation is defined as the nature of the response with human content; *articulation* is defined as the degree to which the response was elaborated; and *integration* is defined as the way the concept of the object is integrated into a context of action and interaction with other objects. Within each of these areas, categories are established along a continuum based on developmental levels. Within each category, ratings range from developmentally lower to developmentally higher levels.

CATEGORIES OF ANALYSIS AND SCORING PROCEDURES

I. Selection of Responses
   A. *Human and quasi-human responses*
      All human and quasi-human [H and (H)] responses are scored. Human and quasi-human details are scored if they (1) involve

SOURCE: Blatt, S. J., Brenneis, C. B., Schimek, J., & Glick, M. (1976). Normal development and psychopathological impairment of the concept of the object on the Rorschach. *Journal of Abnormal Psychology, 85,* 364–373.

human activity (e.g., talking, pointing, struggling); (2) involve a substantial portion of the card and are not just a small rare or edge detail; and (3) contain some description of explicit human or humanoid characteristics. Thus, independent of their location, the following responses would be scored:

> "the face . . . of an old man with wisps of hair on the side"
> "a man with sunglasses on"
> "a girl's head"
> "a baby's face"
> "baby's hands with mittens on"
> "face with a large hooked nose"
> "faces of two angels"

B. *Animal responses*

In some rare instances, animal responses are classified as quasi-human if the animal is explicitly given qualities that only a human could have. The exceptional quality of this classification must be emphasized. It is *not* meant to include all responses scored Animal Movement (FM). Though the following responses might be scored FM, they would not be included as a human or quasi-human response:

1. Humanlike actions that could be achieved as the result of special training and that might, therefore, be expected in the context of a circus act.
2. Activities that humans perform but that can also be performed by animals (e.g., rubbing noses). The human content must be explicit. If, for example, "Bugs Bunny" is given as a response, it is scored only if Bugs Bunny is engaged in a clearly human action. Thus, Bugs Bunny crying or talking would be scored as a quasi-human [(H)] response.

   Applying these criteria, the following animal responses would be scored as quasi-human:

   > "a hookah-smoking caterpillar . . . from *Alice in Wonderland*"
   > "two drunken penguins leaning on a lamppost . . . they're definitely sloshed"
   > "two lobsters coming out of a saloon . . . and they kind of have their arms around one another"
   > "seagull . . . laughing, making fun of somebody"
   > "two frogs . . . tête-à-tête . . . two angry frogs, their mouths are downcast"
   > "spiders (at an insect ball) eating spareribs"

II. Scoring Procedures
  A. *Accuracy of the response*
     Responses are classified as perceptually accurate or inaccurate
     (F+, F±, F∓, F−). F+ or F± responses are classified as accurate,
     and F− responses and F∓ responses are classified as inaccurate
     (Allison, Blatt, & Zimet, 1968/1988); Rapaport, Gill, & Schafer,
     1945).
  B. *Differentiation*
     Here responses are classified according to types of figures
     perceived—whether the figures or subjects of the action are
     quasi-human details (Hd); human details Hd; full quasi-human
     figures (H); or full human figures H.
     1. *Human responses.* To be classified as a human response, the
        figure must be whole and clearly human. Examples:

        "people"
        "men"
        "baby"
        "African natives"

     2. *Quasi-human responses.* Here the figures are whole but less
        than human or not definitely specified as human. Examples:

        "witches"
        "dwarfs"
        "two opposing forces, sticking out arms and hands. Op-
           posing forces, pitted against each other . . . looking at
           each other. With complicated . . . of talons, append-
           ages, arms raised in combat . . . Person maybe . . .
           standing there, being very offensive and attacking."

     3. *Human details.* Here only part of a human figure is specified.
        Examples:

        "hands strangling"
        "faces staring at each other"

     4. *Quasi-human details.* Here only part of a quasi-human figure is
        specified. Examples:

        "angel's face"
        "witch's head"
        "devil face"

  C. *Articulation*
     Here responses are scored on the basis of types of attributes
     ascribed to the figures. A total of seven types of attributes are

considered. These types of attributes were selected because they seem to provide information about human or quasi-human figures. The analyses are not concerned with the sheer detailing of features or with inappropriate articulation. The analyses are concerned only with articulations that enrich a human or quasi-human response, that enlarge a listener's knowledge about qualities that are appropriate to the figures represented. For example, a response that states that a man has a head, hands, and feet does not enlarge the listeners' knowledge about the man. Possession of these features is presupposed by the initial response, "man." An articulation such as "a man with wings" is not scored as an articulation because it is an elaboration that does not add to the specifications of the human or quasi-human features of the figure.[1]

There are two general types of articulation: the articulation of (1) perceptual and (2) functional attributes.

1. *Perceptual characteristics.*

   a. *Size or physical structure.* For this aspect to be scored as articulated, descriptions of the figure must have adjective status. Thus, no credit is given in a response where an examinee only says that a man has feet or that a hand has fingers. Size or structure is scored as articulated only if there is a *qualitative* description of aspects of body parts or the whole body. Descriptions of bodies or body parts as "funny" or "strange" are not scored as indicating articulation of body structure.

   Certain aspects of facial expression can be scored as articulations of size or structure. Included in this category are responses like "eyes closed" or "mouth open" in which the description of facial expression amounts to something more than just a description of physical appearance.

   Applying these criteria, the following responses would be scored as articulations of size or physical structure:

   "slim men"
   "big feet"
   "the top of the body is sort of heavy and her legs are real, real teeny"
   "slanted eyes"
   "chins protruding down from the face"
   "eyes closed"

"mouths open"
"tongue was sticking out"

By contrast, the following responses are *not* scored as articulations of size or structure:

"women with breasts"
"they're shaped like people"
"eyes, nose, mouth"
"woman doesn't have a head"
"a pervert with bunny ears"
"person with wings instead of arms"

b. *Clothing or hairstyle.* For this aspect to be scored as articulated, there has to be a qualitative description of some aspect of *either* clothing *or* hairstyle. It must enrich the description of the figure. Simple mention of items of clothing implied by the response does not enrich one's understanding of the figure and is, therefore, not scored as an articulation. Using these criteria, the following responses are scorable as articulations of clothing or hairstyle:

"some kind of moustache . . . right above its mouth"
"girls with ponytails"
"hair and the things sticking out of them, feathers"
"their pants would have to be skintight and when they lean down, their jackets go pointing out, makes it look like a very tight jacket"
"a couple of witches with red hats"
"wearing a black coat and a homburg hat. Black coat is sort of billowing behind him . . ."
". . . a full-tailed coat"
"two little girls, all dressed up in their mother's things"
"Gay 90s type women . . . both wearing a long bustle and feathers in hair"
"an American Indian in some ceremonial costume with wings and paraphernalia"
"a man . . . with sunglasses on"

By contrast, the following responses would *not* be scored as articulations of clothing or hairstyle:

"two women with skirts on"
"shoes on"

c. *Posture.* Posture is scored if the response contains: (1) a description of body posture that is separate from the verb describing the activity of the figure, or (2) a description of facial expression that goes beyond mere articulation of the physical appearance of features in that it contains a sense of movement or feeling. Posture is *not* scored if body posture is implied in the verb rather than being separately articulated or if it is simply a description of a figure's position in space (e.g., facing outward).

Thus, the following responses are scored as articulations of posture:

"arms flung wide"
"head tilted"
"standing with legs spread apart"
"leaning on a lamppost"
"shoulders hunched"
"somebody hanging . . . dangling down, dropped, formless, shapeless"
"eyes look piercing"
"gritting teeth"
"smiling"

The following responses are *not* considered articulations of posture:

"sitting"
"standing"
"doing a high dive"
"back to back"
"facing outward"
"mouth closed"

2. *Functional characteristics*

a. *Sex.* For sex to be scored, there has to be either a specific mention of sex of the figure or an assignment to an occupational category that clearly implies a particular sexual identity. If the final sexual identity is not decided but alternatives are precisely considered, sex is scored as articulated. If, however, the indecision is based on a vague characterization of the figures with an emphasis on the sexual nature of the figure as a whole, sex is *not* considered articulated. In the following responses, sex is scored as articulated:

"man"

"girl"

"witch"

"mother"

"priest"

"either an old man or an ugly woman"

"two boys putting on a disguise kit or a girl with her makeup kit"

By contrast, sex is *not* scored as articulated in these responses:

"Well, these look like two human figures. I think when you look at the breasts there, they're girls. Then down here could look like phalluses. I don't know. It's rather ambiguous, confusing . . . protrusions from the thorax, you know."

"Looks like two people. Could be a woman or a man. I debated this for a minute. (mean?) Well, this form could be women or the costuming of man. (?) Well, I guess it would be tights and sort of loose shirt. I don't know exactly."

"Two people beating drums in a way like both might be women. In another way, like men. Doesn't seem to be any real indication whether they are male or female. The rather extended chests seem to represent breasts of women and protuberance on bottom seems to be leg. In these respects it has a bisexual appearance. There is something barbaric about the figures. Seems to be something of a representation of gods or something like that. They seem to be wearing high-heel shoes. Both of the figures seem to be very awkward and look as though they're doing some clumsy movements in beating the drums. The heads also don't look human—look as though they're some kind of bird's heads."

b. *Age.* For this aspect to be scored, specific reference must be made to some age category to which the figure belongs. Thus, age is assumed to be delineated in the following responses:

"child"

"baby"

"old woman"
"young girl"
"little boys"
"teenagers"

By contrast, although some indication of age is implied in the following responses, the references are not specific. Thus, age is *not* scored in these responses:

"man"
"girls"
"boys"
"priest"

c. *Role.* When figures are human, a clear reference to the work a figure does (occupation) is scored as an articulation of role. With regard to quasi-human figures, role is scored if the manner in which the figure is represented implies that it would engage in certain activities rather than others. Thus, role is assumed to be articulated in the following responses:[2]

"soldier"
"priest"
"Spanish dancer"
"ballet dancer"
"princess"
"mother"
"witch"
"devil"
"elves"

Role is *not* scored in the following responses because there is no clear indication that they refer to occupation rather than a momentary activity.

"dancer"
"singers"

d. *Specific identity.* Here a figure must be named as a specific character in history, literature, etc.[3] Examples:

"Charles DeGaulle"
"Theodore Roosevelt"

3. *Degree of articulation*. This is the simple enumeration of the total number of types of features articulated. In the preceding section, seven types of attribution were described (size, clothing or hairstyle, posture, sex, age, role, and specific identity). Thus, for any single Rorschach response, a total of seven types of features could be articulated. The average number of features taken into account in each human or quasi-human response constitutes the score for the degree of articulation of individual figures. If, for example, a subject gave four human responses and attributed a total of ten types of attributes to them, his score for degree of articulation is 2.5.

D. *Integration*

Integration of the response was scored in three ways: (1) the degree of internality of the motivation of the action (unmotivated, reactive, and intentional); (2) the degree of integration of the object and its action (fused, incongruent, nonspecific, and congruent); and (3) the integration of the interaction with another object (malevolent–benevolent and active–passive, active–reactive, and active–active). These analyses can be applied only to figures engaged in human activity.

1. *Motivation of action*. The articulation of action in terms of motive implies a developmentally advanced perception of action as differentiated from but related to the subject. Moreover, motive can be ascribed in two ways: as reactive or as intentional. Reactive explanations involve a focus on past events, and behavior is explained in terms of causal factors; one assumes that, for certain prior reasons, an individual *had* to do a certain thing. By contrast, intentionality is proactive and implies an orientation toward the present or future. The individual *chooses* to do something to attain a certain end or goal. The ability to choose between motives and to purposively undertake an activity implies a greater differentiation between subject and action than is the case when an individual is impelled to take an action because of past occurrences. For this reason, the analysis of action will consider whether a motive was provided and whether the motivation was reactive (causal) or intentional.

a. *Unmotivated activity*. Here action is described with no explanation of why it occurs. Examples:

> "two people kissing each other"
> "women looking at each other"
> "men leaning against a hillside"

b. *Reactive motivation.* Here perceived activity is described as having been caused by a prior situation (internal or external), and the subject is seen as having little choice in his reaction. Examples:

> "A German soldier on guard duty. I think he sees something and points his gun at it."
> "Arabs recoiling from an Israeli bomb."
> "A person afraid of a snake, standing on a rocky cliff with arms upraised as if he's going to hit it with something."
> "Two women struggling over ownership of a garment."

c. *Intentional motivation.* For motivation to be scored as intentional, the action must be directed toward some future moment and the subject must be seen as, in some sense, choosing his action rather than having to react. Examples:

> "Halloween witches, making incantations over the fire, in preparation for All Hallows Eve"
> "an orchestra conductor, his arms raised, about ready to begin"

2. *Object–action integration.* In this analysis, four levels of integration of the object with its action are distinguished (fused, incongruent, nonspecific, and congruent).

a. *Fusion of object and action.* For a response to be included within this category, the object must be amorphous and only the activity articulated. In such situations, object and action are fused. The object possesses no separate qualities of its own. It is defined only in terms of its activity. This type of response is exemplified below. In both instances, nothing is known about the object except what it is doing. Examples:

> "Two opposing forces, sticking out arms and hands. Opposing forces, pitted against each other . . . looking at each other. With complicated . . . of talons, appendages, arms raised in combat . . . Person maybe . . . standing there, being very offensive and

attacking."

"Figure there with hands, standing with legs spread apart, reaching out with hands as if trying to grab something."

b. *Incongruent integration of object and action.* For a response to be included within this category, there should be some separate articulation of object and action. Something must be known about the object apart from its activity. Nevertheless, the activity is incongruous, unrelated to the defined nature of the object. The articulation of action detracts from, rather than enriches, the articulation of the object. Examples:

"a great big moth, dancing ballet"
"two figures, one half human and one half animal holding two sponges"
"a little baby throwing a bucket of water"
"a satyr-thing bowling"
"two sphinxes pulling a decapitated woman apart"
"two beetles playing a flute"

c. *Nonspecific integration of object and action.* Inclusion within this category also requires some separate articulation of object and action. However, the relationship between the two elements is nonspecific. The figures, as defined, can engage in the activity described, but there is no special fit between object and action. Many other kinds of objects could engage in the activity described. Thus, while the articulation of action does not detract from the articulation of the object, neither does it enrich it. Examples:

"one big person standing with arms raised"
"a knight, standing ready to do his job"
"cavemen leaning against a hillside"
"two figures dancing"
"two older women trying to pull something away from each other"
"two men fighting"
"a man running away"
"a person, sort of a girl, standing on her toes"

d. *Congruent integration of object and action.* For a response to be assigned to this category, the nature of the object and the nature of the action must be articulated separately. In addition, the action must be particularly suited to the defined nature of the object. By way of contrast with the preceding category, the action not only must be something the object might *do*, it must be something that the object would be especially likely to do. There is an integrated and particularly well-suited relationship between the object and the specified action. Moreover, the articulation of the action enriches the image of the object.[4]

3. *Integration of interaction with another object*
   a. *Content of interaction.*[5]
      (1) *Malevolent:* The interaction is aggressive or destructive or the results of the activity imply destruction or harm or fear of harm.
      (2) *Benevolent:* The activity is not destructive, harmful, or aggressive. It may be neutral, or it may reflect a warm, positive relationship between objects.
   b. *Nature of interaction.* This analysis applies to all responses involving at least two human or quasi-human figures. In addition, this analysis can pertain to situations where a second figure is not directly perceived, but its presence is necessarily implied by the nature of the action.
      (1) *Active–passive interaction.* Two figures can involve a representation of one figure acting on another figure in an active–passive interaction. One figure is active and the other entirely passive, so while acted on, it does not respond in any way.
      (2) *Active–reactive interaction.* In another type of interaction, the figures may be unequal. One figure is definitely the agent of the activity, acting on another figure. The second figure is reactive or responsive only to the action of the other. This is defined as an active–reactive interaction.
      (3) *Active–active interaction.* In a third type of interaction, both figures contribute equally to the activity, and the interaction is mutual.

Scoring Outline

Categories of Analysis

   I. Accuracy of response (F+ or F−)
  II. Differentiation
      A. Types of figures perceived
         1. Human

      2. Quasi-human
      3. Human detail
      4. Quasi-human detail
III. Articulation
    A. Perceptual attributes
      1. Size or physical structure
      2. Clothing or hairstyle
      3. Posture
    B. Functional attributes
      1. Sex
      2. Age
      3. Role
      4. Specific identity
    C. Degree of articulation (number of features articulated/number of responses)
IV. Integration
    A. Motivation of action
      1. Unmotivated
      2. Reactive
      3. Intentional
    B. Integration of object and action
      1. Fusion of object and action
      2. Incongruent action
      3. Nonspecific action
      4. Congruent action
    C. Content of action
      1. Malevolent
      2. Benevolent
    D. Nature of interaction with another object
      1. Active–passive
      2. Active–reactive
      3. Active–active

Composite Scores for the Concept of the Object on the Rorschach

The concept of the human object is assessed for all responses that have any humanoid feature. These responses are evaluated for the *degree of differentiation* (whether the figure is fully human, quasi-human, or a part feature of a human or quasi-human figure); *articulation* (the degree to which the figure is elaborated in terms of manifest physical or functional attributes); *motivation of action* (the degree to which the action of the figure is internally determined—unmotivated, reactive, or intentional action); *integration of the action* (the degree to which the action is a unique attribute of the figure, for example, fused, incongruent, nonspecific, or congruent); *the content of the action* (the degree to which the action is malevolent or benevolent and constructive); and *the nature of any interaction with another figure* (the degree to which the interaction is active–passive, active–reactive, or active–active in which mutual, reciprocal relationships are established). In each of these six categories (differentiation, articulation, motivation of action, integration of the object and its action, content of the action, and nature of the interaction), responses are scored on a developmental continuum. This developmental analysis should be made separately for those humanoid responses that are accurately perceived (F+) and for those that are inaccurately perceived (F−).

Differential weighting for scores within each of the six categories for assessing the concept of the object reflects a developmental progression, with higher scores indicating higher developmental levels. Score values are as follows:

Differentiation: (Hd) = 1, Hd = 2, (H) = 3, H = 4

Articulation: score 1 for each perceptual feature and 2 for each functional feature

Motivation: unmotivated = 1, reactive = 2, intentional = 3

Integration of object and action: fused = 1, incongruent = 2, nonspecific = 3, congruent = 4

Content of action: malevolent = 1, benevolent = 2

Nature of interaction: active–passive = 1, active–reactive = 2, active–active = 3

Reliability estimates for the scoring of these six categories in F+ and F− responses in both clinical and normal samples are quite high, ranging from .86 to .97.

To reduce the number of variables in the measurement of the concept of the object on the Rorschach, a factor analysis was conducted on the 12 object representation (OR) scores. A weighted sum for each of the six categories was obtained for F+ and F− responses separately. Each of these 12 weighted sums was corrected by covariance for total response productivity. The residualized scores for each of these 12 variables (six categories each for F+ and F− responses) were subjected to a common factors (SAS Institute, 1979) factor analysis with communalities less than or equal to 1.00. Using the criteria of λ 1.00, two factors were retained and rotated for an orthogonal varimax solution. These two factors accounted for 53.52% of the total variance. The factor analysis yielded two primary factors: the developmental level of accurately perceived responses (OR+) (percent total variance = 27.19) and the developmental level of inaccurately perceived responses (OR−) (percent total variance = 26.33). All six OR+ scoring categories had factor loadings on Factor I that exceeded .70, and all six OR− scoring categories had factor loadings on Factor I that were less than .20. All six OR− scoring categories had factor loadings on Factor II that exceeded .53, and the loadings of the OR+ categories did not exceed .20 on this factor.

All six residualized scores (that is, weighted sums covaried for total number of responses on the Rorschach) for OR+ scoring categories should be standardized and then summed to give a total residualized weighted sum score for accurately perceived responses. The same should be done for all six OR− scores. The *residualized weighted sum of accurately perceived human responses* (OR+) is viewed as indicating the capacity for investment in satisfying interpersonal relationships. The *residualized weighted sum of inaccurately perceived human responses* (OR−) is viewed as an indication of the tendency to become invested in autistic fantasies rather than realistic relationships.

In addition to the residualized weighted sum OR+ and OR− scores, a *mean developmental level* should be obtained for each of the six categories for F+ and F− responses separately. The six mean developmental level scores for F+ responses should be standardized and then combined into a total mean developmental level score for F+ responses. The same should be done for F− responses. The *mean developmental level for accurately perceived responses* (F+) is viewed as another measure of the capacity to become engaged in meaningful and realistic interpersonal relations. The *mean developmental level of inaccurately perceived responses* (F−) is viewed as another measure of the tendency to become involved in unrealistic, inappropriate, possibly autistic types of relationships.

NOTES

1. Inappropriate articulations were not scored in the initial research with this manual (Blatt, Brenneis, Schimek, & Glick, 1976a). In subsequent research it may prove useful to score both appropriate and inappropriate elaborations.
2. When sexual identity is clearly indicated in a role designation, both sex and role are scored as articulated. Such a situation exists in the following responses: "mother," "witch," "priest."
3. To the degree that age, sex, and occupation are clearly indicated in the specific identity, these features are also scored as articulated. Thus, in the response "Charles DeGaulle," sex and occupation are specified. Such is not the case in the response "piglet."
4. In situations where the role definition of the object amounts to nothing more than a literal restatement of the action, object and action are not considered integrated. Responses like "dancer's dancing," or "singer's singing" are

scored as nonspecific (level 3) relationships. However, responses such as "ballerina dancing" or "character from a Rudolph Falls opera, singing" are classified as congruent (level 4) relationships.
5. Examples for scoring both the nature and the content of interactions are presented below. Notations in the left-hand margin indicate scoring for the nature of the interaction [active–passive (A–P), active–reactive (A–R), and active–active (A–A)]. Notations in the right-hand margin indicate the scoring for the content of the interaction [malevolent (M) and benevolent (B)].

Integration of Interaction

Nature of Interaction		Content of Action
A–P	A couple of undertakers lowering babies into the pit.	M
A–P	A prostitute rolling a drunk.	M
A–P	Crucified man.	M
A–P	A mother holding out her arm and telling her kid never to come back.	M
A–P	Two sphinxes pulling a decapitated woman apart.	M
A–P	Two people kneeling down with hands extended toward and touching other people.	B
A–R	African natives beating a drum; martians applaud.	B
A–R	Eve being tempted by a snake (snake seen on card).	M
A–R	Two people with hands up as if trying to ward off the two people coming to get them. Two guys with black capes . . . coming in to get the other people. . . .	M
A–R	German soldier—thinks he sees something and points gun at it.	M
A–R	An orchestra conductor, arms raised, just about to begin.	B
A–R	A man running away.	M
A–R	A woman crying out for something . . . two forces pulling her apart; one is depression, one is suicide.	M
A–R	A man trying to kill a little girl, who's running away.	M

A–A	A woman with a child looking up at her.	B
A–A	Someone having intercourse, a man child and a woman child, trying to make love but not knowing how.	B
A–A	One person there is pointing and the other is listening.	B
A–A	Two people and two martians fighting.	M
A–A	Two women having a fight, calling each other names.	M
A–A	Two gremlins ready to hit each other.	M
A–A	People placing hands together—like victors, walking along like that.	B

Mutuality of Autonomy on the Rorschach

The Mutuality of Autonomy on the Rorschach developed by Urist (1977) is a scale based on a developmental model that defines various levels or stages of relatedness based on a sense of individual autonomy and the capacity to establish mutuality. Rorschach responses are scored on this 7-point scale if a relationship is stated or clearly implied between animate (people or animals) or inanimate objects. A response is scored even if there is only one animate or inanimate object, but a relationship is clearly implied. Thus, an object that is a consequence of an action (a bear rug cut in half or a squashed cat) or has the potential for an action on another object (a nuclear explosion) is scored in this analysis of Rorschach responses.

Urist (1977) defines 7 scale points for the quality of relations between objects as follows:

Scale Point 1: Figures are engaged in some relationship or activity where they are together and involved with each other in such a way that conveys a reciprocal acknowledgment of their respective individuality. The image contains explicit or implicit reference to the fact that the figures are separate and autonomous and involved with each other in a way that recognizes or expresses a sense of mutuality in the relationship (e.g., "two bears toasting each other, clinking glasses").

At this level, the unique contributions of each individual object to the mutual interaction need to be emphasized. Thus, "two people dancing" would receive a 2, because there is no stated emphasis on the mutuality of their endeavor. To receive a score of 1, a response must have a special emphasis on the mutual but separate nature of a dyadic interaction. Each object must maintain its unique identity and contribution to a relationship in which both objects are mutually engaged.

SOURCE: Urist, J. (1977). The Rorschach test and the assessment of object relations. *Journal of Personality Assessment, 41*(1), 3–9.

Scale Point 2: Figures are engaged together in some relationship or parallel activity, but there is no stated emphasis of mutuality. Despite the lack of direct emphasis on mutuality, the response still conveys the potential for mutuality in the relationship (e.g., "two women doing their laundry"). A response is scored 2 when the integrity of the objects is maintained and there is a potential or an implicit capacity of mutuality, independent of the degree of logic, irrationality, or absurdity to the relationship.

Scale Point 3: Figures are dependent on each other but without an internal sense of capacity to sustain themselves. The objects do not "stand on their own two feet"; rather, they each require some degree of external support or direction. The objects lack a sense of being firmly self-supporting (e.g., "two penguins leaning against a telephone pole").

Scale Point 4: One figure is seen as the reflection, imprint, or symmetrical image of another. The relationship between objects conveys a sense that the definition or stability of an object exists only insofar as it is an extension or reflection of another. Shadows, footprints, and so on would be included here, as well as responses of Siamese twins or two animals joined together.

Scale Point 5: The nature of the relationship between figures is characterized by malevolent control of one figure by another. Themes of influencing, controlling, or casting spells may be present. One figure, either literally or figuratively, may be in the clutches of another. Such themes portray a severe imbalance in the mutuality of relations between figures. On the one hand, some figures seem powerless and helpless, while at the same time, others seem controlling and omnipotent. Themes of violation of an object's integrity through domination, or implied physical damage and destruction, are often present in these types of responses (e.g., puppets on a string, witches casting a spell, or a body cut open).

Scale Point 6: There is a severe imbalance in the mutuality of relations between figures in decidedly destructive terms. Two figures more than simply fighting—such as a figure being tortured by another, or an object being strangled by another—are considered to reflect a serious attack on the autonomy of the object. Literal physical damage is seen as having occurred. Similarly, included here are relationships portrayed as parasitic, where a gain by one figure results by definition in the diminution or destruction of another (e.g., a leech sucking up this man's blood, two people feasting after killing an animal, a compression hammer splitting through rock).

Scale Point 7: Relationships are characterized by an overpowering enveloping force. Figures are seen as swallowed up, devoured, or generally overwhelmed by forces completely beyond their control. Forces are described as overpowering, malevolent, perhaps even psychotic. Frequently, the force is described as existing outside of the relationship between two figures or objects, underscoring the massiveness of the force, its overwhelming nature, and the complete passivity and helplessness of the objects or figures involved (e.g., something being consumed by fire, destruction after a tornado, or God's wrath).

Scales of Premorbid Social Adjustment in Schizophrenia

THE ZIGLER–PHILLIPS SCALE OF PREMORBID ADJUSTMENT IN SCHIZOPHRENIA

(Modified with descriptive criteria by Farina and Garmezy for use with male and female patients)
  I. Premorbid History
    A. Recent Sexual Adjustment (within the year prior to admission)
       (*Note:* Score as sexual contact; when information is not explicitly given, use inference to get at this actual sexual behavior.)
       1. Stable heterosexual relation and marriage 0
       2. Continued heterosexual relation and marriage but unable to establish home 1
       3. Continued heterosexual relation and marriage broken by permanent separation 2
       4. (a) Continued heterosexual relation and marriage but with low sexual drive 3
          (*Note:* If only informant is mother, don't score sexual adjustment. Prorate from rest of Premorbid History section. Look here for evidences of frigidity, distaste, avoidance, infrequency. Don't score on matters of technique.)
          (b) Continued heterosexual relation with deep emotional meaning but emotionally unable to develop it into marriage 3

SOURCES: Zigler, E., & Phillips, L. (1961). Social competence and the process–reactive distinction in psychopathology. *Journal of Abnormal Psychology, 64* 215–222.
Goldstein, M. J. (1978). Further data concerning the relations between premorbid adjustment and paranoid symptomatology. *Schizophrenia Bulletin, 4,* 236–243.

(*Note:* This must involve actual physical contact. Petting behavior is acceptable here. Mutuality of feeling is not necessary but sexual behavior is, that is, no adoration from afar.)

5. (a) Casual but continued heterosexual relations, that is, "affairs," but nothing more 4
(*Note:* "Casual" here implies lack of emotional meaning, although sexual behavior is consistent and regular.)
(b) Homosexual contacts with lack of or chronic failure in heterosexual experiences 4

6. (a) Occasional casual heterosexual or homosexual experiences with no deep emotional bond 5
(*Note:* This differs from 5 [a] on the dimension of frequency. Contacts less often here.)
(b) Solitary masturbation with no active attempt at homosexual or heterosexual experiences 5

7. No sexual interest in either men or women 6
9 = NI

B. Social Aspects of Sexual Life during Adolescence and Immediately Beyond (to the end of age 18)

1. Always showed a healthy interest in the opposite sex—with a "steady" during adolescence 0
(*Note:* "Steady" implies the exclusiveness of the dating relationship [neither partner dates anyone else] as well as frequency and emotional attachment.)

2. Started dating regularly in adolescence 1
(*Note:* This implies twosomeness, pairing off into couples, distinguished from 3, below.)

3. Always mixed closely with boys and girls 2
(*Note:* This involves membership in a "crowd"—interest in and attachment to others, but without the initiative factor for males, the selection factor for females.)

4. Consistent deep interest in same-sex attachments with restricted or no interest in opposite sex 3

5. (a) Casual same-sex attachments with inadequate attempts at adjustment or going out with opposite sex 4
(*Note:* This differs from 4 on the basis of the consistency and meaningfulness of the same-sex attachment.)
(b) Casual contacts with boys and girls 4
(*Note:* This differs from 3 in that the person was not a regular member of a crowd and just associated with others on occasion.)

6. (a) Casual contacts with same sex, with lack of interest in opposite sex 5
   (b) Occasional contacts with opposite sex 5
7. No desire to be with boys and girls; never went out with opposite sex 6

   9 = NI

C. Social Aspects of Recent Sexual Life—Below 30 Years of Age
1. Married, living as family unit, with or without children 0
2. (a) Married, with or without children, but unable to establish or maintain a family home 1
   (b) Single, but engaged or in a deep heterosexual relationship (presumably leading toward marriage) 1
3. Single, has had engagement or deep heterosexual relationship but has been emotionally unable to carry it through to marriage 2
4. Single, consistent deep interest in attachments to persons of either sex 3
   (Note: This implies a habitual interest in object relations, a consistent desire for human intimacy, but person has never settled into a meaningful, continued relationship with one partner in particular.)
5. Single, casual relationships with persons of either sex . 4
   (Note: Has dated more often than implied by 6 below, less often than implied by 4 above. Differentiated on the basis of frequency, regularity of social–sexual activity.)
6. Single, has dated a few persons casually, but without other indications of a continuous interest in object relationships 5
   (Note: Dating here is the exception rather than the rule. Person has had occasional social–sexual contact but doesn't actively seek out other persons. This behavior has not been consistent, nor an important part of his life. His contacts have been solely casual, i.e., with prostitutes to satisfy sex drive; no warmth or capacity to establish human relationships.)
7. (a) Single, never interested in or never associated with either men or women; asocial 6
   (b) Antisocial; destructive, belligerent, acting out against others 6

   9 = NI

D. Personal Relations: History (to the end of age 18)
(Note: Score here is determined by the time at which person

withdraws, narrows his range of social contacts. The earlier this occurs, the higher the score will be.)

1. Always has been a leader and has always had many close friends 0
   (*Note:* Score for "closeness" if record states close friends or describes frequent contact, shared activity.)

2. Always has had a number of close friends but did not habitually play a leading role 1
   (*Note:* From childhood until breakdown, person had extensive social contacts.)

3. (a) From adolescence on had a few close friends 3
   (*Note:* This may involve a drop in the number of close friends after adolescence, but person has retained relationships involving mutual give-and-take with several people through this period.)
   (b) From adolescence on had a few casual friends 3
   (*Note:* Person maintains relationships with several persons, even though these relationships may lack real emotional depth. Throughout life he has kept contact with others.)

4. From adolescence on stopped having friends 4
   (*Note:* Cultivated human relationships during childhood but has withdrawn since puberty.)

5. (a) No intimate friends after childhood 5
   (*Note:* Withdrawal began earlier—before puberty.)
   (b) Casual, but never any deep, intimate, mutual friendships 5
   (*Note:* Implies no close friends, even during childhood, but did maintain contacts on a superficial level, as distinguished from 6 below.)

6. Never worried about boys or girls; no desire to be with boys and girls 6

   9 = NI

E. Recent Adjustment in Personal Relations
   (*Note:* Score here the period prior to the noticeable change in behavior that *preceded* symptoms and hospitalization. Any changes noted within 6 months to a year prior to hospitalization will constitute a "change" by this definition. Score period *prior* to these changes.

   1. Habitually mixed with others, was usually a leader 0
      (*Note:* Again, this involves extensive social contacts.)

   2. Habitually mixed with others but was not a leader 1

   3. Mixed only with a close friend or group of friends 3

(*Note:* Distinguished from 4 below on the basis of consistency and frequency of contacts.)
4. No close friends or very few friends or had friends but was never quite accepted by them 4
5. Quiet or aloof or seclusive or preferred to be by self 5
6. Antisocial, actively avoided contact, acted out against others 6

9 = NI

PREMORBID ADJUSTMENT SCALE—UCLA SOCIAL ATTACHMENT SURVEY

The following ratings are based on adolescent social adjustment (16–20 years).
I. Same-Sex Peer Relationships
Number and closeness of relationships with youngsters his own age. Do not include in this rating transient relationships, those with younger or older individuals, or relationships with relatives.
1—No friends his own age
2—One or two casual friends only
3—Several casual friends or close relationships with one individual only
4—Several casual friends with one or two close relationships
5—Several casual friends with three or more close relationships
6—No information

II. Leadership in Same-Sex Peer Relations
Frequency with which patient assumed a leadership role with youngsters his own age. How often did he seek out others or make plans or decisions for his group?
1—Never assumed leadership. Almost always waited for others
2—Rarely assumed leadership
3—Sometimes assumed leadership
4—Often assumed leadership
5—Usually assumed leadership role. Actively showed initiative in making plans and decisions with others every day
6—No information

III. Opposite-Sex Peer Relations
Involvement with and emotional commitment to a member of the opposite sex. The extent to which the patient extended himself for another, showed concern for their needs and interests.
1—No emotional involvement with an opposite sex peer
2—Mild emotional involvement
3—Moderate emotional involvement

      4—Strong but intermittent emotional involvement

      5—Strong, continuous involvement and commitment to an opposite-sex peer

      6—No information

IV. Dating History

      1—Never dated

      2—Dated a few times

      3—Occasionally went out on dates

      4—Dated often but never had a lasting steady association

      5—Dated regularly and went steady

      6—No information

V. Sexual Experience

      1—No interest in sex

      2—Interested but no sexual play or intercourse

      3—Sexual play only on one or two occasions

      4—Sexual play or intercourse on one or two occasions

      5—Sexual intercourse and sexual play on several occasions

      6—No information

VI. Outside Activities

Number of activities outside the home the patient initiated on his own, e.g., movies, dances, parties, shopping, picnics, hobbies, camping, riding, hiking.

      1—Initiated no activities outside the home

      2—One or two outside activities

      3—Several outside activities

      4—Moderate number of outside activities

      5—Initiated many outside activities

      6—No information

VII. Participation in Organizations

Attendance and participation in activities of organizations or social clubs on his own initiative, e.g., church, scouts, YMCA, school sport, or social club. Do not rate involvements of less than 6 months.

      1—Did not attend any of these activities

      2—Belonged to none but occasionally attended

      3—Belonged to at least one organization and sometimes attended but rarely participated

      4—Belonged to at least one organization and sometimes participated

      5—Belonged to at least one organization, attended regularly, and participated actively

      6—No information

Synopsis of Anaclitic and Introjective Configurations of Psychopathology

ANACLITIC CONFIGURATION

The anaclitic configuration is object oriented and involves themes of relatedness and intimacy. These issues of interpersonal relationships are expressed in concerns about trust, closeness, affection, and the dependability of another, as well as the capacity to give and to receive love in a context of security, cooperation, and mutuality.

Psychopathology within the anaclitic configuration involves concerns and conflicts around themes of interrelatedness; symptoms are expressions of exaggerated attempts to compensate for disruptions in interpersonal relations. These disturbances are manifested in conflicts around establishing satisfactory intimate relationships and around feeling loved and being able to love. The basic wish is wanting to be loved. Conflicts within the anaclitic configuration revolve around libidinal issues such as deprivation of care, affection, love, and sexuality. The basic issues appear to be the reliability and dependability of care and affection. The development of the self may be interfered with by intense preoccupations and struggles to establish satisfying interpersonal relationships.

CHARACTERISTIC ANTECEDENT RELATIONSHIPS

Depriving, rejecting, inconsistent, or unpredictable care of overindulgent relationships.

SOURCE: Blatt, S. J., & Shichman, S. (1983). Two primary configurations of psychopathology. *Psychoanalysis and Contemporary Thought, 6,* 187–254.

ANACLITIC DEFENSES

Primarily *avoidant* maneuvers—denial and repression. The defenses may be bolstered by acting out, externalization, and displacement. At times, one may also see a hypomanic search for substitute objects and for comfort. Defenses are used to manage fears of abandonment, to defend against intense rage over deprivation and frustration, or to avoid intense erotic longings and competitive strivings that are seen as potentially compromising or threatening one's interpersonal relationships. Primary conflictual situations include the threat or experience of a loss of care, love, and affection. Feelings of helplessness and hopelessness are likely.

The following disorders would be considered types of anaclitic psychopathology: nonparanoid schizophrenia, infantile syndrome, anaclitic depression, various hysteroid organizations, and hysterical disorders.

INTROJECTIVE CONFIGURATION

The primary concerns in the introjective configuration are around issues of self-definition, self-control, self-worth, and identity. The focus is on defining the self as an entity separate from and different from another, with a sense of autonomy and control of one's own mind and body, and with feelings of self-worth and integrity.

Psychopathology within the introjective configuration involves exaggerated attempts to achieve a sense of self-definition, self-control, and self-worth. The development of satisfying interpersonal relationships is interfered with by an exaggerated struggle to establish an acceptable self-definition and identity. Preoccupation with issues of self-definition dominate and determine the nature and quality of interpersonal interactions. The basic wish is to be acknowledged, respected, and admired. Conflicts within the introjective configuration revolve around the management and containment of affect, especially aggression, toward others and the self. The basic issue is the struggle to achieve a sense of separation, definition, and independence.

CHARACTERISTIC ANTECEDENT RELATIONSHIPS

Struggles to achieve separation, definition, and independence from controlling, intrusive, punitive, excessively critical, and judgmental figures.

INTROJECTIVE DEFENSES

Primarily *counteractive* maneuvers—projection (splitting, externalization, disavowal, and reversal), doing and undoing, abstinence, negativism, reaction formation, isolation, intellectualization, introjection and internalization, identification with the aggressor, reversal, rationalization, and overcompensation. Defenses involve efforts at overcompensation for feelings of inadequacy, guilt, and/or failure rather than a denial or object loss. Themes of grandeur and power may occur. Primary conflictual issues include the threat of the loss of super-ego approval. Feelings of inferiority, worthlessness, and guilt are likely.

The following disorders would be considered types of introjective psychopathology: paranoid schizophrenia, paranoia, obsessive–compulsive disorders, introjective (guilt-laden) depression, and phallic narcissism.

Manual for Scoring Defenses on the Thematic Apperception Test

This manual presents procedures for assessing the use of three defense mechanisms—denial, projection, and identification—as revealed in stories told to standard TAT cards. The scoring for each defense is based on seven categories, each designed to reflect a different aspect of the defense. Each category is scored as often as necessary, with the exception of a direct repetition in the story; in cases of repetition, the category is scored only once.

Although examples are provided to aid in deciding whether a category should be scored, questions inevitably arise. Knowledge of the nature of defense mechanisms will help in answering these questions. Beyond this, the general rule should be, "When in doubt, leave it out." If there is a serious question about whether the story segment is an example of the defense, do not score it.

PRIMITIVE DENIAL

In the categories of primitive denial, the storyteller assumes that the stimulus card is something, and the defense is expressed in the avoidance or changing the nature of that thing including:

1. Omission
2. Misperception
3. Reversal
4. Statements of negation
5. Denial of reality

SOURCE: Cramer, P. (1991). *The development of defense mechanisms, theory, research and assessment*. New York: Springer-Verlag.

1. *Omission of major characters or objects.*   This category refers to the failure to perceive major or obvious segments of the card usually perceived by nearly all subjects. Do not score, however, if reference is made to the function of a critical object. For example, the knife in TAT 8BM may be implied by the mention of an operation; or on TAT 1, reference to the object, even if not named, is sufficient. (If it is named incorrectly, however, score under misperception.)

2. *Misperception.*   This may come about because the perceptual process itself is distorted or because the name of the object is not known and the individual defensively calls it something it is not, rather than referring to it as a "thing" or an "object," in which case no score for denial is given. In this latter case, the point is whether, in a situation in which the individual does not have all the necessary information, he is able to cope adaptively or whether he must distort the situation to fit his inadequate knowledge.

Examples of adaptive coping are seen in the following two stories for TAT. In both cases, the person is uncertain about how to identify the violin:

> This person is thinking what to do with something that is in front of him. He might use it for something, or something might happen. The thing that might happen is that he might think of something to do with the thing. (What happens?) He's going to do something with it. He's thinking that he will use it for what it is supposed to be used for; on some kind of material, which is called paper.
>
> That's a little boy. He's down on his work bench, and he's looking this over, and he's wondering what it is. And he's wondering if he'll ever find out. He can't wait till his father comes home so he can ask his father. And he's kind of sitting there wondering when his father will come home.

(a) Any unusual or distorted perception of a figure, object, or action in the picture, which is without sufficient support for the observation, is scored for denial if, and only if, the projected image is not of ominous quality, in which case it should be scored under projection.

(b) Perception of a figure as being of the opposite sex from that usually perceived.

Note: If the storyteller misperceives an object, and then corrects the misperception, score denial. If, after the correction, he continues to use the misperception as the basis for the story, then denial is scored again under category 5.

3. *Reversal.*   Reversal may be either in terms of the usual perception of the card or in the story itself, especially when the reversal is normatively unusual.

(a) Score transformations such as weakness into strength, fear into courage, passivity into activity, and vice versa.
(b) Score any figure who takes on qualities previously stated conversely in the story, including a change of the sex assigned to the figures.

Reversal should be scored if it involves both ends of a continuum (e.g., weak–strong) rather than just one end (e.g., weak–not weak) that is negated or overly stressed. Reversal may also be scored where one end of the continuum is implied but not explicitly stated (strength–weakness, implied by growing old).

Do not score "growing old" by itself or if a character doesn't know how to do something and then learns how. Denial (reversal) is also not scored if the character was strong, became weak through tiredness, but in the end won, or was strong again. Denial is not scored if the character was sad but, through doing something, becomes happy.

4. *Statements of negation.* Simply stating something in the negative (e.g., "He didn't do it") is not sufficient to be scored in this category. Whether a negative statement should be scored depends on whether the negation is defensive. Sometimes this can be determined by the fact that the negative statement is unusual or unexpected (e.g., "He didn't stuff peanuts up his nose")—that is, that no one would have expected this event to happen anyway, so why point out that it didn't happen? At other times the defensive nature of the negation is more straightforward (e.g., "He didn't get hurt"). Often, only the context makes it clear if the statement is defensive or not. Negation is scored if a character does not get involved in any action, wish, or intention that, if acknowledged, would cause displeasure, pain, or humiliation, or if the storyteller negates or denies a fact or feeling. Negation is also scored when doubt is expressed about what the picture is or represents. "What is it? I don't understand the picture." This should be distinguished, however, from references to difficulty in formulating a story ("I can't think of what to say"), which is an example of repression. The difference lies in the fact that denial generally operates on a more concrete level, whereas repression is seen in the person's inability to think of something.

Denial (negation) is not scored when "I don't know" is used to end a story or is stated in response to a question by the examiner. Negation is also not scored if a character wants to or tries to do something but can't or isn't able to, or doesn't know how to, or if a character doesn't like something, or doesn't want to do something that is neutral or pleasant in nature (e.g., do not score "He doesn't want to practice the violin" or "He doesn't want to get hurt"). Denial (negation) is scored, however, for

"He doesn't get hurt." Denial (negation) is not scored if subject asks, at the end of the story, if the story was "right" or "correct."

A statement such as "He does not reveal it" (a secret, a clue, etc.) is scored as projection.

5. *Denial of reality.* Denial of reality (this overlaps with negation) is scored for the use of such phrases as "It was just a dream"; "It didn't really happen"; "It was all make believe"; or when the picture is described as part of a movie. Denial of reality is scored for the use of sleeping, daydreaming, or fainting as a way of avoiding something unpleasant or for references to avoidance of looking, hearing, or thinking something that would be unpleasant.

Denial of reality is also scored for any perception, attribution, or implication that is blatantly false with regard to reality as generally defined in the picture.

Themes of running away from or avoiding "society" are not scored as denial of reality.

Pollyannish Denial

Pollyannish denial of reality frequently involves a saccharine, "life is beautiful" attitude, often characterized by a note of unfounded optimism.

6. *Overly maximizing the positive or minimizing the negative.* Any gross exaggeration or underestimation of a character's qualities, potency, size, power, beauty, or possessions. Exaggerations of physical objects (e.g., "the highest mountain"; "he fell thousands of feet"), however, are not scored.

7. *Unexpected goodness, optimism, positiveness, gentleness.* This is a difficult category to score and should be scored only when it is beyond doubt. It is often seen in instances of revenge, when the revenge is built up to, but not consummated when the opportunity arises. Building up to a theme of harm and then concluding without justification that all is well is scored here. It is also scored when a character "takes his lumps" or takes his punishment or bad luck completely in stride when all previous indications were of an avenging "righteous indignation" attitude. It is also scored for any sort of drastic change of heart for the good; references to natural beauty, wonder, awesomeness; nonchalance in the face of danger, and acceptance of one's (negative) fate or loss, with the justification of not really wanting it anyway (a "sour grapes" attitude).

Clichés such as "they lived happily ever after," used at the end of a story, are not scored.

Projection

Projection includes the following:

1. Attribution of aggressive or hostile feelings, emotions, or intentions to a character, or other feelings, emotions, or intentions that are normatively unusual
2. Addition of ominous people, ghosts, animals, objects, or qualities
3. Magical, autistic, or circumstantial thinking
4. Concern for protection from external threat
5. Apprehensiveness of death, injury, or assault
6. Themes of pursuit, entrapment, and escape
7. Bizarre or very unusual story or theme

1. Attribution of aggressive or hostile feelings, emotions, or intentions to a character, or any other feelings, emotions, or intentions that are normatively unusual. This category is scored either when such emotions are attributed by the storyteller to a character in the story or when one character attributes them to another character, but only if such attribution is without sufficient reason. References to a character's *face* looking a certain way (e.g., anguished, puzzled) are scored here.

2. Addition of ominous people, ghosts, animals, objects, or qualities. This category is scored only if the details added to the situation are of an ominous or potentially threatening nature, especially the addition of blood or mention of serious and uncommon illnesses, including mental illness, comas, and nightmares. References to people, animals, or objects being decrepit, falling apart, or deteriorating are also scored as projection.

3. Magical, autistic, or circumstantial thinking. This category is scored for unusual powers or control of one character over another (e.g., hypnosis), including animals banding together to accomplish some herculean task; attribution of human thoughts or emotions to objects other than animals and people; circumstantial reasoning that has a paranoid flavor such as a hyperalert search for flaws and misleading cues (implying a mistrust of others); efforts to find hidden or obscure meanings; or criticism of the way in which the pictures are drawn.

4. Concern for protection from external threat. This category includes fear of physical assault or injury and the need for protection, as seen in the building of walls (real or imaginary), the use of masks, disguises, shields, armor, locking of doors or windows, or the creation of other protective barriers. Included here are references to suspiciousness, to people or animals hiding or "lying in wait," concern about being "taken by surprise," spying on others, anticipation of kidnapping that does not occur, or statements that "others are against you." This would also include references to having seen something one should not have seen or that will get one into trouble; the necessity for hiding incriminating evidence, oneself, or one's property; and the fear of being seen. Also scored here are themes indicating a defensive need for self-justification on the part of the storyteller, but not in response to a question from the examiner.

5. *Apprehensiveness of death, injury, or assault that actually occurs or has occurred in the story.* Unexplained or unjustified punishment is scored here, as are completed suicide and fear of going to sleep. Justified punishment by authority or parents, or justified self-protection or vindication is not scored.

6. *Themes of pursuit, entrapment, and escape.* This category is scored for themes involving one character pursuing another, one character trapping another, kidnapping or unjustified incarceration; themes of escape from a physical imprisonment or physical danger; or the anticipation of pain or punishment, when the anticipation is not justified by the story. Pursuit–entrapment and escape can both be scored.

"Being put in jail" is scored under projection only when the character has not committed a crime but is put there because of jealousy, fear, or the whim of someone else—that is, only when the incarceration is not (legally) justified, such as for political or military reasons. If the character is already in jail or prison at the beginning of the story, projection is scored only if it is clear that this is not due to criminal activity. If it is not clear why he is in prison, do not score.

Escape is not scored if it is only mentioned at the end of the story, or after the examiner's inquiry, unless the need for escape has been implied throughout. Also escape is not scored when the hero is running away from home or escaping from "society" or "the world."

7. *Bizarre story or theme.* This category is a subjective judgment about the extent of bizarreness in the story, but it should be scored for negative themes that occur very rarely, especially if they have a peculiar twist, or for instances of unusual punishment, including unusual self-punishment (spanking is not an unusual punishment unless it continues for a very long time).

IDENTIFICATION

1. Emulation of skills
2. Emulation of characteristics

3. Regulation of motive or behavior
4. Self-esteem through affiliation
5. Work: Delay of gratification
6. Role differentiation
7. Moralism

1. *Emulation of skills.* This category is scored for references to imitating, taking over, or otherwise acquiring a skill or talent of another character, or trying to do so. This is often seen in a younger character emulating an older one.

2. *Emulation of characteristics.* This category includes references to imitating, taking over, or otherwise acquiring a characteristic, quality, or attitude of another character, or trying to do so. "Identification with the aggressor" is scored here. References to being like or the same as another, or, in an extreme case, merging with another are scored here, but not the acquisition of another's physical property (e.g., money, jewels).

3. *Regulation of motive or behavior.* This category includes indication that the storyteller has internalized regulatory mechanisms that are attributed to a character in the story. References to demands, control, influence, guidance, or prohibitions of one character over another, or through societal mores, or the active rebelling against these, including running away from the pressures of the family or society, or being caught doing something one should not be doing, are scored here. Also scored are indication of self-criticism or self-reflection on the part of either the storyteller or a character in the story, and references to justified punishment by parents or authority as a way of controlling or regulating a character's behavior.

Magical control and unjustified punishment are scored under projection, as is escape from physical danger, or demands that are of an ominous nature or suggest an ominous outcome.

4. *Self-esteem through affiliation.* This category is scored with themes of affiliation with someone external to one's family or the expressed need for such an association such as adoption by a foster family (if pleasant), or for being part of a special group from which special pleasure or help is derived.

5. *Work: Delay of gratification.* This category includes references to a character working, or the implication that a character is about to work or has been working, such as at homework, or extensive practicing, or studying very hard. Also scored are references to delay (e.g., waiting, biding one's time, planning ahead) to attain some future gratification, and recognition that success will not be immediate.

References to exercising or to being tired from athletic endeavors, or to thinking about work but not doing it, are not scored.

6. *Role differentiation.* This category includes mention of current or historical characters in specific adult roles, other than mother or father or other relatives. Mythical, comic book roles, or roles indicated only by the addition of the word "man" or "woman" to a noun or adjective (e.g., trapezemen, violinman, strongman), are not scored unless the term is a commonly accepted designation of that role (e.g., mailman, businessman, fireman).

7. *Moralism.* This category includes stories that have a moralistic outcome, in which good conquers evil, wrongdoing is punished (by other than parents), goodness begets goodness, justice triumphs, a (moral) lesson is learned, or justified punishment is administered by teacher, judge, policeman, or other authority figure (excluding parents or guardians). Included here are stories in which someone breaks (or has broken) the law and is apprehended and put in jail. Usually, this will occur near the end of the story. If a character is in jail at the beginning of the story, score only if it is explained that he is in jail for having committed a crime.

Standard Deviation for All Variables Derived from Clinical Case Records and Psychological Test Protocols at Time 1 and Time 2

TABLE A.1
Standard Deviation for Clinical Case Record Variables at Time 1 and Time 2

	Total (n = 90)		Anaclitic (n = 42)		Introjective (n = 48)	
	Time 1	Time 2	Time 1	Time 2	Time 1	Time 2
Menninger Scales						
Factor I (Interpersonal relatedness)	2.65	3.66	2.70	2.92	2.62	4.09
Motivation for treatment	9.07	15.18	9.88	13.34	8.39	16.38
Sublimatory effectiveness	11.14	13.49	11.25	12.45	10.64	14.10
Superego integration	7.76	9.15	7.91	7.36	7.65	10.35
Object relations	7.43	7.77	7.31	6.15	7.62	8.71
Factor II (Impulsivity)	15.64	14.96	16.52	13.08	14.82	16.10
Fairweather Scale						
Interpersonal communication	.22	.24	.23	.25	.21	.23
Strauss–Harder symptoms						
Neurotic	2.98	2.55	2.93	2.63	3.05	2.41
Psychotic	2.04	1.54	1.50	1.52	2.37	1.56
Labile Affect	1.30	1.19	1.28	1.34	1.33	.93
Flattened Affect	.96	.59	.30	.73	1.09	.41

TABLE A.2
Standard Deviation for Psychological Test Variables at Time 1 and Time 2

	Total (n = 90)		Anaclitic (n = 42)		Introjective (n = 48)	
	Time 1	Time 2	Time 1	Time 2	Time 1	Time 2
Rorschach						
Composite thought disorder	27.32	23.00	24.38	24.51	29.85	21.86
Inaccurate Object Representation (OR−)						
Developmental Index	6.53	3.78	2.46	2.53	8.63	4.47
Developmental Mean	4.67	4.74	4.60	4.15	4.59	4.80
Accurate Object Representation (OR+)						
Developmental Index	4.37	5.50	4.27	5.30	4.51	5.73
Developmental Mean	4.16	4.32	4.38	4.16	4.00	4.48
Mutuality of Autonomy (MOA)						
Mean Score	1.12	1.08	1.25	1.21	1.01	1.03
Most Malevolent Score	1.81	1.75	1.88	1.71	1.76	1.78
Most Benevolent Score	.90	.91	1.12	.93	.65	.91
Traditional Measures						
Reality Testing (F+%)	15.36	15.81	15.89	16.69	15.05	15.13
Affective Liability (Sum C)	2.85	2.80	3.05	3.02	2.70	2.59
Adaptive Fantasy (M+)	1.72	2.17	1.79	1.97	1.68	2.35
Maladaptive Fantasy (M−)	.62	.56	.64	.44	.59	.65
Total Responses (R)	17.06	16.03	13.32	15.89	19.61	16.22
Thematic Apperception Test (TAT)						
Defenses						
Total Score	3.82	3.25	4.23	3.67	3.45	2.86
Denial	2.17	1.60	2.48	1.40	1.87	1.77
Projection	2.12	2.03	1.97	2.43	2.23	1.63
Identification	1.66	1.56	2.01	1.72	1.24	1.43

(*continued*)

TABLE A.2
(Continued)

	Total (n = 90)		Anaclitic (n = 42)		Introjective (n = 48)	
	Time 1	Time 2	Time 1	Time 2	Time 1	Time 2
Intelligence Test						
Full Scale IQ	10.27	9.80	9.13	9.58	11.05	9.63
Verbal IQ	10.47	11.18	10.75	11.68	9.98	10.58
Performance IQ	11.55	10.42	9.17	9.41	13.37	11.01

	Total (n = 32)		Anaclitic (n = 15)		Introjective (n = 17)	
	Time 1	Time 2	Time 1	Time 2	Time 1	Time 2
Human Figure Drawings						
Goodenough–Harris						
Total Score	1.81	1.98	1.46	2.14	2.08	1.89
Female Figure	1.00	1.00	.85	1.11	1.12	.92
Male Figure	.91	1.07	.70	1.11	1.07	1.06
Robins Balance-Tilt						
Total Score	2.65	2.97	2.08	3.46	2.94	2.54
Female Figure	1.62	1.35	1.66	1.01	1.58	1.62
Male Figure	1.42	2.16	1.19	2.95	1.56	1.10

Index